2nd edition

Babies and Young Children

Book 2: Early Years Care and Education

Marian
Beaver

Jo
Brewster

Pauline
Jones

Anne
Keene

Sally
Neaum

Jill
Tallack

Stanley Thornes (Publishers) Ltd

Text © Marian Beaver, Jo Brewster, Pauline Jones, Anne Keene, Sally Neaum, Jill Tallack 1999

Original line illustrations © Stanley Thornes (Publishers) Ltd 1999

The right of Marian Beaver, Jo Brewster, Pauline Jones, Anne Keene, Sally Neaum and Jill Tallack to be identified as authors of this work has been asserted by them in accordance with the Copyright, Designs and Patents Act 1988.

First published in 1995 by:
Stanley Thornes (Publishers) Ltd
Ellenborough House
Wellington Street
CHELTENHAM
GL50 1YW
United Kingdom

Second edition 1999

00 01 02 03 / 10 9 8 7 6 5 4 3 2

A catalogue record for this book is available from the British Library.

ISBN 0 7487 3975 0

Illustrated by Phil Ford and Oxford Illustrators
Typeset by Columns Design Ltd, Reading
Printed and bound in Italy by Vincenzo Bona, Turin

Contents

Introduction

This book has been written for both child-care students and practitioners with the intention of examining the principles, practice and context of the child-care worker's role in providing for care and education of children from birth to 8 years. The book relates to the syllabus requirements of the CACHE Certificate in Child Care and Education and the CACHE Diploma in Nursery Nursing as well as the BTEC National Diploma in Early Childhood Studies. The book also covers the requirements for underpinning knowledge for NVQ awards in Level 3 Child Care and Education. Students on any of the many other courses that require a knowledge and understanding of child development will also find the book useful. Child-care establishments may find the book a valuable addition to their reference shelves and helpful in supporting in-service training.

The book is divided into seven parts, each part containing a number of chapters covering an important aspect of working with children. This is presented in a way that is accessible to the reader, identifying the responsibilities of the child-care worker and examining their role in caring for children in the family and in the child-care setting in the wider context of present-day society. Case studies help the reader to relate theoretical points to real-life situations. Throughout the chapters there are questions and tasks to recall knowledge and develop understanding.

Although the book is complete in itself, some references are made to chapters in the companion volume, *Babies and Young Children 1: Early Years Development*, 2nd edition, so that readers can extend their understanding of a particular point, perhaps relating it to an aspect of development. The index also contains full page referencing to the companion volume.

Since the first edition, the book has been substantially revised. Every chapter has been examined and extended or updated as necessary and there are some additional chapters. A number of new features have been introduced to help readers relate theory to practice and to check and develop their own learning. Throughout the book there are cross-referenced exercises and tasks which provide the reader with opportunities to gather evidence for Key Skills at level 2 in Communication, IT and Application of Number.

About the authors

Marian Beaver has worked in social work, teaching and early years care and education. She has taught for many years on child-care courses in FE. She continues to work in FE at New College Nottingham, Basford Hall and as an external verifier for CACHE, as well as writing and inspecting nursery provision for Ofsted.

Jo Brewster has practised as a nurse, midwife and health visitor. She has taught for many years on child-care courses in FE at New College Nottingham, Basford Hall, as well as writing, inspecting nursery provision for Ofsted and working as an external verifier for CACHE.

Pauline Jones worked in residential child care and as a social worker before lecturing in FE, including Doncaster College for the Deaf. She developed the Diploma in Nursery Nurse Training for profoundly deaf students. She now manages the Child, Health and Social Care curriculum area at West Nottinghamshire College.

Anne Keene comes from a background of nursing, midwifery and Health Visiting. Until June 1998 she managed child-care programmes at Basford Hall College. She has recently established MTW International, a child-care training and recruitment agency, which aims to recruit high quality child-care workers for families, child-care establishments, out-of-school clubs and playschemes, as well as businesses seeking to meet child-care needs of their employees.

Sally Neaum has taught in nursery classes and across the infant age range. She has taught a range of child-care courses in a college of FE. She now works freelance, writing, teaching and as an Ofsted inspector of nursery provision.

Jill Tallack has taught in schools across the whole primary age range. She has worked for some years in a college of FE, teaching on child-care programmes. As well as writing, she also inspects nursery provision for Ofsted.

How to use this book

The new edition of this book and its companion volume, *Babies and Young Children Book 1*, have been written and designed to be even more effective and informative than their enormously popular first editions. The features have been changed to update their relevance. The design has been altered to make the books more open, and a second colour added to make each page more attractive and easy to use. The range of features used in both books is described below.

Introduction to each part

Both books are divided into a number of parts, each of which has a title and comprises several chapters linked by a common theme.

Chapter introduction

Every chapter begins with a summary of its contents, and a list of other chapters that may be relevant for additional reading.

Definitions

Students can be surprised by some of the technical language included in what they read. Where significant new words are introduced in the text, you will find a clear definition of each word in a box in the margin alongside.

Case studies

New case studies have been developed, showing how an issue can be dealt with in a practical environment. Each is followed by two or three questions to give you practice in problem-solving.

Do this!

These are activities that require you to do something. Each one is numbered and by looking up the number in the Key Skills grids on pages x–xi you will find out the Key Skills evidence that may be generated if you complete the activity.

Think about it

These are ideas for thought and reflection. You may wish to think these through on your own, or discuss them with others. Many make ideal subjects for whole class discussion.

Progress check

At the end of each major section within a chapter you will find a short list of questions. Answering these will confirm that you have understood what you have read.

Key terms

At the end of each chapter you will find a list of all the words that appear in the definition boxes throughout the text. You can read through to check that you understand each one.

'Now try these questions'

Each chapter finishes with a number of short-answer questions. If you answer these, you will show that you understand the key concepts in the chapter and are able to write about them in your own words.

Glossary

At the end of the book you will find a comprehensive glossary. It explains all the key terms used in both Books 1 and 2 of *Babies and Young Children*.

Index

Like the glossary, the index covers both Books 1 and 2. If a word has an entry in both books, then both page references will appear, with the references to this book in blue, and to Book 1 in black.

Key skills

Many students studying child care also need to demonstrate their competence in Key Skills. You will find guidelines to five of the level 2 Key Skills on pages vi–ix (more detailed coverage will be available from your tutor, assessor or supervisor). The *Do this!* activities in these books provide evidence for the Key Skills units Communication, Number and Information Technology. You will also find a grid on pages x–xi showing you which *Do this!* activities provide evidence for which Key Skills units and elements.

This book and its companion has been written to support a variety of CACHE, City and Guilds, Edexcel (BTEC), RSA early years education, child-care and health awards at level 2 and level 3. It aims both to provide knowledge and understanding and to enhance practical skills for a range of workers including NVQ candidates and DNN (NNEB) students. We are sure that you will like it – and wish you good luck in your studies.

Communication

Effective communication is at the heart of good working practice. There are many ways in which we communicate at work, through conversations, discussions and presentations. These may be direct, over the telephone, by fax, letter or email. They may involve colleagues, managers, children, their parents and others in the community. When you are caring for children what you say and what you understand can have serious consequences for children's well being. Communication includes each of the following areas.

Taking part in discussions

Child-care workers need to be able to speak clearly and listen carefully. In any discussion it is helpful to:
- keep to the subject
- express yourself clearly (and say if you do not!)
- keep the discussion moving forwards.

Discussions take many forms: informal conversations with colleagues, formal meetings such as staff meetings, planned presentations to groups of people or telephone conversations with, for example, a child's parent or carer.

Producing written material

The benefit of written communication is that the opportunity for misunderstanding may be reduced and accurate records kept. Information can also be shared between several people when direct contact is not possible. Once something is written down, however, it is more difficult to amend. Written information needs to be accurate, legible, easy to understand and in a suitable format.

There are many ways in which written material can be produced. You may need to complete a child's record card, send a letter to a parent, produce a report for a nursery manager, apply in writing for a job as a nanny or complete surveys and questionnaires when helping to set up a local playgroup. Spelling, grammar and punctuation should be checked to ensure accuracy.

Using images

You have probably heard the saying that a picture is worth a thousand words. There will be many opportu-nities in your work in early years care to use pictures and images to communicate.

Choose clear images that are relevant to what you want to say and:
- suited for those who will need to understand them
- recognise and value diversity
- promote equality of opportunity and anti-discrimi-natory practice.

Images may be nursery floor plans, illustrations for a monthly newsletter for parents, graphs and charts of attendance for use in an annual report or eye-catching photographs for advertising your facilities. Images can equally well be used to clarify a point in one-to-one or group discussion.

Reading and responding to written materials

We are surrounded by written materials: magazines, reports advertisements, timetables, signs, books and leaflets – the list is endless. It is important to be able to choose the right source of material for your purpose and to be able to get the information you want from it. Once you have chosen your source, you need to be able to extract the relevant information, check that you understand it and are able to summarise it.

As a child-care worker you need to understand documents such as the important written policies and procedures of your workplace, the timetable for the children's day, letters from parents or the statutory bodies and agendas and minutes for meetings. You also need to be able to interpret any pictures and images accompanying written information.

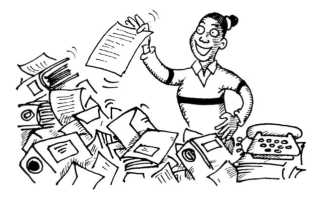

Application of number

It may surprise you how often you will be dealing with numbers, data and mathematical problem-solving in your work with children. Dealing with numbers is more straightforward when you understand why you are doing it. Accuracy is important. Application of number includes the following areas.

Collecting and recording data

Data is numerical information; you need to be able to collect and record such information. Once you know what kind of information you need, you will have to decide how you are going to collect it, conduct your tasks in the right order and record your results clearly and accurately. You may wish to record information from parents at an enrolment interview or record attendance levels at a nursery over a period of weeks. You may need to plan a new home corner, measure up the space available and draw up an accurate plan of your proposals. You may be involved in collecting money from parents and keeping accurate records of how much has been paid to you.

One question you do need to ask yourself when collecting data is how precise you need to be. If you are surveying the arrival times of children at a nursery you may need to be precise only to the nearest five minutes. If you are collecting money from parents, you cannot afford any mistakes at all!

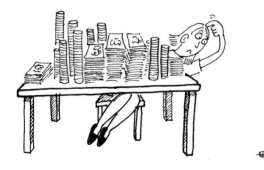

Tackling problems

From time to time you will come across problems at work which will need to be solved using numerical techniques. It is important to choose the correct technique to start with and to make sure that you do everything in the right order. Any calculations need to be accurate and you should check your work to make sure that there are no errors and that your results make sense.

You may need to:

- work out amounts of disposable materials such as paper, paints or clay that will be required for an activity
- account for how money has been spent during a certain period
- help in conducting local surveys for the opening of a new nursery.

All these require their own techniques and the results of each need to be presented appropriately.

Interpreting and presenting data

Large amounts of data are impossible to understand unless presented clearly; just as a picture can speak a thousand words, so a graph can present a thousand numbers. It is almost certain that you, or someone else, will be making decisions based on the information you present, so the graphs, charts, tables, pictograms, plans, diagrams or drawings used should be clear and appropriate. You should outline the main features of your data, ensure appropriate axes or labels are clear and explain how your results are relevant to the problem.

The outcome of a nursery survey may best be presented in graphs, charts an tables, while proposals to change the use of nursery space, for example, will probably use plans and diagrams.

Information technology

Most information is now stored electronically, on an information technology (or IT) system. The strength of such systems is that they can also reorganise, manipulate and provide information and (in theory at least!) reduce the amount of paper used in the workplace. Information technology includes the following areas.

Preparing information

Output information is only as good as the information put in, so all information should be accurate. It is important to plan carefully so that the information you put in is in an appropriate form, and once entered, can easily be edited. You should also save all your information in well organised files and folders and make back-up copies in case something goes wrong with your centrally stored files.

The names, addresses and postcodes of parents, for example, should be organised so that the information can be easily used for mailings; survey and questionnaire findings should be carefully recorded so that they can be transferred to a spreadsheet and source information for a termly newsletter (text, pictures, tables or graphs) entered so that it can be electronically merged into a single file.

Processing information

Entering information onto a system is not, in itself, particularly useful. It is the computer's power to access and select information in different ways, to combine information from different sources and to provide user-friendly output that makes it such a useful tool. Finding, retrieving, editing, combining and reorganising information will help you shape raw data to your needs.

Once properly organised, parental addresses can be used, for example, for mail shots, individual letters, reaching the parents of children within a specific age range or within a particular postal district. The raw data from the survey can be processed into graphs, charts or tables and the individual parts of the newsletter put into an appropriate format.

Presenting information

Presenting information clearly and professionally is in your own interest as well as your employer's. Even the best ideas may go unnoticed if poorly presented; people may simply not understand your point. A professional approach is particularly important in working with children, as you may need to win the approval, confidence and support of parents, the local authority and the wider community – and your employer.

You should be able to present your processed information in an appropriate way and choose the most effective software to do so. Consistency is important and you should always save your finished work in carefully organised files and make regular back-ups.

You will develop a reputation for thoroughness and professionalism by doing the following:

- consistently and accurately fulfilling and updating your mailings
- producing surveys and other reports in a recognisable form in a common format
- publishing your newsletters to the same high standard every term.

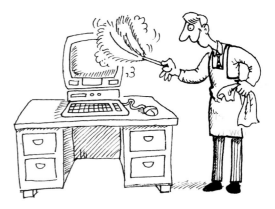

Evaluating the use of information technology

It is important that you know when information technology can make your life easier – and when it cannot! It is also important to understand the range of software available to you and what its functions and limits are.

A computer and its software is like any other machine. It needs to be carefully maintained, and faults and problems logged so that thay can be dealt with. It is also important that your working practices are healthy and safe and that you protect yourself and your machine by correctly positioning the keyboard and screen, keeping cables tidy, keeping food and drink away from where you are working and storing equipment away from sources of heat and other electrical equipment.

Improving own learning and performance

We all have strengths and weaknesses, and to improve our own learning and performance it is important that we can identify them. Setting targets and reviewing progress will help you to focus more clearly on what you need to do. Improving own learning and performance includes the following areas.

Identifying targets

You should be able to identify your strengths and weaknesses and provide evidence to support what you say. You will also need to be able to help in setting short-term targets for your own improvement, in conjunction with your teacher, assessor or workplace supervisor. When targets have been set, make sure that you understand what is required of you!

Following schedules to meet your targets

Once your targets for improvement are agreed, you should be able to follow them without close supervision, within the specified time scale. You will, of course, receive support in your work and you should know how to put this to good use in improving your work and meeting your targets.

Being SMART!

Be	**S**pecific in setting your targets and schedules!
Tackle learning in	**M**anageable chunks!
Make sure your targets are	**A**chievable!
Keep your targets	**R**elevant.
Track progress so you are on	**T**ime in meeting your targets!

Working with others

When you work in child care, you are unlikely to work alone. Learning with other people can be a great challenge, but also bring great rewards. Working with others includes the following areas (see also Chapter 3, *The nursery nurse in employment* in this book).

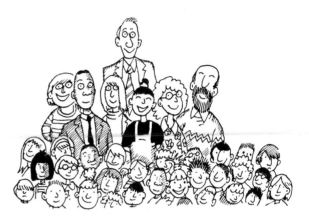

Identifying collective goals and responsibilities

When you work with others you need to be able to identify and agree group goals. You also need to be clear about who is responsible for what and how you are going to organise working together.

Working to collective goals

Once you understand your responsibilities you should set about organising your work so that you will be able to achieve your goals on time. You will need to stick to the working methods agreed by the whole group.

Key skills grid

The following grid indicates key skills coverage provided by *Do this!* activities in this book.

Do this!	Communication				Information Technology				Application of Number		
	2.1	2.2	2.3	2.4	2.1	2.2	2.3	2.4	2.1	2.2	2.3
1.1					x	x	x		x	x	x
1.2			x				x		x	x	
1.3						x					
2.1	x			x							
2.2		x					x				
3.1		x		x			x				
3.2	x										
3.3	x			x							
3.4				x							
3.5		x									
3.6	x	x		x			x				
4.1	x			x							
4.2				x							
4.3		x	x				x				
4.4	x	x	x				x				
4.5	x	x									
5.1					x	x	x				
5.2		x		x							
5.3		x		x							
5.4		x									
5.5		x									
5.6	x	x									
6.1				x			x				
6.2		x	x								
7.1	x	x									
7.2		x									
7.3	x			x							x
7.4				x							
7.5		x	x	x							
7.6		x	x								
7.7		x							x		
7.8		x									
7.9		x									
8.1						x	x		x		
8.2									x		
8.3		x									
8.4				x							
8.5				x	x	x	x				
8.6				x							
8.7									x	x	
9.1		x	x								
9.2									x		x
9.3	x		x								
9.4									x		x
10.1	x										
10.2									x		x
10.3				x							
10.4	x						x		x		x

Do this!	Communication				Information Technology				Application of Number		
	2.1	2.2	2.3	2.4	2.1	2.2	2.3	2.4	2.1	2.2	2.3
10.5				X							
10.6									X	X	X
10.7					X	X	X				
10.8		X							X		
11.1							X				
11.2					X	X	X	X			
12.1	X										
12.2									X		X
12.3											X
13.1	X			X							
13.2	X			X							
13.3		X									
13.4	X	X									
13.5		X		X							
13.6							X				
14.1	X										
14.2					X						
14.3				X							
14.4		X									
14.5		X								X	X
14.6									X	X	X
15.1	X	X	X	X	X	X	X				
15.2	X	X	X	X	X	X	X				
16.1	X	X							X	X	X
16.2	X	X	X	X			X		X		X
17.1			X	X	X	X	X		X	X	X
17.2		X	X						X	X	X
17.3				X	X	X	X		X	X	X
17.4		X		X			X				
17.5									X	X	X
18.1									X		
19.1	X	X	X	X							
19.2		X	X								
19.3			X								
19.4		X									
19.5		X									
20.1		X		X							
20.2	X	X	X	X	X	X	X		X	X	X
20.3	X	X	X	X			X		X		
20.4	X										
21.1			X								
21.2				X							
21.3				X							
22.1			X	X							
22.2	X										
23.1		X									
23.2			X								
24.1											
24.2									X	X	X
24.3	X		X	X							

Acknowledgements

The authors and publishers would like to thank the following people and organisations for permission to reproduce photographs and other material:

The University of Sheffield for an extract from *Ways of Working with Parents to Promote Early Literacy Development* in USDE Papers, by J. Weinberger, P. Hannon and C. Nutbrown; Jacky Chapman/Format; The National Medical Slide Bank, The Wellcome Trust, St John's Institute of Dermatology, Great Ormond Street Hospital for Children, The National Eczema Society; Val Jackson, Irene Tipping, Juliette Khan and Sue Didcott; and Sterling Associates for the cover photograph.

Every effort has been made to contact copyright holders and we apologise if any have been overlooked.

Part 1: Aspects of Professional Practice

The first part considers some important features of good, professional child-care practice. The role of the child-care worker in providing an environment for children that is safe, stimulating and secure is examined in some detail. The rights and responsibilities of the child-care worker in employment are identified in the context of a commitment to ongoing professional development. The authors recognise that the needs of children are met most effectively if child-care workers work alongside the child's primary carers. This part looks at the ways in which this crucial relationship can be established and fostered.

All good child-care practice should be viewed through the perspective of equality of opportunity. A chapter on this subject raises issues that are developed throughout the rest of the book.

1 The care and education environment

This chapter includes:

- **The physical environment**
- **Creating a stimulating environment for children**
- **A reassuring environment**

Child-care workers should plan and create an environment that is caring, stimulating and attractive to children and one that best meets their needs at different ages. There are many factors involved in creating a stimulating and caring environment for children. It can be achieved by providing a range of age-appropriate equipment and resources, giving careful consideration to the layout and decoration of a room, including safety, through good teaching skills and a caring approach. Displays and interest tables are also an effective way of creating a stimulating and attractive environment for children and enhancing their self-esteem.

The child-care and education environment may be the only place outside the child's home that a child is left without their main carer. Child-care workers need to provide a reassuring setting for the children in their care. If their needs are met in a friendly and nurturing environment, it will increase their feelings of security and well-being.

You may find it helpful to read this chapter in conjunction with:

- **Book 1, Chapter 7**   An introduction to language and cognitive development
- **Book 1, Chapter 14**   The development of self-image and self-concept
- **Book 1, Chapter 15**   Bonding and attachment
- **Book 2, Chapter 5**   Play

The physical environment

Arranging the area

Child-care settings are located in a variety of types of accommodation. Some will be modern and purpose-built, but others will be sited in buildings which were not designed with the needs of children in mind. In a large area, such as a village hall, several activities can be in progress at the same time. In a home environment, the activities may be restricted to one or two at a time, but with changes of scene and other everyday activities, like shopping, planned throughout the day.

Choosing furniture and equipment and planning the layout is important to make the setting welcoming, safe, reassuring and stimulating for the children.

When deciding how to arrange the area, the following factors are important.

> **regulations**
> Formal rules that must be followed

■ *Local authority* **regulations** In order to comply with the Children Act 1989, all social services departments issue guidelines for providers of day care, including childminders. These guidelines cover aspects of child care such as safety, heating, ventilation, hygiene and outside play spaces. Regulations also cover the amount of space required for each child and the number of adults required to care for the children.

The prescribed **ratios** of adults to children for these age groups are:

> **ratio**
> The numerical relationship or proportion of one quantity to another

    0–1 years – 1 adult to 3 children
    1–3 years – 1 adult to 4 children
    3–5 years – 1 adult to 8 children.

These numbers are the minimum requirements. You would expect to have fewer children per adult if some of the children had special needs. Children also need to get out and about to enjoy local outings to the shops or park and you would need more adults in these circumstances.

The required amount of space for each child in these age groups is:

    0–2 years – 40 square feet (3.72 square metres)
    2–3 years – 30 square feet (2.79 square metres)
    3–5 years – 25 square feet (2.32 square metres).

■ *Safety requirements* There should be adequate space, heating, ventilation and lighting. Heating appliances should be properly guarded. Local authority regulations should be adhered to with regard to the physical space provided and the number of adults caring for the children. Exit doors should be securely fastened and not be capable of being opened by any of the children. Doorways, emergency exits and fire escapes should be kept clear at all times. Staff should be aware of the procedure for emergencies, such as fire, and there should be regular drills and practices.

■ *Feeling secure* Welcoming children into an attractive and thoughtfully arranged environment will help to reassure an insecure child. Child-care settings should be geared to the needs of the children with child-sized equipment, attractive displays and a quiet, calm atmosphere.

■ *Attractiveness* Furniture carpets and curtains will all help to make the environment a pleasant place for the children to work in. In a child-centred environment, these items should be chosen with children in mind, particularly with regard to size and durability.

■ *Space* Children need plenty of space to play, but often a large open space is not conducive to the most purposeful types of play. Large spaces should be broken up by moving furniture into smaller areas which offer different types of activities for example, sand/water/painting/home corner/book area. This will enable the children to concentrate more readily and allows for flexibility in the overall makeup of the space.

- *Outdoors* The outdoor area provides for an important aspect of children's learning and should be planned with care. Eliminate obvious hazards with regard to large equipment, like slides and climbing frames, by paying particular attention to where they are placed and providing adequate supervision. A tarmac or paved space should be available and, where possible, a grassy area and space for growing things.
- *Comfort* Ensure that the temperature of the setting is kept between 16–24° C (60–75° F) and that there is adequate fresh air circulating. Lighting in each part of the setting should be adequate for the activities provided. A quiet area with carpet and/or cushions to settle and look at books or to do a puzzle will encourage children to pick up and look at books and engage in quieter activities.
- *Working as individuals, in pairs or groups* The environment can be modified to encourage children to work alone, with partners or in groups. A carpeted area is a good idea for bringing the children together for registration, sharing news and at story time. Children may also be encouraged to work in groups by setting small tables with chairs. Individual work, such as reading to the carer and using the computer, can also be managed in this way.
- *Movement between activities* Adults and children need to be able to access all parts of the setting. Planning the layout of the environment should allow for sufficient space between activities and free access to the cloakroom, toilets, kitchen and outdoor areas.
- *Access to equipment* Children thrive on responsibility and being allowed to make their own decisions within a safe framework. Resources should be as accessible as possible to the children so that they can choose which materials they are going to use.
- *Providing a variety of activities* Child-care workers will need to change the activities on offer, perhaps with the help of the children – access to storage areas is necessary. Children can be encouraged to be responsible for parts of the setting, putting equipment away, tidying areas of the setting and clearing litter from the outdoor area. Children can also be involved in helping to prepare and give out snacks.

Ensuring accessibility

accessible
Easy to reach or approach

All activities and areas of the setting must be **accessible** to all children. Children with special needs can be welcomed into any setting where thought and consideration is given to their needs. Children with a physical disability may need wider doorways, ramps, larger toilet area and space to manoeuvre around classroom furniture.

Children with a sensory impairment may need equipment to help to increase their sensory awareness. For example, a deaf child may need a hearing aid, good lighting, use of British Sign Language. A visually-impaired child will need the floor to be kept clear and the furniture and activity areas to be arranged in the same way. Any changes to the physical environment should be planned and explained to the child in advance. Large print books may be helpful and it is important to provide rich and varied tactile experiences.

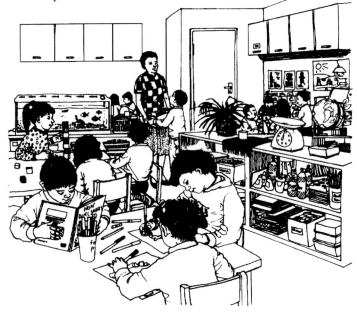

Group activities can be encouraged in a child-centred environment

A child-orientated environment

There are several ways of making a child-care environment that is not purpose-built, such as a family home, safer and more child-friendly. Provide:

■ small tables and chairs
■ small toilets or toilet seats
■ steps to make sinks accessible and to enable children to reach things
■ stairgates and fireguards
■ high handles on doors where you need to prevent children gaining access to other areas
■ locks on cupboards not to be used by the children, and on fridges and upstairs windows
■ low cupboards for storing creative equipment/books/activities for the children to select themselves.

Outdoor play area

Children need to be able to be out in the fresh air as much as possible and to be involved in vigorous play activities. The external environment may need to be adapted to allow this, or there may be no garden or outside play space so the children will need to go out on walks or to local parks or playgrounds. The outdoor play space should be safe and secure. It should provide a variety of surfaces, areas that are covered for when the weather is wet, shady areas to provide cover on hot days. If possible, there should be trees and plants within the outdoor area. The activities should be planned within the outdoor area to allow for space to run around and use the wheeled toys safely, while still allowing an area to be used for more restful activities.

Case study: Playing outside in hot weather

Maria is a childminder and cares for three children each day – Tom and Venus, both aged 3, and Damon who is 4. It is a very hot and sunny day, too hot to be indoors. Maria's house has a garden that the children like to play in; there is some shade in one part of the garden under the tree. Maria is very careful to put high-factor sun cream on the children's skin and she reapplies this regularly. She also makes sure that the children have plenty to drink.

1 How can the outdoor play be arranged to make it suitable for the children on days like this?
2 List three activities that would be suitable for the garden of a family home on a hot day?
3 How could you, quickly, create more shade in the garden?

The natural world

Children learn from and enjoy activities involving growing plants and investigating the living world. Participating in gardening activities has many benefits for children, if there is an awareness of their level of development and if expectations are adjusted accordingly. Safety will be an important consideration, and fences and gates must be secure.

The benefits of these activities include:

- an increased knowledge of biological processes and cycles as seeds develop into plants
- a sense of achievement as the children see the plants grow
- an increased awareness of the care of plants, for example the need for regular watering and feeding
- developing language as new words are used to describe the plants, stages of their development and gardening activities
- learning new skills, such as planting, digging, watering, pruning
- an awareness of time during the growth cycle
- learning about safety issues, for example not eating berries or flowers, taking care with gardening tools, hygiene after gardening.

Pets

There may also be an opportunity to keep pets in the child-care setting. This can be an enjoyable way for children to learn about animals and to take responsibility for their care. However, it is important to find out whether any child or member of staff is allergic to any type of pet.

Do this!   *1.1*

1 Draw a plan to scale of a large village hall which is 50 feet long and 25 feet wide (15.24 metres by 7.62 metres). The hall is used every morning as a pre-school playgroup for children aged 3–5 years old. On your plan show:
  - the measurements of the hall
  - the total surface area in square feet and in square metres
  - the number of children that could be accommodated under the local authority regulations
  - the number of adults that would be needed under the Children Act regulations
  - the kitchen
  - the exit(s)
  - the toilets
  - how you would divide up the space available for the playgroup
  - where you would position the activities.

2 Devise a checklist that could be used to check the safety of the outdoor play area. Present this in chart form using information technology.

✓ Progress check

1 What factors are important when deciding the layout of a child-care setting?
2 What type of equipment would make the environment more child-centred?
3 How can a child with a physical disability be made to feel welcome and secure in the child-care setting?
4 How can the environment be adapted to enable a visually-impaired child to make full use of all facilities?
5 What are the benefits for children of exploring the natural world?

Creating a stimulating environment for children

Displays and interest tables are an effective way of creating a stimulating and attractive environment for children and of enhancing their self-esteem.

The values of display

Why display? Display has many values. It can:
- be used as a stimulus for learning across all areas of the curriculum

- encourage children to look, think, reflect, explore, investigate and talk and respond to their interests
- act as a sensory and imaginative stimulus
- give children ideas, and promote further investigation and research
- encourage parental involvement in their children's learning, and reinforce links with home
- encourage self-esteem by showing appreciation of children's work
- encourage communication with children
- make the environment attractive, and attract children's attention
- encourage awareness of the wider community, reflect the rich cultural diversity of society and reinforce acceptance of difference.

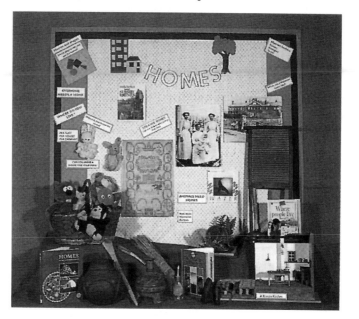

Displaying work encourages children's interest

Where display?

Displays should be placed wherever they can be seen easily, or touched if appropriate. It is worth an adult getting down to the child's eye level and viewing the surroundings from that position. The position of the display will affect the size and type of display. A flat wall can be made into a three-dimensional display if there is enough space in front of it. A corner can be made into an imaginative play area with appropriate decoration; the display may be on a table, cupboard or screen.

What to include in a display

Variety makes displays interesting, so it is important to change styles, techniques and content. Displays can include paintings, items of children's individual work, co-operative efforts, natural materials and plants, objects of interest, photographs, pictures, collage, real objects, use of different colours, textures and labelling.

All children should be able to contribute to the displays in their environment. When looking around their room, it is preferable for every child to have at least one piece of their work displayed, or have taken part in a group display.

Children should be involved in the choice of work that will be displayed and where possible in the mounting of work and the creation of the display.

Any labels must be clear, of an appropriate size, in lower case letters except at the beginning of sentences and proper nouns, and include the home languages of the children in the setting.

Displays that include people should, wherever possible and appropriate, reflect a **multicultural**, **multiability society** and be without gender bias. Displays should project positive images in any setting. Black people, women and people with disabilities are usually under-represented in the wider visual environment. When planning displays, workers should choose images that challenge stereotypes, such as a black barrister, a disabled doctor, or a woman police officer.

Children should be given the opportunity to represent themselves accurately. Workers should provide mirrors, and paints and crayons that enable children to match their own skin tones.

The entrance to a centre gives the first impression that parents, children and visitors gain of your work. A welcoming entrance with displays of children's work will contribute to giving a positive impression and demonstrate your professional standards.

> **multicultural society**
> A society whose members have a variety of cultural and ethnic backgrounds

> **multiability society**
> A society where people have a variety of differing abilities and disabilities

Display techniques

It is important to plan displays, thinking everything through first. Having decided the position, consideration should be given to the appropriate colours, backing, drapes and borders that are appropriate.

Good presentation is essential, including good mounting and well-produced lettering. Staples and adhesive materials should be used discretely.

The use of colour should be carefully considered. There are no rules – bright colours can be effective, but black and white may also be appropriate.

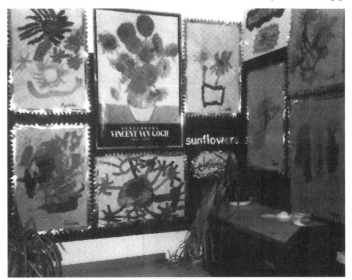

Good planning and presentation are essential for successful displays

Case study: An outing to the theatre

It is December and the staff of a rural infant school plan to take the children to see a performance for schools of a pantomime at a theatre in a nearby town. On their return a variety of cross-curricula work is planned, including a display showing both the stage and the audience at the theatre.

The outing is very successful for the children. On their return the teacher first discusses what and who they have observed, and establishes they have understood the story of the pantomime. She also finds that they have noticed there were children from different ethnic backgrounds in the audience, and also some children with special needs. As part of the display, in order to make a collage, the children are encouraged to paint a small figure of themselves and also a few paintings of other children in the audience. The children enjoy painting themselves and others, and then cutting around them and helping to stick them onto the display. The result is a colourful, multiethnic, multiability picture that is a source of much discussion both between the children, and with their parents and other visitors to the classroom.

1 Why might it be particularly relevant to take children from a rural environment to the theatre in a town?
2 Why is it valuable for children to paint pictures of themselves for the display?
3 What is the value of the discussion about the people the children had observed in the audience?
4 What do you think the children gained from painting other children in the audience?
5 Why do you think this display was such a valuable resource for discussion?

How long to display?

The length of time a display remains should be considered and planned. Any display that has become old or faded should be replaced. A display should remain only while it bears relevance to the curriculum and is still being referred to. Displays can be used as an integral part of the curriculum, especially to reflect aspects of topic work. Once a new topic is begun, it is important to plan and make new displays.

Interest tables

Interest tables can be used to follow a theme or the class topic, or display work/collections from a recent outing. They should be at the child's height, used to display three-dimensional objects and sited in a quieter area of the setting. The table should be covered and any objects that are not intended to be touched should placed in a protective container, such as a plastic tank.

Helping children to learn about the natural world is vital – seeing how things grow and develop is part of learning about the world. Children can collect and display their findings – from autumn leaves to sea-life. Health and safety is important when displaying such objects – be aware of the dangers of displaying poisonous berries and plants, or sharp objects. Food on display should be fresh and changed regularly.

Reference books should be available on the table for children to look up areas of their interest.

Adding interest to displays

Interest can be added by good use of:

- colour – a co-ordinated backing and border can be used to display the children's work to its best advantage, drapes may add interest
- texture – include things that are interesting to touch and contrast with each other, for example smooth, shiny pebbles and rough sandpaper
- movement – consider hanging displays and windmills that spin in the breeze
- sound – crackly paper, shakers and musical instruments made by the children all make appealing displays
- characters that the children are familiar with from books read at story time, people they have met on a trip or who have visited the establishment.

Benefits to child development of display work

- *Physical development* – Fine motor skills in creative work, such as cutting, sticking, drawing, painting
  Gross motor skills in co-ordination, reaching, stretching, bending, balancing
- *Cognitive (intellectual) development* – Encourage problem-solving, decision-making and thinking skills, stimulate memory
  Mathematical skills – patterns, shapes, angles, measuring
- *Language development* – New words and vocabulary, use of reference books, discussion and listening skills, asking questions
- *Emotional development* – Sense of achievement and increased self-esteem, children feel proud of their work displayed for parents to see. Displays which are pleasant and stimulating to look at help children to feel comfortable with their environment
- *Personal and social development* – Encourage team work and co-operation between adults and children, sharing of resources and ideas. Opportunity to experience new materials and textures, sensory stimulation. Increase awareness and knowledge of cultural diversity

> ### Do this! 1.2
>
> Choose an area for a display. Measure the entire surface. Calculate the proportion of the surface that the display will cover. Calculate the amount of backing paper that will be needed. Work out the length of the border that must be made to surround it.
>
> Create a display using children's work. Ensure that it is appropriate to the curriculum or stage of development of the children. You should include appropriate handwritten or word-processed labels.

✓ Progress check

1 What are the values of good displays?
2 Why is it important to display children's work?
3 What do you need to think about before planning a display?
4 How can interest tables be used?
5 What are the benefits of display to development?

A reassuring environment

The child-care and education environment may be the only place outside the child's home that a child is left without their main carer. Child-care workers therefore need to provide a reassuring setting for the children in their care. If children's needs are met in a friendly and nurturing environment, it will increase their feelings of security and well-being.

Providing a secure environment

In order to provide adequate and appropriate reassurance for children, child-care workers need to have a knowledge of typical social and emotional development. Looking at the world from the child's point of view will help to identify their fears. Most babies up to the age of 6 months are usually afraid of loud noises and sudden movements. Those commonly experienced by toddlers and older children include fears of separation, loud noises, the dark, spiders, strangers, animals, blood, and other anxieties.

All children should be kept physically safe from harm, but they also need to feel safe and secure emotionally. This will be helped by adapting the physical environment; large areas can be divided into smaller spaces for quieter activities. Pre-school children who are in day care should be offered experiences which are similar to those they would have at home, such as visiting the shops, the park and posting letters. Adopting similar sleep times and daily routines and offering familiar foods will also help a child to feel more secure.

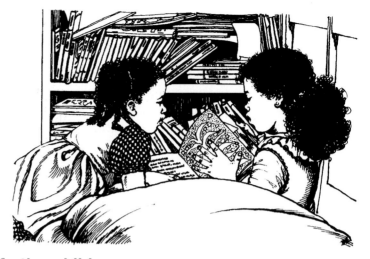

Children feel secure with familiar objects

Comforting children

Most children who are afraid will cry and seek comfort from a caring adult. Some fears are shown in more subtle ways and a child may show signs of being generally anxious. Children in an unfamiliar environment may react in a variety of ways. They may show their fears by crying, clinging to their parent/carer, being unwilling to try new experiences, loss of appetite, sleeping problems. As children cannot always tell the adult what the source of their anxiety is, the child-care worker must try to identify the cause.

Dealing with the problem depends on the cause of the anxiety. Some children may need more reassurance than anticipated in certain situations, so it is important to know about any special methods for helping individual children. Listening to what parents and carers tell you about this will help. Generally children will respond positively to:

- clear and honest explanations about what is going to happen. You may need to repeat these explanations, as young children may not remember or understand what you have said
- in the case of an unexpected incident, clear explanation of what has just happened
- a reassuring cuddle – although some children may not appreciate physical comfort
- stress-reducing activities like playdough, looking at books, painting
- having their preferred comfort objects, such as a special blanket or soft toy. This is especially important for the under 2s. Young children should not be discouraged from having their preferred comfort objects as they help to bridge the gap between the home setting and the care environment. They also play an important part in helping children to become more confident and independent in new situations. Comfort objects should be readily available to children. It may be advisable to keep all comforters, labelled with the children's names, in a central location until they are needed. A list of comforters and particular remedies will be useful if it can be displayed where staff can see and refer to it.

Changes and unexpected events

Children can easily become unsettled and upset if there are changes to their routine or environment. This can be more upsetting if the changes are unexpected or not explained, so it is important that, wherever possible, children have advance warning of any changes that you know about. Telling the children what is going to happen in simple and understandable terms will help to prevent anxiety. It is important for child-care workers to be positive and cheerful about any changes as this will be reassuring for the children. It will also be necessary to repeat and remind the children about what is going to happen. One of the most upsetting changes for children can be when their child-care worker leaves or is absent because of sickness or holiday. Whenever possible, children should be prepared for changes, but it is not possible to plan for unexpected events so the children will need to be reassured and comforted if they become distressed.

Case study: An unexpected visitor

The children at Fir Tree Pre-School were happily enjoying their mid-morning snack of fruit and milk. Helen, the leader, had opened the outside door as it was a warm day. The children were gathered on the carpet happily discussing the morning's events and sharing news from home. Helen was talking with the children when she noticed that Tom and Tanya were laughing and pointing at the doorway. Helen stood up and at that moment a large dog appeared, barking loudly. Some of the smaller children began to cry and the older ones looked anxious. Leanne, one of the other helpers, rushed to the door and managed to close it, leaving the dog outside. However, the dog continued to bark very loudly and more of the children got upset. Helen and Leanne comforted the children, but they were very relieved when the dog's owner arrived. He apologised saying that the dog had run off and explained that it was noisy but friendly. He put the dog on a lead and made it stop barking.

1 What would you do to help the children after the dog had gone?
2 What activities might help the children retell the event?
3 How would you help the children learn more about dogs and when it is safe to touch them and be friendly?

Belonging

Children need to develop a sense of belonging and will feel more at home in a setting that contains objects that are familiar to them from their homes and reflect their culture. For example:

■ The home play area should contain a range of types of cooking equipment – woks, griddles, chop-sticks, as well as saucepans, kettles, knives and forks.

■ Dressing up clothes should reflect a diversity of cultures and include saris, head-dresses, veils.
■ A wide selection of books should be available showing positive images of different races, cultures and sexes and reflecting equality of opportunity (see Chapter 2).
■ Displays should promote all cultures in society. Children can be encouraged to produce art and/or written work about their homes and families for display.
■ Visitors should be invited to come and talk to the children and help them to experience and appreciate social and cultural diversity.
■ Coat hooks should be labelled with names and/or pictures.
■ Equipment should be personalised – names on cups, flannels, work trays, etc.

Offering reassurance

Child-care workers should be warm, caring and responsive. Children easily recognise those who value and appreciate their company and those who have no real interest in them. The following points can help if you are not confident and will give positive messages to the children in your care.

■ Be calm and try to speak softly.
■ Maintain eye contact when speaking to children and try to get down to their eye level, sit with them or squat down to them if they are playing on the floor.
■ Meet their needs quickly. Pick up the non-verbal clues and anticipate their needs, for example the child hopping from one foot to another may need the toilet.
■ Be ready to cuddle a young child who is unhappy or upset. On the other hand, never force physical comfort on a child who does not welcome it.
■ Encourage conversation and give children time to speak. Ask open questions that will encourage a child to answer with more than a yes or no.
■ Always be cheerful, positive and polite. Enjoy your contact with the children in your care.

Do this!	*1.3*
Word-process an information sheet for parents and carers that explains how you will help new children to settle into the setting. Describe how you will ensure that the environment will be reassuring for the children and how you will anticipate and deal with any fears that the children may have.	

✓ *Progress check*

1 How can child-care workers help children to feel secure?
2 What are some common fears in young children?
3 How can adults comfort children who are distressed?
4 How can a sense of belonging be encouraged in a child-care setting?
5 Describe how you would explain to a group of children that the fire service will be coming to test the fire hydrants that morning.

Key terms

You need to know what these words and phrases mean. Go back through the chapter and find out.
accessible
multiability society
multicultural society
ratio
regulations

Now try these questions

1 When planning the indoor and outdoor play areas and putting out the equipment, what are the main factors you will need to take into account?

2 Describe some tasks that would be suitable for children, aged 2 to 5 years, to encourage a sense of responsibility towards the environment.

3 How can display work promote children's all-round development?

4 In what ways can displays be used to promote positive images of society?

5 Describe the behaviour of a child who is new to your child-care setting and who is anxious about the unfamiliar surroundings. How would you be able to help this child and allay the anxieties?

2 *Equality of opportunity*

This chapter includes:

- **Attitudes and discrimination**
- **Understanding equality**
- **Providing for equality**

This chapter examines why equality of opportunity is a key issue for child-care workers and one that is central to good, professional practice. It attempts to explain what is meant by the term and then looks generally at how child-care workers can promote equality of opportunity in their practice.

It is important to bear in mind that this chapter is only an introduction to the area: all of the following chapters will address aspects of equal opportunities as an integral part of their content.

Attitudes and discrimination

It is important that child-care workers demonstrate positive attitudes towards the children and families that they work with. Children and their families need to feel that they are valued for themselves, for who they are. Negative attitudes on the part of child-care workers can lead to discriminatory practices which affect feelings of self-worth. This may result in children failing to achieve their potential in later life and in families becoming disaffected with the child-care centre and its workers.

Positive and negative attitudes

Attitudes reflect our opinions. These can be both positive and negative. Our attitude to people affects the way we act and behave towards them. If we demonstrate a positive attitude towards someone, it enables that person to feel good, valued and have high **self-esteem**. A negative attitude towards a person is likely to lower their self-esteem and to make them feel worthless and rejected.

self-esteem
Liking and valuing oneself

Stereotyping

Stereotyping contributes to the development of negative attitudes. It involves making assumptions about people, without any evidence or proof, because, for example, they are of a particular race, gender or social origin. Stereotypes are harmful because they perpetuate negative, unthinking attitudes: they are limiting because they influence expectations.

stereotyping
When people think that all the individual members of a group have the same characteristics as each other; often applied on the basis of race, gender or disability

We give specific names to some negative attitudes.

- *Racism* describes when people of one race or culture believe that they are superior to another.
- *Sexism* is the term used when people of one gender believe that they are superior the other.

Stereotypical assumptions are often made about people with disabilities, those in the lower **socio-economic groups**, gay men and lesbian women, and other groups.

Where one group in society is powerful and holds stereotypical views about other groups, **discrimination** and **oppression** are likely to occur. This can reduce the choices, chances and, ultimately, the achievements of that group.

Institutionalised discrimination

Discrimination can occur even when individual workers have positive attitudes. If the institution does not consider and meet the needs of everyone involved in it, **institutionalised discrimination** can occur. This can happen when, for example:

- children with disabilities are not given access to the full curriculum
- the meals service does not meet the dietary requirements of certain religious groups
- a uniform code does not consider the cultural traditions of certain groups concerning dress.

Child-care workers are often not aware of how powerful the institutionalised practices of their organisation are in discriminating against certain groups of children and their families. Institutionalised discrimination is not necessarily a conscious policy on the part of the organisation, more often it occurs because of a failure to consider the diversity of the community. Whether conscious or unconscious, institutionalised discrimination is a powerful and damaging force.

The effects of stereotyping and discrimination

Children may suffer the effects of stereotyping and discrimination in a number of ways.

- Research by Milner (1983) shows that children as young as 3 attach value to skin colour, with both black and white children perceiving white skin as 'better' than black. This indicates that children absorb messages about racial stereotyping from a very early age. These messages are very damaging to the self-esteem of black children and may result in a failure to achieve their potential. Harm is done to white children too, and to society in general, unless this perception of racial superiority is confronted and challenged effectively. These findings underline the need for all settings, including those in all-white areas, to provide a positive approach that challenges stereotyping.
- Even very young children can hold fixed ideas about what boys can do and what girls can do. Observation of children's play shows that some

socio-economic group
Grouping of people according to their status in society, based on their occupation, which is closely related to their wealth/income

discrimination
Behaviour based on prejudice which results in someone being treated unfairly

oppression
Using power to dominate and restrict other people

institutionalised discrimination
Unfavourable treatment occurring as a consequence of the procedures and systems of an organisation

activities are avoided because of perceptions of what is appropriate for girls or for boys. This can result in boys and girls having a very limited view of the choices available to males and females in our society. This is particularly significant when, despite advances in recent years, many women still under-achieve.

■ Children with disabilities and their families are subject to many forms of discrimination. Even a caring environment may neglect the ordinary needs of the disabled child out of a concern to meet their special needs. This may mean that the disability is seen first, rather the child, and that the child's development is affected because of limited opportunities and low expectations.

■ Statistically, children from lower socio-economic groups under-achieve academically. As there is a strong connection between educational success and subsequent economic well-being, this is a worrying link which government policy is keen to address.

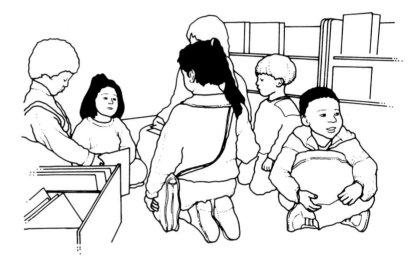

Child-care practice must meet the needs of a culturally diverse community

---

✓ *Progress check*

1 Why is important that child-care workers demonstrate positive attitudes towards the children and families that they work with?
2 What are the effects of stereotyping and discrimination?
3 What is institutionalised discrimination?
4 Which are the main groups that are likely to be affected by discrimination?

---

equal opportunities
All people participating in society to the best of their abilities, regardless of race, religion, disability, gender or social background

Understanding equality

Promoting **equal opportunities** means giving everyone an equal chance to participate in life to the best of their abilities, regardless of race, religion, disability, gender or social background. This will not be achieved by treating everyone the same, but by recognising and responding to the fact that people are *different* and that different people will have different needs and requirements. If these needs and differences are not recognised, then people will not receive equality of opportunity.

Case study: Responding to difference

Dinh started at playgroup when he was 3. His family had recently moved to the small town where the playgroup was located. His mother and father spoke some English, but Dinh understood and spoke only Vietnamese. The playgroup staff had little experience of working with non-English-speaking children, but they contacted the local educational authority who were able to provide them with some support from a peripatetic English as a Second Language teacher and access to some specialised resources. Together with the teacher, the staff were able to support Dinh who gradually gained competence and confidence in English, and was soon able to join in and enjoy all the playgroup activities.

1 What were Dinh's needs?
2 What would have happened to Dinh if the playgroup staff had not responded to him in this way?
3 Think of some other situations where failing to respond to difference would result in needs not being met?

Equality of opportunity is promoted in a number of ways.
- At government level, laws exist that are aimed at combatting oppression and discrimination.
- At institutional level, many organisations have policies and codes of conduct that promote equality.
- On a personal level, equal opportunities are addressed as the awareness of individuals is raised and they examine their own attitudes and values.

Equal opportunities and the law

Laws in themselves do not stop discrimination, just as speed limits do not stop people speeding. However, the existence of a law does send out a very clear message that discrimination is not acceptable and that penalties exist for those who flout the laws.

Race legislation
- The Race Relations Act 1965 outlawed discrimination on the basis of race in the provision of goods and services, in employment and in housing. Incitement to racial hatred also became an offence under this Act.
- In 1976 the Commission for Racial Equality was given power to start court proceedings in instances of racial discrimination.

■ The Children Act 1989 required that needs arising from children's race, culture, religion and language be considered by those caring for them.

Gender legislation

■ The Equal Pay Act 1970 gave women the right to equal pay with men for work of the same value.
■ The Employment Protection Act 1975 gave women the right to paid maternity leave.
■ The Sex Discrimination Act 1975 outlawed discrimination on the grounds of sex in employment, education, provision of goods and services and housing.
■ The Equal Opportunities Commission was set up in 1975 to enforce the laws relating to discrimination on the grounds of sex.

Disability legislation

■ The Education Act 1944 placed a duty on local education authorities (LEAs) to provide education for all children, including those with special needs.
■ The Disabled Persons (Employment) Act 1944 required larger employers to recruit a certain proportion of registered disabled people into their workforce.
■ The Education Act 1981 laid down specific procedures for the assessment and statementing of children with special educational needs. This was superseded by the Code of Practice for Special Educational Needs which was introduced as part of the Education Act 1993.
■ The Chronically Sick and Disabled Persons Act 1970 and the Disabled Persons Act 1986 imposed various duties on local authorities towards disabled people.
■ The Children Act 1989 defined the services that should be provided by the local authority for 'children in need'. Children who are disabled are included in this category.
■ The Disability Discrimination Act 1995 was passed to ensure that any services offered to the public in general must be offered, on the same basis, to people with disabilities.

Although there appears to be a substantial amount of legislation here, it should be remembered that it is up to the person who feels that they have been discriminated against to make a case and start proceedings. Successful prosecutions are comparatively rare.

Equal opportunities and the organisation

Many organisations have developed and adopted their own equal opportunities policies which they apply to matters involving both staff and clients. Operating against the policy will often have serious disciplinary implications for staff involved. As with all policies, equal opportunities policies are only effective in promoting their aims if staff are committed to implementing them, if they are properly resourced and if they are regularly evaluated, reviewed and updated.

Do this! 2.1

Examine your workplace equal opportunities policy. Find out who was responsible for writing it and if it is reviewed and evaluated on a regular basis. What evidence can you find that the policy has been effective in influencing practice?

Equal opportunities and the individual

As individuals, people contribute to promoting equality of opportunity by:

- examining their own attitudes and values – this can sometimes be a difficult and disturbing experience
- challenging behaviour and language that is abusive or offensive
- increasing their knowledge and understanding of people who are different from themselves
- undertaking training to increase their ability to provide for the needs of all.

✅ Progress check

1 What do you understand by the term 'equality of opportunity'?
2 Why is treating everyone the same unlikely to provide equality of opportunity?
3 Why is it important to have laws that deal with discrimination?
4 How can equal opportunities policies promote equality?
5 What can an individual child-care worker do to promote equality?

---

non-judgemental
Not taking a fixed position on an issue

anti-discriminatory practice
Practice that encourages a positive view of difference and opposes negative attitudes and practices that lead to unfavourable treatment of people

Providing for equality

The first step in providing for equality is to recognise the diversity of our society and to value this diversity as a positive rather than a negative factor. In order to be able to do this, child-care workers will need to adopt an approach that is **non-judgemental** when working with families. This means that differences in family style, beliefs, traditions and, in particular, ways of caring for children should not be judged as being better or worse but should be respected. Different families will provide for their children in a number of different ways and child-care practice that is **anti-discriminatory** will seek to meet the needs of all families within a framework that respects their individuality.

Valuing diversity

The clearest indication that child-care workers value diversity will be in a positive environment provided for the care and education of children. In this context, the environment comprises the attitudes and behaviour of everyone associated with the centre, as well as the physical environment of buildings, displays and equipment and the day-to-day implementation of care and the curriculum. An approach that values diversity enriches the experience of all children and prepares them for adult life in today's society. The following should be considered:

- demonstrating, through a positive approach, that you value families and children for themselves
- providing resources, including books and displays, that present **positive images**, particularly of under-represented groups
- ensuring that the environment and activities presented are accessible to all children in the group, including those with disabilities
- giving consideration to the wishes and customs of parents concerning the care of their children. This may include preferences concerning diet or dress or any other matter
- having an equal opportunities perspective as an integral element of curriculum planning
- encouraging all children to participate in a full range of activities that avoid gender and cultural bias
- taking **positive action** when one child or group of children seems to be at a disadvantage. Intervention and another approach will often solve the problem
- encouraging staff to question their own attitudes and values. Is rough play more readily accepted from boys than from girls? Do staff have lower expectations of children from some socio-economic groups, of children from ethnic minority groups or of children with disabilities?
- showing a commitment to monitoring and evaluating provision to ensure that it meets the needs of all groups.

> **positive images**
> Images that challenge stereotypes and that extend and increase expectations

> **positive action**
> Taking steps to ensure that a particular individual or group has an equal chance to succeed

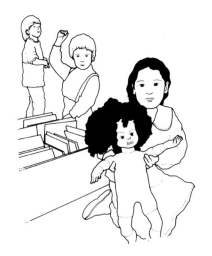

Provide resources that reflect the cultural diversity of the community

> ### *Do this!* 2.2
>
> Look carefully at the provision in your workplace. For each of the areas of race, gender and disability, evaluate how what is provided promotes equality of opportunity. Consider the building, displays, resources, activities and the physical space, as well as aspects such as policies and staff awareness. Present your findings as a matrix.

Opposing discrimination

There are occasions when, despite taking the positive steps outlined above, child-care workers will have to deal with instances of discrimination. This is likely to be a difficult and challenging experience. It may be helpful to consider some strategies in advance.

- Challenge abusive behaviour or language. This could be the sexist joke you overhear in the lift or the racist remark someone makes in the staff room. If you allow the incident to go unchallenged, you will appear to be condoning it. If this occurs at work, you may need to discuss the incident with your manager.
- Take seriously any incidence of name calling or bullying. It is not enough to comfort the victim; the behaviour must be challenged and be seen to be unacceptable.
- Remember that language has a powerful influence in shaping children's self-esteem and identity. Be aware of the terms that you use. Sexist comments about 'strong boys' and 'pretty girls' reinforce stereotypes. Avoid terms that associate black with negative connotations, such as 'black mood', 'black magic', 'accident black spot', rather than in a descriptive way, such as 'black paint', 'black trousers', 'black coffee'. Challenge abusive words such as 'nigger', 'spastic' and 'cripple' when you hear them used by children and by adults.

Case study: Responding to discriminatory behaviour

Luke and Callum both attended a busy inner-city nursery. They lived on the same street and were often dropped off at nursery together. The nursery staff were puzzled when they stopped playing together and, in fact, began to avoid one another. One afternoon it became clear what had happened. At home time, their mothers started arguing outside the nursery entrance. They had fallen out about one of them playing loud music late at night and disturbing the neighbours. The argument became very heated and culminating in Callum's mother shouting abuse and calling Luke and his mother a pair of 'black bastards'. The nursery staff heard what was going on and tried to calm things down by separating them and taking them into other rooms, away from the children. The teacher asked them both to come and see her the next day. When she spoke with Callum's mother, she made it clear to her why her remarks were unacceptable and asked for an assurance that it would not happen again or she would not be welcome on nursery premises in future.

1 Why was this a difficult situation for the nursery staff to deal with?
2 How did they manage to diffuse the situation?
3 What would the needs of the children be in this situation?

Everyone who works with children is very influential in the formation of their attitudes and values. Children will take their cue from adult responses and reactions, and it is therefore important that staff do not skate over issues of equality.

✓ *Progress check*

1 Why is important to value diversity?
2 How can child-care workers show that their commitment to promoting diversity?
3 What can child-care workers do to oppose discrimination?
4 Why is language an important aspect of anti-discriminatory practice?
5 Why should you always take a stand when you witness abusive or discriminatory behaviour?

Key terms

You need to know what these words and phrases mean. Go back through the chapter and find out.

anti-discriminatory practice
discrimination
equal opportunities
institutionalised discrimination
non-judgemental
oppression
positive action
positive images
self-esteem
socio-economic group
stereotyping

Now try these questions

1 Why is a consideration of equal opportunities an important issue for child-care workers?

2 What laws exist to counter discrimination? Why are successful prosecutions rare?

3 As officer-in-charge, you are responsible for ensuring that the nursery reflects the cultural diversity of the community. How would you do this?

4 Within your day-to-day work as a child-care worker, how can you oppose discrimination?

5 What kinds of training activities do you think would be helpful for child-care workers who are committed to implementing anti-discriminatory practice?

3 The nursery nurse in employment

This chapter includes:

- **Employment in child care**
- **The responsibilities of a professional child-care worker**
- **Contributing to the work of a team**
- **Seeking employment**

This chapter aims to develop your understanding of employment opportunities for child-care workers. It covers the structure of organisations and the child-care worker's role. It gives guidance on discharging the responsibilities of a professional worker and how to contribute to the work of a team. There are practical suggestions about seeking and preparing for employment.

You will gain most from this chapter if you put some of the theory in to practice and, following the *Do this!* suggestions, undertake some research into your own and other's workplaces. Job search skills should be practised well before applying for actual posts. Simulation and role-play will help you to practise many of the skills you will require.

You may find it helpful to read this chapter in conjunction with:

▶ **Book 2, Chapter 8**   Early years care and education

Employment in child care

Patterns of employment

Patterns of employment change over time. Child-care workers now work in a wider range of settings than ever before.

Whilst some opportunities in the **statutory sector** remain static, or have declined, there are increasing opportunities within the private and **voluntary sectors**, both in establishments such as private day nurseries and in play facilities linked to leisure opportunities. Due to the expansion in tourism, many tour operators employ child-care workers abroad in holiday destinations.

Disabled children are now more likely to be included in all settings. Consequently, there are more employment opportunities for child-care workers, to support an **inclusive** approach to their care and education.

The UK government's commitment to after-school clubs, and other opportunities to support carers to return to employment, may provide additional employment opportunities for child-care workers.

statutory sector
Care establishments provided by the state

voluntary sector
Care establishments provided by voluntary organisations

inclusive
Organised in a way that enables all to take a full and active part; meeting the needs of all children

Nannies and childminders

Opportunities for employment of nannies in private families continue to increase, both for residential and daily nannies. Many families choose childminders to care for their children.

This chapter relates largely to those working in settings as part of a team. Some of the needs of nannies, childminders and others working in isolation may be rather different. It is important that those in this type of employment seek ways of accessing feedback on their practice, support and professional development. Discussion with others in a similar role can be supportive. There are a number of nannying networks developing in various parts of the country. Opportunities for updating and further training should be considered.

The workplace

Structure and roles

Your workplace may be owned and managed by a statutory, voluntary or private organisation. This will influence its aims and objectives and the structure, including staff roles and **line management**.

In order to function effectively within the organisation you need to be aware of the people who work there, their role, responsibilities and accountability including their line management. You need to be clear about your own role, responsibilities and who you are accountable to.

Do this! 3.1

a) Find out who owns and runs your workplace.
b) Draw and label a diagram showing the structure of the establishment, including lines of management, responsibility and accountability.
c) Describe the roles and responsibilities of the staff, including your own.

Aims and objectives

Each workplace is likely to have its own specified aims and objectives to influence and inform its practice. These, together with supporting policies and procedures, should be underpinned and influenced by the rights and needs of young children.

Do this! 3.2

In your workplace find out:
a) the aims and objectives of the organisation
b) what is considered to constitute good practice
c) how staff seek to develop relationships with children and parents or carers.

Policies and procedures

Within your workplace there are likely to be policies and procedures (codes of practice) concerning the following:

- equal opportunities: this means that no adult or child receives less favourable treatment on the grounds of their sex, race, colour, nationality, ethnic or national origins, age, disability, religion, marital status or sexual orientation
- admissions
- financial arrangements
- premises and health and safety
- medical emergencies
- child protection
- health, nutrition and food service
- staff rights and responsibilities, qualifications, management, training and development
- ratio of staff to children
- record-keeping
- partnerships with parents
- liaison with other agencies
- fire evacuation
- behaviour
- children with special educational needs
- off-site visits
- administration of legal drugs
- liaison with other professionals.

Do this! 3.3

In your workplace find out the policy and/or procedures applicable to each of the following:

a) allocation of places
b) equal opportunities
c) administration of first aid
d) prevention of illness and maintenance of health
e) safety of outdoor play
f) food hygiene
g) provision of a balanced diet
h) ratio of staff to children
i) staff qualifications, supervision and training
j) roles and responsibilities of senior staff and managers
k) daily routine within the establishment
l) outings for children
m) supply of materials and equipment
n) authorisation of expenditure
o) fire evacuation procedures

p) methods of keeping records of:
- income and expenditure
- assessments of children's development in all aspects
- accidents
- attendance
- information concerning family background and emergency contact
- stock levels.

Statutory requirements

Some policies and procedures result from statutory requirements (i.e. they are laid down in legislation). Aspects of the following legislation (laws) will have implications for policy and practice within all establishments:

- Children Act (1989)
- Education Act (1988)
- Education Reform Act (1993)
- Race Relations Act (1975)
- Sex Discrimination Act (1975, 1986)
- Equal Pay Act (1970)
- Employment Protection Act (1978)
- Disabled Person's Act (1986)
- Offices Shops and Railway Premises Act (1963)
- Health and Safety at Work Act (1974)
- Food Safety Act (1990)
- Food Hygiene Regulation (1970)
- Food Hygiene Amendment Regulation (1990).

Do this 3.4

Find out which legislation has implications for the policies and procedures in each of the 16 areas outlined in *Do this! 3.3*.

✅ *Progress check*

1 What has led to increased employment opportunities for child-care workers?
2 What areas can policies and procedures cover?
3 What lays down and governs statutory requirements?

The responsibilities of a professional child-care worker

Policies can increase awareness, but will not, in themselves, change attitudes or practice. Good practice will depend on staff commitment to the needs and rights of children and to their ability and willingness to carry out their duties in a professional way.

The rights and needs of children

The following statements, taken from *Young Children in Group Day Care: Guidelines for Good Practice* by the Early Childhood Unit of the National Children's Bureau, outline a challenging set of beliefs about the needs and rights of young children. They apply equally well to any care or educational setting.

paramount
Of first importance

- Children's well-being is **paramount**.
- Children are individuals in their own right, and they have differing needs, abilities and potential. Thus any day-care facility should be flexible and sensitive in responding to these needs.
- Since discrimination of all kinds is an everyday reality in the lives of many children, every effort must be made to ensure that services and practices do not reflect or reinforce it, but actively combat it. Therefore equality of opportunity for children, parents and staff should be explicit in the policies and practice of a day-care facility.
- Working in partnership with parents is recognised as being of major value and importance.
- Good practice in day care for children can enhance their full social, intellectual, emotional, physical and creative development.
- Young children learn and develop best through their own exploration and experience. Such opportunities for learning and development are based on stable, caring relationships, regular observation and ongoing assessment. This will result in **reflective practitioners** who use their observations to inform the learning experiences they offer.

reflective practitioners
Workers who think about what they have done/said with a view to improving practice

- Regular and thorough evaluation of policies, procedures and practices facilitates the provision of high quality day care.

Think about it

1 Why is it important to document and publicise the rights and needs of children?
2 For each of the statements of principle, think of an example from your workplace that shows how these needs and rights are:
   a) met in practice
   b) denied in practice.
3 Why are the following so important in practice:
   a) stable, caring relationships?
   b) equality of opportunity and anti-discriminatory practice?
   c) regular evaluation of policies, procedures and practices?

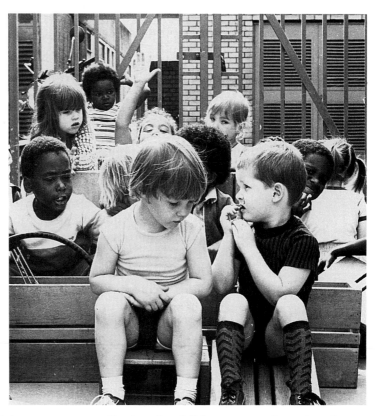

Young children learn and develop best through their own exploration and experience

Practising as a professional child-care worker involves several commitments:

■ putting the needs and rights of children and their families before your own needs
■ respecting the principles of confidentiality
■ demonstrating responsibility and accountability
■ being willing to plan, do, record and review
■ working in partnership with parents or carers
■ being committed to personal development and further training.

We will look at each of these in turn.

Putting the needs and rights of children and their families first

You will need to meet the needs of children, according to the limits of your work role, irrespective of your personal preferences or prejudices. This will involve recognising the value and dignity of every human being, irrespective of their socio-economic group, ethnic origin, gender, marital status, religion or disability. This is particularly important with young children who may be unable to understand or express their rights and needs fully.

Working with young children may give you a deep sense of satisfaction, but children are not there to provide this for you; you are there to provide for their needs.

> **Think about it**
>
> 1 Why is it important to put the needs and rights of children and their families before your own needs?
> 2 Are there children in your workplace you find it difficult to work with? Think about why this is and strategies for overcoming your personal preference or prejudice.

The principles of confidentiality

Sensitive information concerning children and their families should be given to you only if you need it in order to meet effectively the needs of the child and family concerned. It should not be given, or received, to satisfy your curiosity or to make you feel superior or in control.

Although the principles of confidentiality may be easy to understand, the practice can be complex and will require self-control and commitment to the welfare of the child and their family.

> **Think about it**
>
> 1 Why is respecting confidentiality complex and sometimes difficult to carry out?
> 2 Why does respecting confidentiality require self-control?

Responsibility and accountability

Showing responsibility and accountability involves doing willingly what you are asked to do, if this is in your area of responsibility. You may need to jot down instructions to make sure that you are able to follow them accurately. You must then carry out the tasks to the standard required, and in the time allocated, making sure that you are aware of the policies and procedures of your workplace.

Ask your line manager or someone in a supervisory role if you do not understand what to do, or if you think the task is not your responsibility. You may need to refuse to do some tasks until you have been shown how to do them by someone in a supervisory role, or until you have received appropriate training.

If you have any suggestions for changing things, make them to an appropriate person, rather than grumbling or gossiping behind their back. Open communication of positive and negative issues helps staff to develop positive relationships with each other. Assert a point of view, but also be open to the views of other people.

> **Think about it**
>
> 1 Think of an occasion when you should have refused to carry out a task because you did not understand what you were supposed to do.
> 2 Why does open communication of positive and negative issues help staff develop positive relationships with each other?
> 3 What is the difference between being assertive and being aggressive?

Think about it

How can you encourage your colleagues to make comments on your work and give you feedback?

Plan, do, record and review

You will need to spend time thinking and planning in advance for your work with young children. A useful way of doing this is to *plan, do, record* and *review*. Encourage your colleagues to make comments on your work, as this will give valuable feedback and help you to improve your working practice.

Your aim when planning will be to include all children and make sure that they have full access to the curriculum or activity, whatever their cultural background, socio-economic group, religion or disability. A further aim will be to avoid repetitive, adult-centred tasks, but rather to help children to develop their creativity and achieve their full learning potential.

Working in partnership with parents or carers

Professionals recognise the importance of partnership with parents or carers. To carry out *your* duties in a professional way, you will need to show that you believe in the importance of working with parents or carers. You must respect their views and wishes and recognise that, in many instances, they are the ones who know their own children best. In order to do this it is essential to understand and value individual children's **cultural background**, and take account of their **customs**, **values** and **spiritual beliefs**.

cultural background
The way of life of the family in which a person is brought up

customs
Special guidelines for behaviour which are followed by particular groups of people

values
Beliefs that certain things are important and to be valued, for example a person's right to their own belongings

spiritual beliefs
What a person believes about the non-material world

Professionals recognise the importance of partnership with parents or carers

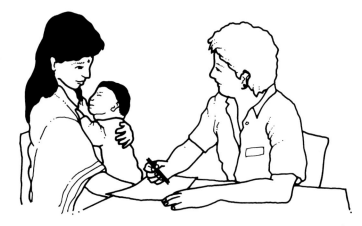

If you have any religious or cultural issues which may affect your work, you will need to discuss them with your line manager. An example might be if you were unwilling to work on particular days because of your religious practices.

conscientious objections
Not to do something on the grounds of belief

Think about it

1 Why is it important to understand and value individual children's cultural background?
2 Which parental actions and choices are not legitimate?
3 What relevant **conscientious objections** may child-care workers have?

Think about it

How can a nanny in a private family receive feedback on their work and continue to develop professionally?

Personal development and further training

As a professional child-care worker, you will want to receive further training, and you also need to be open to suggestions for changing your methods of working. You should find that your self-awareness increases through the supervision you receive from experienced workers. In-service staff development and further training will also help to keep you up-to-date with new developments and improve your working practice.

> ### ✓ *Progress check*
>
> 1 According to the statements of the needs and rights of children, what must always be the most important consideration in the care or education of young children?
> 2 Why must day-care facilities be flexible?
> 3 Why is it important to observe and assess young children regularly?
> 4 When should a child-care worker be given sensitive information about children and their families?
> 5 Why may it be necessary to jot down the instructions you are given?
> 6 Why may child-care workers need to refuse to do some tasks?
> 7 What should you do if you have a suggestion for changing something in your workplace?
> 8 Why should you encourage colleagues to give you feedback on your work?
> 9 What should be one of your main aims when planning?

Contributing to the work of a team

Working with colleagues in a team

multi-disciplinary
Made up of different professionals

In the workplace, child-care workers usually work with colleagues as part of a team. This may be a **multi-disciplinary** team, with representatives from a number of other professional groups, for example teachers and social workers. Those who work as nannies or childminders may find it helpful to see themselves as part of a team with the child's family.

The advantages of team work

The potential advantages of working in a team include:
- individual staff weaknesses are balanced by other people's strengths
- members stimulate, motivate, encourage and support one another
- the skills of all members are used to arrive at the best solutions
- a more consistent approach to the task of caring for children and their families is possible
- individual staff feel a sense of belonging and can share problems, difficulties and successes
- responsibility, as well as insight, is shared

- individuals often become more willing to adopt new ways of thinking or working
- team membership satisfies a need to belong and be respected, and have ideals and aims that are confirmed and shared by others
- the children see the benefits of people working together and co-operating with each other.

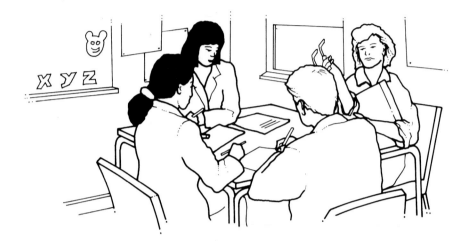

In the workplace, child-care workers usually work with colleagues as part of a team

---

Think about it

1 Why may team work enable a more consistent approach to caring for children?
2 Why are members more likely to adopt new ways of thinking or working as a result of belonging to a team?

What makes a team effective?

Effective teams will have the following:
- clearly defined aims and objectives (clarified and redefined regularly) that all members can put into words and agree to put in to practice
- flexible roles that enable individuals to work to their strengths, rather than in **prescribed roles** where they must conform to pre-determined or stereotyped expectations (for example, the teacher always does story time, the child-care worker always clears up)
- effective team leaders who manage the work of the team, encourage and value individual contributions and deal with conflict
- members who are committed to:
  - developing self-awareness
  - building, maintaining and sustaining good working relationships
  - demonstrating effective communication skills, expressing their views assertively rather than aggressively
  - understanding and recognising their contribution to the way the group works
  - carrying out team decisions, irrespective of their personal feelings
  - accepting responsibility for the outcome of team decisions.

prescribed roles
Duties laid down by others

Think about it

1 Why is it important for a team to have clearly defined aims and objectives?
2 What communication skills do you need to demonstrate to facilitate team work?
3 Why is individual self-awareness important?
4 Why is it important to implement and accept responsibility for the outcome of group decisions?

Dealing with conflict in a team

Within any team there is likely to be conflict. It is important to deal with this constructively rather than try to ignore it. The following guidelines for behaviour are likely to encourage the resolution of conflict.

- Join with the other person so that you can both 'win': people in a conflict often tend to be against rather than with each other. Keep a clear picture of the person and yourself, separate from the issue. The issue causing the conflict may be lost by the strength of bad feeling against the other person. You need to be committed to working towards an outcome that is acceptable to both parties.
- Make clear 'I' statements: take responsibility for yourself and avoid blaming the other person for how you feel and what you think.
- Be clear and specific about your view of the conflict and what you want, and listen to the other person's view.
- Deal with one issue at a time: avoid confusing one issue with another and using examples from the past to illustrate your point. Using the past or only telling part of the story to make your own point can lead to a biased version of what happened. The other person is likely to have forgotten or may remember the incident very differently.
- Look at and listen to each other: deal directly with each other and the difficulty.
- Ensure that you understand each other: if you are unclear and confused about the issue, ask open questions and paraphrase back what you think you hear.
- Pool your ideas for creative ways of sorting out the conflict: make a list of all the possible solutions and go through them together.
- Choose a mutually convenient time and place: it is useful to agree on the amount of time you will spend.
- Acknowledge and appreciate one another: think of the other person's attributes separately from the conflict issue and acknowledge and appreciate them.

Think about it

Why is it important to deal with conflict?

Group dynamics

Groups and team meetings in the workplace

Within the workplace there will be many groups meeting formally and informally: staff team meetings, groups of parent/carers, children and other professionals. Groups can be very effective at stimulating new ideas, managing projects, making decisions, monitoring and reviewing progress, and supporting group members. However, they can also be unproductive. It can help group members to consider their behaviour and the characteristics that may enhance or detract from the aims of the group.

Behaviour and characteristics of group members

The following are behaviours and characteristics observed in members of a group.

- *initiating* – getting and keeping things going
- *informing* – volunteering information, ideas, facts, feelings, views or opinions
- *clarifying, summarising or paraphrasing* – helping the group to sort things out, bring things together or round things off
- *confronting* – an important function if groups are to be effective, but requiring some skill and concern for the feelings of others. Did the person upset anyone?
- *harmonising* – working to reconcile disagreements, to relieve tension, and helping to explore differences
- *encouraging*
- *compromising* – admitting an error or modifying a view or position
- *time-keeping* – ensuring the group keeps to time
- *aggressive behaviour* – attacking others or belittling their contribution or putting them down
- *blocking* – preventing the group from getting on with the task
- *dominating* – dominating, interrupting, asserting authority or interfering with the rights of others to participate
- *avoiding* – preventing the group from facing issues
- *withdrawing* – displaying a lack of involvement.

> **Think about it**
>
> Identify the positive and negative behaviours and characteristics from this list?

✓ *Progress check*

1 Name the professionals who may be part of a multi-disciplinary team.
2 What do the following people need to do in order to facilitate effective team work:
   a) the team collectively?
   b) members individually?
   c) the leader?
3 What is meant by having a flexible role?
4 What do team members need to be committed to?
5 What is the desirable outcome in dealing with conflict?
6 What groups may operate in the workplace?

> **Do this!**   **3.5**
>
> Think of any group of which you are a part. Next time you meet, analyse the way the group works by:
> a) noting any of the behaviours or characteristics listed
> b) considering what effect these behaviours and characteristics were having
> c) thinking why people were demonstrating them
> d) noting if and how they were managed.

> **Think about it**
>
> Why do you think child-care workers need to avoid sentimentality and glamorising the role?

Seeking employment

Job search

The same considerations apply to seeking and obtaining work with young children as for any other profession. Child-care workers need to avoid sentimentality and glamorising the role.

Finding out what is available

Employment opportunities may be advertised in magazines, journals, local newspapers or national newspapers, in the Job Centre or in some areas by the local authority in a job sheet. Alternatively, employment may be sought through an agency.

Remember to use all channels open to you to find out about possible employment opportunities. Your family and friends and the staff and students where you have undertaken training are all useful contacts.

> **Think about it**
>
> What are the advantages of using an agency when seeking employment?

Mutual expectations

One of the most crucial aspects of obtaining and retaining employment is ensuring clarity of expectation on the part of the employer and the job seeker. Employment by a statutory, private or voluntary organisation is likely to be covered by a *job description* and *conditions of service*. A *person specification* may have been drawn up to indicate the requirements of the employer, the qualifications, experience, skills, knowledge and attitude required in any applicant. However, this is less likely to be the case when seeking employment as a nanny in a private family

> **Think about it**
>
> Why is it important to clarify mutual expectations when considering employment? Why is this especially important for a nannying post?

Applying for employment

The information that follows is necessarily brief and in summary form. If possible, seek expert help with the process of applying for employment. At each stage in the process you will need to make the most of yourself, your qualifications, experience, skills and knowledge, if you are to move successfully to the next stage and ultimately obtain employment.

Preparing a curriculum vitae (CV)

The following guidance, taken from *A Practical Guide to Child-Care Employment* by Christine Hobart and Jill Frankel, outlines the points to remember:

- The CV should be typed (or word processed) and presented tidily on white A4 paper.
- Some people think an imaginative and unusual presentation will have more impact. It may, but it could put as many people off as it interests. Ask friends, colleagues or tutors for their response.
- Spelling and grammar *must* be correct (have it checked).
- Keep it brief. It should be no more than two pages long.
- Avoid solid blocks of script
- Use space to emphasise points and make sections stand out.
- Get a tutor or friend to check it for any ambiguity. It may be clear to you but muddled to an outsider
- Update it regularly

Your basic CV should include:

- personal details
- education and qualifications
- work experience and career history
- personal interests and hobbies
- other relevant details.

Think about it

How could you get support and help with preparing your CV?

Completing an application form

You may be required to complete an application form instead of sending a CV. Read any information sent with it thoroughly. Ensure it is completed neatly and clearly. All questions should be answered honestly. Use your CV as a guide.

Think about it

How can you ensure your application form is neat with no crossing out or Tippex?

Covering letter

Use the information sent by the prospective employer to guide you. Again ensure it is neat and legible, brief and to the point.

Statement of suitability for the post

This may be requested separately. Try to draw out points from your CV to match the job description.

Interviews

Preparation and practice are vital. Prepare by learning about the specific post and about interviews in general. This can be achieved through reading text, accessing Information and Learning Technologies, and through training programmes. Practise your communication skills in formal and informal settings. Undertake a mock interview with feedback from the interviewers.

Think about it

What communication skills do you need at interview?

Finding out about the post

As well as a potential employer finding out about you, you will need to check out that you actually want the employment offered. You will obviously need to consider the terms and conditions, but you should also ensure that you are in agreement with the aims and objectives of the setting. You should also seek to find out the style of management that you would have to work with. Is the service run on democratic lines where decisions are made by the team? Are all the decisions made by managers without the team being consulted? Is there strong direction evident or does there appear to be a lack of leadership? If you do not know the setting, read any information sent to you and request a pre-visit.

Think about it

1 What questions should you ask at interview or on a pre-visit?
2 Consider the advantages and disadvantages of working in the following positions:
   a) A nanny in a wealthy private family, living in a rural area
   b) A nursery officer in a day nursery or family centre run by the local authority social services department
   c) A special needs support assistant in an infant school run by the local authority education department, employed to support a child with special educational needs
   d) A play worker in the paediatric department of a general hospital
   e) A residential child-care officer in a residential special school for children with autism, run by a voluntary organisation.

Case study: Helen's first job

Helen was delighted to be the first student in her group to get a job. She had seen an advertisement in the local paper. It sounded great – own room with en-suite and use of a car. She had to share a room at home and couldn't wait to leave. The children's parents seemed really nice. They were too embarrassed to talk about money and hours, but she thought they would sort all that out when she started.

Helen came back to visit her tutor at college six months later. When her tutor asked how she was getting on, Helen said she had left. She explained that whilst the eldest child was at nursery, they had expected her to do more and more housework. They were so busy themselves that she couldn't say no. All that training to do the housework!

Then they expected her to baby-sit without any notice and told her to take time off in the day, when it suited them. She ended up doing split shifts and could never plan anything. The home was in the middle of nowhere and the last bus back was at 7 p.m!

The money was OK, but she never got chance to go out and spend any of it! She was really lonely. The parents did their best, but they were a lot older than her. She said she actually enjoyed sharing a room when she finally came home.

She got really attached to the children though and, when she said she

> wanted to leave, she felt really guilty for leaving them. The family offered her more money to stay, but it wasn't the money that was the problem. She wanted to make a clean break and finally just packed her bags and left without warning the parents. She felt she could never go back now even to visit and didn't think they would give her a reference
>
> 1 How could this situation have been avoided?
> 2 What should Helen have clarified and asked for, before accepting the job?
> 3 What was wrong with the job as far as Helen was concerned?
> 4 How will the family feel now? What may the children have thought?
> 5 Draw up a job description and a contract for this post. (You will need to read the next section first.)

Conditions of employment

Contracts of employment

Think about it

Why is a contract of employment essential?

The Employment Protection Acts require that all employees who work for more than 16 hours a week have a contract of employment – a document stating their terms and conditions of employment.

Rights and responsibilities

Once employed, both you and your employer will have entitlements and responsibilities laid down in employment law. You will need to consider your responsibility for paying income tax and National Insurance contributions. You may also want to contribute towards a retirement pension.

> **Think about it**
>
> 1 Who is responsible for the payment of:
>   a) income tax?
>   b) National Insurance contributions?
>   c) retirement pension contributions?
> 2 How can you find out about the contributions you and employer have to make to each of the above?

Trade unions and professional associations

You may wish to consider joining a union and/or a professional association. You will need to research and be clear about the role of each and what membership entails.

Trade unions and professional associations may offer the following to their members:

- access to legal protection
- negotiation of pay and conditions

- inexpensive insurance cover
- collective efforts to improve working conditions
- protection of its members through health and safety practices, pension and entitlements issues.

✓ *Progress check*

1 Where may employment opportunities be advertised?
2 What does a person specification indicate?
3 What should be included in a basic CV?
4 How can you prepare for an interview?
5 What will you need to know about the post you are applying for?
6 What should be included in a contract of employment?
7 What are the advantages of belonging to a trade union/professional association?

Do this! 3.6

1 Find out the benefits and costs of belonging to the various trade unions and professional associations for child-care workers.

2 Prepare an up-to-date CV for yourself.

3 Take part in a mock interview.

4 Select a post and prepare a statement outlining your suitability for it.

5 Prepare a job description and person specification for a post as a nursery officer in a social services family centre.

Key terms

You need to know what these words and phrases mean. Go back through the chapter and find out.

conscientious objections
cultural background
customs
inclusive
line manager
multi-disciplinary
paramount
prescribed roles
reflective practitioners
spirtual beliefs
statutory
values
voluntary

Now try these questions

1 In practice, how can child-care settings encourage partnership with parents?
2 Describe and explain six aspects of professional practice.
3 What are the needs and rights of young children?
4 Explain the advantages of working with colleagues in a team.
5 How can staff deal with conflict in the workplace?
6 Describe the behaviours and characteristics that make groups effective.

4 Working with parents

This chapter includes:

- **Why work with parents?**
- **Making parents welcome**
- **Keeping records**
- **Difficult situations**
- **Getting parents involved**

All those who work with young children will recognise that the relationship between the child-care establishment and the parents (or primary carers) of the child is very important. A good relationship will benefit the child, the parent and those who work with the child. This chapter will look at issues surrounding working with parents and will examine ways of establishing and maintaining an effective partnership between the child-care centre and parents.

It is recognised that not all children are cared for by their parents. This term has been used for ease of reading and includes others who take on the parenting role.

You may find it helpful to read this chapter in conjunction with:

▶ **Book 2, Chapter 3**   The nursery nurse in employment

Why work with parents?

Until quite recently the practice of actively involving parents in the child-care setting was relatively uncommon. You may remember seeing notices that positively discouraged parents from crossing over the threshold into school or nursery. A notice that proclaims 'No parents beyond this point' is hardly likely to foster good relationships between parents and those who care for their children, and should be harder to find these days. There are a number of reasons why working with parents is considered to be important and necessary.

- Parents have the most knowledge and understanding of their children. If they are encouraged to share this with staff, the child will benefit.
- Children need consistent handling to feel secure. This is most likely to occur if there are good channels of communication between parents and staff.
- Recent legislation contained within the Education Reform Act 1988, the Children Act 1989, and the Special Educational Needs Code of Practice 1993, places a legal responsibility on professionals to work in

partnership with parents. Services provided for children in the public, private and voluntary sector must take this into account.

- Initiatives such as the Parents' Charter emphasise parents' rights to make choices and be consulted in decisions concerning their children's education.
- Research has demonstrated conclusively the positive effect that parental involvement in the education process has on the progress of children. If parents become involved early on in the child's education, they are likely to maintain this involvement throughout the the child's educational career.
- Children's learning is not confined to the child-care setting. An exchange of information from centre to home and from home to centre will consolidate learning, wherever it takes place.
- Parents have a wealth of skills and experiences that they can contribute to the child-care centre. Participation in this way will broaden and enrich the programme offered to all the children. Many playgroups rely on a parents' rota to complement their staffing.
- An extra person to work at an activity, to help out on a trip or to prepare materials can make a valuable contribution to a busy setting. Parents who are involved in this way will gain first-hand experience of the way that the centre operates and an understanding of the approach.
- Some centres may operate with regulations that require a parent representative on the management committee or governing body. The responsibilities here can be quite significant and will include financial management and accountability, selection and recruitment of staff, as well as day-to-day running of the centre.
- Parents who are experiencing difficulties with their children may be able to share these problems and work towards resolving them alongside sympathetic and supportive professionals.
- Child protection procedures may require that professionals in the child-care centre observe and supervise parents with children as part of an access or rehabilitation programme. (Such situations need workers with experience and sensitivity.)
- Parents may experience a loss of role when their child starts nursery or school. Being involved and feeling valued may help them to adjust to this change.
- Provision for young children is often underfunded. Many centres have parent groups that organise social activities and raise funds. This enables parents who are not available during working hours to become involved.

Do this! 4.1

1 a) Read through the preceding section again. Think of other reasons why child-care centres should work with parents. Add them to the list.

b) Choose what you think are the three most important reasons for working with parents from the list above and link these with your own experiences in the workplace. Discuss your choices with another student. Did you agree? Now choose the reason that you think is the least important and compare your choices.

2 Look at your workplace, talk to your colleagues and write about how the centre makes links with parents.

All centres develop ways of working with parents, but naturally there are differences, depending on the emphasis of each particular establishment. For example, a family centre where many of the children are referred by social services, perhaps as a result of some crisis, will work with parents in ways that are quite different to those used in, say, a workplace day nursery that cares for children during parents' long shifts, or a playgroup where parents operate a daily rota. Nevertheless, there are general principles that will always apply.

- Be friendly and approachable. Remember that parents might feel uneasy in an unfamiliar setting and it is up to staff to make the right kind of approach.
- Be courteous and maintain a professional relationship (see Chapter 3, pages 30–5).
- Encourage a meaningful exchange of information between the home and centre.

✓ Progress check

1 Why is it important for child-care professionals to work with parents?
2 What legislation requires that professionals work in partnership with parents?
3 How does partnership benefit:
  a) children?
  b) parents?
  c) child-care workers?
4 Why do centres need to develop their own particular ways of involving the families that they work with?

Making parents welcome

It is the responsibility of those who work with children to do everything that they can to make parents feel welcome and valued. The needs and feelings of all parents should be considered. This may include some who have less than positive memories of their own childhood experiences and who need particular encouragement to feel comfortable. Parents who are unfamiliar with the methods and approaches used may require extra explanation and reassurance. Parents from some minority ethnic groups may be concerned that their child's cultural and religious background is understood. Provision should be made to ensure that parents who do not use the language of the setting are provided with the full range of opportunities to be involved in their children's care and education.

First impressions

First impressions count for a great deal and can make the difference between a parent choosing a particular centre for the child or going elsewhere. Most establishments will recognise this and take particular care to make the way into the building clear, with signs directing visitors to an appropriate person. Noticeboards and displays in entrance halls and foyers give an immediate impression of the philosophy of the centre. Carefully mounted and imaginatively displayed children's work demonstrates professional standards and shows what the children do and that you value their work. Named photographs of staff and their roles give parents an indication of how the centre operates. A well-maintained noticeboard giving information about current activities and topics may attract a parent's attention and encourage them to become involved. The physical condition and upkeep of the building also creates an impression; no parent would choose a gloomy, unsafe or unhygienic environment for their child.

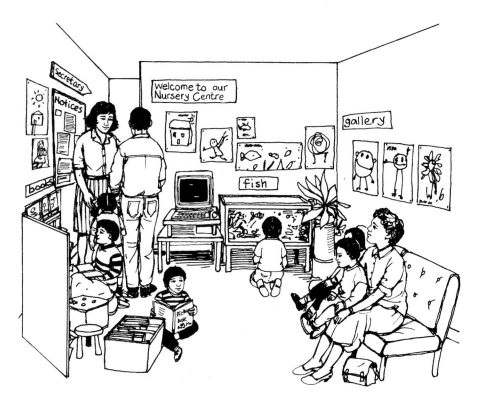

A welcoming entrance creates a positive impression

Think about it

Consider the entrance to your workplace. Does it make parents feel welcome? Could you suggest any ways to improve it?

Perhaps even more important than the welcome communicated by the physical environment is the response of the staff. In most establishments there will be a particular person with responsibility for dealing with enquiries and settling in new children and families, but this does not mean that other members of staff should not be involved. Everyone should have time for a greeting and a smile while the required person is found. Remember that parents may feel ill at ease in an unfamiliar setting. Leaving a child for the first time is almost certainly going to be stressful and they will need your support. Remembering the following may help you to put parents at their ease.

- Smile or nod when you see a parent, even if they are making their way to another member of staff.
- Make time to talk with parents. If they have a concern that requires time and privacy, try to arrange a mutually convenient appointment.
- Try to call people by name. 'Ellen's mum' may do in an emergency but might not be the most appropriate way to address someone.
- Remember that family patterns change and that it is not at all unusual for parents to have a different surname from that of their child or of their partner. In our culturally diverse society, be aware that communities have their own naming customs and may not follow the western naming custom of personal names followed by family names. Ask colleagues or consult records to find out parents' preferred forms of address. If you are unsure of the correct pronunciation, ask the parent.

Case study: A good impression

Marcia took a career break from her job when her daughter, Imogen, was born. When the time came for her to return to work, she visited a number of day nurseries that were conveniently situated between her home and workplace. Many of her friends had children at local nurseries, so she listened to what they had to say and chose some to visit. When Marcia telephoned the nursery that she eventually chose, she arranged a visit for a time when the senior nursery nurse would be free to show her around. She was encouraged to bring Imogen.

Marcia had no difficulty in finding the nursery. A sign directed her to the main door which opened into a bright entrance hall. It was clear that the nursery were expecting them as the member of staff who opened the door greeted her and Imogen by name. She was asked to sit down and wait in the hall while the senior nursery nurse was found. She had time to look at the displays of children's work and the prominent parents' noticeboard which was full of information about what was going on at nursery, alongside reminders for parents. Marcia and Imogen were taken on a tour of the nursery. The organisation of the rooms and the routine were explained and they were introduced to the staff. Imogen was shown the room that she would be based in and she met the staff who worked with that age group.

Marcia was offered a cup of tea in the nursery office and given an opportunity to ask about anything that she had seen and to raise any other points. She was given plenty of time and all of her questions were answered fully. As she left, she was given a copy of the nursery brochure and encouraged to get in touch if she had any questions or concerns.

1 What do you think made Marcia choose this nursery?
2 Why do you think the nursery encouraged Imogen to visit with her mother?
3 What might a parent want to find out on a first visit to a nursery?

Skills for talking and listening

Thinking about your own communication skills and how these might have an effect on your relationships with parents can be helpful. When talking with or listening to parents, consider the following points.

- Make eye contact but be careful – a fixed stare can be very off-putting.
- Don't interrupt and make comparisons from your own experiences. Encourage further conversation with phrases such as 'I see...', 'Tell me...'
- Make sure that you are at the same level. Do not sit down if the parent is standing, or vice versa. This will make communication less equal.
- If the parent seems upset or wants to discuss something in private, find somewhere suitable to talk.
- Make the limits of confidentiality clear. Assure the parent that you will deal with any information shared professionally but that you may have to pass some things on.
- Summarise the points that have been made during and at the end of a discussion. This recap will be particularly helpful if the parent has come to discuss ways of dealing with a problem.
- Keep your distance. Everyone needs a space around them. If you get too close, the person you are speaking to may feel uncomfortable. (On the other hand, people from some countries might have a different view of personal space and could interpret your distance as hostile.)
- You may feel that a parent is worrying over something quite unimportant. Do not dismiss these concerns as insignificant as the parent may be reluctant to confide in you in future. Try to be reassuring.
- Avoid using **jargon** (terms that only someone with your professional background would understand). This is off-putting and limits the effectiveness of your communication.
- If you have parents at your centre who do not speak English, try to organise someone to interpret for them. Some local authorities will provide this service or you might find someone locally. All parents, not just those who speak English, will want to share information and be consulted about their children's progress.

jargon
Terminology that is specific to a particular professional background

Think about it

When were you last in a stressful situation in an unfamiliar setting? Was it an interview for a job? Your first day in a work placement?

Think about what made you feel uncomfortable and what (or who) put you at your ease. How was this done?

■ Remember (particularly if you are a student) that you will usually need to discuss with colleagues and your line manager any requests that a parent might make. Don't make agreements that you might not be able to keep!

Do this! 4.2

Using the previous section as a guide, note down some of the factors that encourage communication between parents and staff. When you are next in your workplace, take notice of how staff interact with parents. How do they encourage communication? Is there anything that hinders communication? Do staff go out of their way to ensure that they talk with all parents, not just those who come forward? (You will need to ask permission before you begin as this task would not be possible to do unobtrusively.)

Written communications

All centres will have a brochure that they provide for parents which will give them initial information about the service offered. Of course, these will vary, though there will be common factors. These will probably include:

■ location, including address, telephone number, person to contact
■ the times that the centre is open and the length of sessions
■ the age range of children catered for
■ criteria for admission (for example, a workplace nursery may require the parent to work in the establishment; many social services establishments require children to be referred through a social worker or health visitor)
■ information about meals and snacks provided
■ information about the facilities and accommodation available
■ schedule of fees (if any) to be charged
■ reference to any policies, especially those relating to special educational needs and equal opportunities
■ the qualifications of the staff and staff roles and responsibilities
■ an example of the daily or sessional programme for the children
■ what parents are expected to provide, for example nappies, spare clothing, sun cream
■ details of any commitments the parent must make, for example rota days, notice of leaving, regular attendance
■ details of any approach to learning followed such as learning through play, Highscope and the curriculum followed, for example the Desirable Outcomes, the National Curriculum (see Chapter 6)
■ in some settings, information about the complaints procedure.

The brochure provides the parent with a great deal of information which is also useful for reference once the child has started at the centre.

> ## *Do this!*   *4.3*
>
> 1 Collect two or three brochures from different types of establishment and compare them, giving each a rating for content, clarity and presentation. Consider the tone of the brochure. Does it patronise parents? Does it bewilder with jargon? Does the it genuinely welcome the involvement of parents?
>
> 2 Design your own brochure for the child-care centre of your choice. Use appropriate computer software to present it in a suitable format. Include all the necessary information and give a clear message to parents that you value their involvement.

Think about it

What are the limitations of written communications? Think about how you might pass on information to parents who speak and read another language or to those who have limited literacy skills.

Parents can expect to receive a whole range of written communications once their child has started at a centre. Some centres produce their own booklets, for example, about their approach to reading or other areas of the curriculum, indicating to parents how they can be a part of their children's learning. Parents might also receive regular newsletters, invitations to concerts, parents' meetings, requests for assistance and support, information about the activities provided for children, advance notice of holidays and centre closures, and so on. These will often be reinforced with notices and verbal reminders. It is important that these notices and letters communicate the information in a clear and friendly manner.

Sometimes there will be a need for a more individual exchange of information, for example if a child has an accident during the session. This might be written in a note to the parent or it might be explained at pick-up time. Parents need to know what has happened and someone needs to have responsibility for passing on this information.

> ### ✔ *Progress check*
>
> 1 Why is it important that the entrance to a centre is welcoming and inviting to parents?
> 2 What should child-care staff do to ensure that their conversations with parents are positive and rewarding?
> 3 How can you ensure effective communication with parents who do not use English as their first language? Give examples.
> 4 What information should be included in the brochure?
> 5 What other kinds of written information might parents expect to receive?
> 6 What should you have in mind when preparing written information to circulate to parents?

Keeping records

All establishments are required to keep records of the children and families that they work with. The content of these records will vary depending on the type of care that is being provided. They will always include personal data about the child supplied by parents. There will also be records that document the child's progress and achievements during their time at the centre and parents will be asked to contribute to these too.

Initial information

Usually parents are asked to complete a form that includes the following:

- personal details about the child: full name, date of birth, etc.
- names, addresses and phone numbers of parents and other emergency contacts
- medical details that will include the address and telephone number of the child's doctor and any information about allergies and regular medications
- details about any particular dietary needs
- details about religion which might have a bearing on the care provided for the child.

Additionally, there may be sensitive information that is necessary for the centre to have; for example, are there any restrictions on who may collect the child from the centre? Are social services involved with the family?

Parents will need to be assured that such information will be confidential and stored securely. Centres need to make sure that this essential information is correct and up-to-date.

Other types of information will also be very helpful to staff. These might include the following:

- any comfort object the child might have
- food likes and dislikes
- any particular fears
- special words the child might use, for example for the lavatory.

It is particularly important that parents have confidence in staff and feel that they are able to pass on information about events at home that might affect the child. Illness in the family, a new baby or a parent leaving home will all have an effect on the child. The more that the exchange of this type of information is encouraged, the smoother the process of sharing care is likely to be. Some centres use a **key worker** system where one member of staff has a responsibility for particular group of children. This can be helpful to parents as they can build a relationship with their child's key worker.

Remember that some parents may have difficulty with filling in forms and with written information. They may not be literate, or they may be literate in another language and might need oral support or access to translated information.

key worker
Works with, and is concerned with the care and assessment of, particular children in a setting

---

Case study: Expressing concerns

Shamila had been coming to nursery for over a year. She was a bright and outgoing child who had plenty of friends and joined in with all the activities. One morning she came in looking very pale and tired. She spent the whole of the session curled up in the book corner, often with a rug over her, pretending to be asleep. At home time, the nursery nurse made a point of having a word with Shamila's mother and described her behaviour. Her mother seemed very upset. She explained that Shamila's grandmother, who lived with them, was seriously ill and had been admitted to hospital the previous day and the whole of the family had been affected.

1 What do you think was wrong with Shamila?
2 Why is it helpful for the staff to know what's upsetting her?
3 What opportunities do parents in your setting have to share this kind of individual information?

Progress and achievements

A great deal is to be gained from sharing record-keeping with parents. This does not mean merely making children's records available to parents, but encouraging parents to contribute by offering their own observations of their children, thus putting the child into the wider context of home and community. Parents can be involved in the process of recording their children's progress and achievements in a number of ways.

■ Parents will often help staff to compile a profile of their child at admission. This is usually organised around areas of development and shows what the child can do. It may also include space to refer to the child's preferences, for example 'likes painting', and any other related information, including concerns. These initial profiles serve as a starting point and will be added to as the child progresses and achieves new skills.

■ An exchange of information about a child's achievements or concerns will usually take place on an informal basis at the beginning and end of sessions and can be very useful.

■ Most settings and parents would agree that there is a place for a regular, more structured exchange of information where records can be updated by parents and by staff and progress discussed. This will give parents the opportunity to add to the records compiled by staff and supplement these with additional information from their own observations. Plans for continuing progress should also be discussed with parents, emphasising the partnership between parents and staff and recognising the parents' key role in promoting their children's development.

■ Checklists that break down a certain area, for example reading, are quick and easy to fill in. Children and parents will enjoy filling these in and recording progress together (see the example on page 54).

■ Diary-type booklets that are regularly written up and sent home with children for parents to read and comment on provide another useful channel for exchanging information, particularly for those parents who are unable to get to the centre on a regular basis.

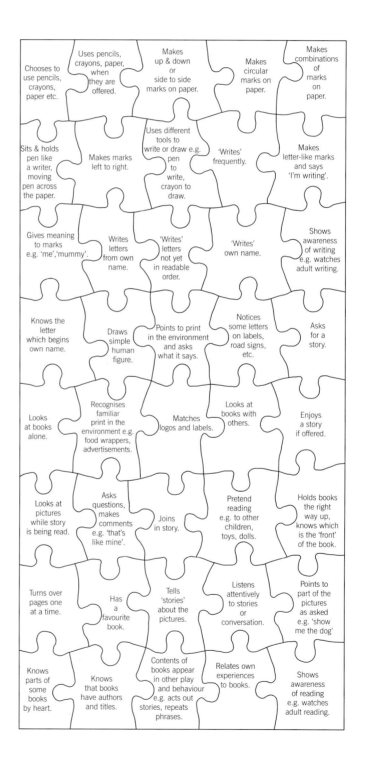

As reading skills develop, parents can record progress with their children

✓ Progress check

1 What kind of information will centres keep on the children they care for?
2 Why is important that this information is stored securely and kept up-to-date?
3 How can child-care workers ensure that parents have an opportunity to share individual or sensitive information that concerns their children?
4 How can parents contribute to records of their children's progress and achievements?
5 Why is this beneficial to parents and to the staff?

Difficult situations

There may be times when there is conflict between the child-care centre and workers and parents. Understanding and resolving this conflict can be a demanding task for staff to manage. Difficulties that arise out of a simple misunderstanding, for example a child coming home with the wrong coat, are usually fairly easy to sort out in a good humoured way. Below are some examples of situations that might not be quite so straight-forward.

- The values of the centre, for example methods of disciplining children, may sometimes be quite different from those of the home.
- Parents who are experiencing stresses and strains in their lives may appear to react angrily and aggressively to what seems to be a minor incident, for example a tear in the child's clothes.
- Where there are child-protection procedures in operation and a centre has a role in monitoring and reporting on contact between parents and children, the relationship between child-care workers and parents may be strained.
- There may be agreements over, say, collecting children at the agreed time, paying fees in advance, that are not kept to.
- Parents may disagree with the methods of the centre, for example challenging a learning through play approach.
- Rules such as no smoking on the premises may be broken and challenged.
- Parents may have complaints and concerns directed at particular members of staff. This could result in an official complaint being lodged against the centre.

Think about it

1 Read through the above examples again. Have you had any experience of observing or handling a disagreement with a parent? How was it managed?
2 Think of any other situations where there might be misunderstandings or disagreements with parents.

There is no magic formula for resolving difficulties of any type and there is a clear need for regular training to equip staff with the skills that enable them to cope with challenging and difficult situations. A centre that values its partnership with parents will work hard to maintain the confidence of parents by attempting to resolve difficulties to the satisfaction of all concerned. This is most likely to happen if:

- staff deal seriously and courteously with parents' concerns
- anger and aggression are dealt with calmly and not in a confrontational manner
- parents' skills, feelings and opinions are acknowledged and valued
- the centre has a consistent and well thought out approach to the way that it works with parents and all staff are aware of and supportive of it
- any concerns the staff have are communicated promptly and honestly with parents.

To sum up, to work most effectively with parents, child-care workers need to take a non-judgemental approach, that is one that recognises that parents have a great deal to contribute to the shared care of their children, and where professionals value and act on these contributions.

Case study: A difficult situation

Helen had been having a difficult time with her partner. Staff at the family centre who cared for her son, Liam, were aware that there were problems at home and had noticed how worn and tired Helen looked recently. One afternoon Helen stormed into the centre shouting abuse at Julie, Liam's key worker. When Julie asked her what was wrong, she grabbed Liam and then tried to leave the centre. Julie stood by the door and asked Helen to come and have a word with her in the office. Helen was reluctant but Julie remained calm and firm and eventually she agreed. Julie asked Helen what was wrong and Helen explained that she had arrived home to find that her partner had left her. She said that she'd been worried that he might try to take Liam away with him. Julie suggested what she might do and who she should contact if she felt that there was a risk that Liam would be snatched. After she had calmed down, Helen apologised and said that she would to stay with Liam for the rest of the session to put her mind at rest.

1 Why did Julie feel that she needed to talk with Helen, rather than let her storm off?
2 What did Julie do to minimise confrontation?
3 Why was it helpful to go into the office?

Progress check

1 What kinds of issues might give rise to conflict between the child-care centre and parents? Give some examples.
2 Why is it important that staff try to resolve these difficulties?
3 How can staff help to minimise the effects of this conflict?
4 Why is a non-judgemental approach important?

Getting parents involved

All parents will have some involvement with the centre that their child attends. Just what form this involvement takes depends on the type of centre, on the way that the staff interpret their brief to work with parents and on the parents themselves. The following are some examples of ways in which child-care centres can work together with parents to the benefit of their children.

Settling in

Everyone recognises the importance of the settling-in period for both the child and the parent and will encourage parents to play a full part. Centres will use some or all of the following to make this transition a positive experience.

- Parents will often stay with their child until, with the encouragement of staff, they feel comfortable about leaving. At this stage the exchange of information is vital: staff will want to know all about the child and parents will want to know all about how their child is doing during these early days. Parents who have full-time jobs may find it difficult to stay during these sessions but will be just as concerned; giving them plenty of notice of arrangements for starting may mean that they can organise other commitments and be there.
- Day nurseries who cater primarily for working parents will often have a programme for introducing parents and children to the setting, providing evening sessions where children and parents can meet staff and visit the building. When the child starts, there is usually someone at the end of a telephone to report back and reassure parents.
- Some centres will have their own pre-school (or pre-nursery) club where children come with their parents for a number of sessions before they start officially.
- Some centres will make home visits to families prior to their children starting nursery or school. Parents often feel more comfortable in their own homes rather than in a strange, perhaps intimidating environment.

It is important to remember that the settling-in period can sometimes be more stressful for the parents than for the child. Parents may take some time to adjust to a new role.

> ### Do this! 4.4
>
> You have been asked to organise an open afternoon in your nursery for new parents. You want parents to find out about the way that the nursery operates, meet staff and generally have their questions answered. Talk to your colleagues about what your aims for this session are. Plan what you would do and present this as a schedule for the afternoon. Prepare an information pack for parents to take away with them which you will refer to during the meeting.

After the settling in period, parents can be involved in a variety of ways.

Working with the children

Here parents are encouraged to stay and become involved in activities with the children, sometimes committing themselves to a regular session – as with a playgroup rota – more often on an occasional basis. The children benefit from the presence of another adult, parents have a chance to see the setting at work and the child is aware of the link between home and the centre. Cooking, craft and swimming sessions are often provided in this way and many schools rely on parent help for reading activities. Outings with groups of children would neither be possible nor safe without parent volunteers to accompany them. Parents might also be able to contribute in a more specific way, for example by talking about their job, telling a story in another language or playing an instrument.

Case study: Giving a talk

The reception class had been working on a topic about 'Ourselves'. The children had examined their own features and compared them with those of their friends and taken part in many other linked activities. The school had a good relationship with its parents and they were often involved in classroom activities. At the beginning of every topic, class teachers displayed their plans on the parents' noticeboard and asked parents for contributions, either of materials or ideas. One parent noticed that some work was planned on joints and the skeleton. As a radiographer, she had access to X-rays which she thought might be useful for the project. After a chat with the class teacher, she was persuaded not only to donate the X-rays but to come and give a talk to the class. Although she had some misgivings, she came along in her hospital uniform and talked to the children about her job. There were lots of questions after she'd finished, with many from children who'd had their own experiences of X-rays after accidents. When she came in next to pick up her children, she saw the follow-up work that the children had done after her visit was displayed on the classroom noticeboard.

1 What do you think the children gained from this experience?
2 What do you think the parent gained from participating in this way?
3 Do you think all parents would be happy taking on this role? What would it depend on?

Working behind the scenes

Not everyone feels comfortable or is able to work alongside the children. Making, mending and maintaining equipment is a task that can involve parents. Also in this category of involvement will be the fund-raising and organisation of social events that many parent groups take responsibility for. These social events that bring together staff and parents are usually very successful in promoting good relationships and often raise funds too. Parents who are not available during the day may be able to become involved in these ways.

Special occasions

Most centres have occasions when parents are invited along to parties, concerts, sports, open days or stay and play sessions. Such events are usually very popular indeed. More parents will be able to take advantage of the invitation if other commitments are taken into account, for example if babies and toddlers are welcome at an afternoon concert, or if there are occasional evening events so that those who are out at work during the day can attend.

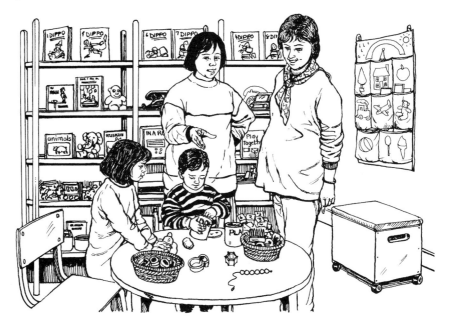

Stay and play sessions can be very popular

Support for parents

In some day nurseries and most family centres the staff have a special brief to work with parents. This is probably because there is some difficulty in the family that affects the child and the parent needs some support. Staff work alongside parents and children in individual programmes. For this kind of work to be successful, it is crucial that the member of staff has the trust and confidence of the parent. Some centres might also offer 'drop-in' facilities and parents' groups as part of their programme.

Taking the curriculum home

Most parents will expect to play a part in helping their children to read. Home–school reading diaries, in which parents and staff exchange comments on books and reading, provide a link and show children that everyone is involved. Other schemes such as Impact Maths and Science are popular in some areas. In these, children and parents are guided through a practical, problem-solving activity using a prepared pack. Such schemes recognise and emphasise the important role that the home and parents have in children's learning.

Official roles

Some parents will be involved with the child-care centre in an official capacity. All state schools will have parents, elected by other parents, on their governing bodies and they have an important role defined in law. Playgroups are usually run by a committee of parents for the benefit of the local community. Other types of centre may have parent representatives on their management committees. Sometimes parents may be reluctant to become involved in this way and need to be assured that they have a necessary and valuable contribution to make.

Do this! 4.5

Read the section above again. Think of any other ways to involve parents. What might prevent parents from becoming involved?

Suggest ways to overcome this. Make a list of your suggestions and discuss them with a colleague.

✅ Progress check

1 Why is settling in a key time for involving parents?
2 Why is it important to be flexible when making arrangements for children to settle in?
3 Does being involved mean that the parent has to help out in the classroom? Explain your answer.
4 How can parents participate in the curriculum?
5 List ways in which parents can work 'behind the scenes'.

Key terms

You need to know what these words and phrases mean. Go back through the chapter and find out.
key worker
jargon

Now try these questions

1 Why is it important that child-care staff should work in partnership with parents?

2 How can you make it clear to parents that you welcome them and that you value their participation?

3 How might you meet the needs of:
   a) parents who are not fluent in English?
   b) parents who feel uneasy or intimidated in the setting?

4 Design a settling in programme for children who are about to go to nursery. Explain how it will meet the needs of both children and parents.

5 Why is it helpful to children's learning if record keeping is shared with parents?

Part 2: Play and the Early Years Curriculum

It is important that child-care workers understand *how* children learn so that they can provide an appropriate learning environment for the children in their care. An understanding of *what* children need to learn enables staff to focus the activities and their interaction with the children to develop necessary early skills and concepts.

Studies of *how* children learn – Piaget's work in particular – show that children learn best through developmentally-appropriate first-hand experiences. This approach is evident in most early years settings. Typically the children will be active, selecting activities, following their interests and interacting with the other children and staff. They will be *learning by doing*. This learning by doing, or play environment, is the best vehicle for teaching young children. It provides the opportunity for children to be actively involved in their learning. It is familiar, repetitive and enjoyable. It is appropriate across the early years as it can be something as simple as the soothing experience of kneading playdough or as complex as a board game involving addition, subtraction and multiplication.

It is also important for all child-care workers to realise that the curriculum contains more than its academic subjects. Teaching transmits the values of the setting and of the people who work there, for example what is appropriate male and female behaviour. So, as well as the academic curriculum, these aspects of the 'hidden curriculum' need to be carefully considered in what children learn.

5 Play

This chapter includes:

- **The value of play**
- **What children learn through playing**
- **The adult's role in play**

Play is the way in which young children find out about their world and acquire, practise and refine their emerging skills. Play occurs naturally in children. Through their play, children develop physical, intellectual, linguistic, social and emotional skills and concepts.

Adults can use children's eagerness to play to create an effective learning environment. A well-planned, rich and stimulating play environment will provide opportunities for children to explore the world, and to adapt and refine their understanding of it.

You may find it helpful to read this chapter in conjunction with:

- ▶ **Book 1, Chapter 7** An introduction to language and cognitive development
- ▶ **Book 1, Chapter 8** Language development
- ▶ **Book 1, Chapter 9** Cognitive development
- ▶ **Book 2, Chapter 6** Philosophy and approaches
- ▶ **Book 2, Chapter 7** Curriculum components

The value of play

Young children and babies need to acquire many skills and to find out about the world they live in. They do this through relentless exploration of their environment and constant practising of their developing skills. Adults call this *play*. To enable children to get the most out of their play, it is important that people who are involved with children understand the value of play and how to organise play opportunities.

Why is play a good way of meeting young children's needs?

- Play occurs naturally in young children. It is therefore familiar to the child, a link between home and the establishment. It is a way to harness what the child is already able to do to help their learning.
- Play cannot be wrong. It therefore provides a safe situation for the child to try out new things without the fear of failure. This is important for the child's development of a positive **self-esteem**.

self-esteem
Liking and valuing oneself

■ Play provides the opportunity for repetition. One of the important ways that learning takes place is through repetition. Play provides the opportunity for the child to practise and consolidate new skills in a enjoyable, familiar and interesting way.

■ Play provides the opportunity for extending learning. A carefully structured play environment will provide opportunities for learning across a wide ability range. For example, sand can be a soothing, sensory experience and also provide the opportunity for a child to begin to learn about capacity and volume. A child's skills can therefore develop in a familiar situation, one where there is no competition between the physical skills and the intellectual and language skills.

■ Play provides the opportunity for a child to practise and perfect their skills in a safe environment. Through play situations, children can also try out new skills. This can be done within a safe environment as the child can opt out of the play situation when they want.

■ Play is always at the child's own level, so the needs of all children within the group can be met. It is important therefore to make sure that there is a range of play materials and equipment to enable all children to participate at their own level. Adult intervention in a child's play is necessary to move them onto the next developmental level.

> ✓ **Progress check**
>
> 1 How do children and babies find out about the world?
> 2 Why is play familiar to children?
> 3 Why is play safe for children?
> 4 Why is repetition in play important for children?
> 5 How can play meet the needs of all the children in the group?

What children learn through playing

Young children need to develop a whole range of skills. These need to be practised and developed through the opportunity to repeat them in concrete situations. The skills that a child needs to develop can be categorised into a number of areas to make them easy to understand and learn (see the diagram opposite), but it is important to remember that children's development cannot be divided up in the same way. All the areas of development are dependent upon one another.

Play provides the opportunity for all these skills to be developed. It also has the advantages of being familiar to the child, secure in that mistakes are not permanent and always at an appropriate level. It is also enjoyable and provides the opportunity for the repetition of skills necessary to learning.

Social development
The development of skills needed to interact with other people in both individual and group settings.

Emotional development
Concerned with the development of healthy expression and control of feelings and emotions. This includes feelings about self. This is called self-esteem.

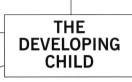

THE DEVELOPING CHILD

Physical development
The development of bodily movement and control. It can be divided into two main areas: gross motor and fine motor skills.

Language (linguistic) development
The development of communication through speaking or British Sign Language; this includes non-verbal communication. It is also the development of early reading and writing skills.

Cognitive (intellectual) development
The development of thinking and learning skills; it includes the development of concepts, problem-solving skills, the imagination, creativity, memory and concentration.

Physical development

Physical development is the growth, development and control of bodily movements. Children need to practise these skills by repeating them over and over again. Physical development includes:

- **gross motor skills** – whole body and limb movements, co-ordination and balance
- **fine motor skills** – small finger movements, manipulative skills and hand–eye co-ordination.

---

physical development
The development of bodily movement and control

gross motor skills
Whole body and limb movements, co-ordination and balance

fine motor skills
Small finger movements and manipulative skills, hand–eye co-ordination

---

Do this! 5.1

Prepare, process and present a chart to show how the skills listed above are practised and/or used in the following activities:
a) building with large bricks
b) playing with wet sand with buckets and spades of various sizes
c) junk and box modelling
d) doing large floor jigsaws.

Case study: Developing fine motor skills

As part of their ongoing assessment of the children, staff in the nursery noted that, overall, the children in the group needed to work at their fine motor skills. The staff decided to work towards doing some sewing with each child. They planned a series of activities, linked to the sewing, to develop the children's manipulative skills and their hand–eye co-ordination. Over a term, alongside all the other activities, the children were encouraged to:

- play with lacing boards and tiles
- thread beads, cotton reels and buttons
- play with peg boards
- do some weaving
- complete simple sewing boards, with laces and bodkin needles.

Finally, when staff felt that they were likely to succeed, each child was introduced to sewing.

1 Why is sewing a good way to develop fine motor skills?
2 Why did the staff plan activities linked to sewing for the children to attempt first?

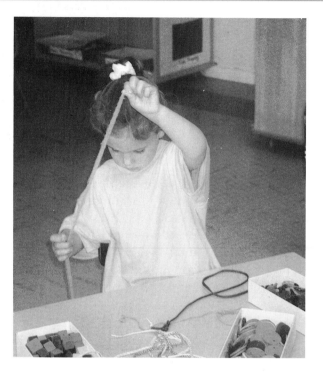

Threading activities contribute to the development of fine motor skills

Outdoor play

Outdoor play is an important aspect of physical development. It provides the opportunity for a range of physical skills to be practised and developed, but there are many other benefits:

- fresh air and exercise that aid growth and development
- space, which allows children to release energy; this provides a contrast to indoor areas within an establishment where physical movement needs to be restricted
- the opportunity to make a noise; indoors low levels of noise need to be maintained. Outdoors children can make far more noise, which may help them to adapt to the usual necessary restrictions
- a different time scale; more space may result in longer play sequences. The space is usually not required for other activities and fewer restrictions are necessary
- adjustment to the school environment; play outside is familiar to most children. It allows a feeling of freedom. Nursery children can get used to playtime
- discovery of the environment; children can experience different materials (leaves, twigs, pebbles, stones). Outdoor play provides a rich sensory experience where children can develop awareness of many

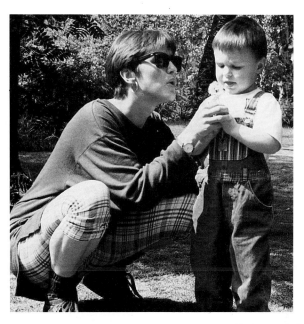

Children can experience different materials in an outdoor environment

concepts, for example wind, rain, temperature, light and shade, smell, water, heat and cold.

Outdoor play needs to be as carefully planned as all other play activities. Issues that need to be considered include safety, staffing, space, storage, opportunities for all skills to be developed and all children to be involved over a range of abilities and needs.

Think about it

1 What are the differences in planning indoor and outdoor play?
2 How may these issues be resolved?

Do this! 5.2

1 List outdoor equipment or activities that promote the development of physical skills.

2 For each piece of equipment or activity that you have listed, identify where each skill can be practised and developed.

3 From your list of equipment and activities, draw up a floorplan of a day's outdoor play for a group of young children. Make sure that you consider issues of space, safety, staffing, a balance of skills and a range of abilities.

cognitive development
The development of thinking and understanding, which includes problem-solving, reasoning, concentration, memory, imagination and creativity; also called intellectual development

Cognitive development

Cognitive development (or intellectual development) is the development of thinking and learning skills. It includes the development of concepts, problem-solving skills, creativity, imagination, memory and concentration. Play provides the opportunity for the early stages of all these skills to be developed.

A painting activity, for example, may develop the following skills:

- concepts of colour, size, shape, properties of water, mixing, thick, thin, wet and dry
- an opportunity to work through problems of how to stop the paint running, how to mix colours, how to stop the paintbrush dripping, what size to draw to fit everything onto the page. These may seen like simple problems, but the child is developing skills that can be applied elsewhere
- an opportunity to use creative and imaginative skills. Children choose what to paint and develop their own ways of representing their ideas. Again, the skills necessary to enable them to do this can be transferred to other situations where the child needs to think through ideas or problems and develop personal responses to them
- encourages children, by being an absorbing and enjoyable activity, to use their memory and develop their skills of concentration by finishing what they started.

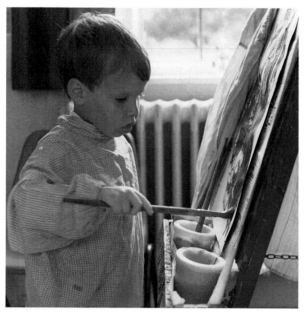

Children choose to paint and develop their own ways of representing ideas

Through play, therefore, children have the opportunity to acquire, practise and consolidate intellectual skills that form the basis of later learning. This can be done in a secure, familiar and enjoyable environment.

Language development

Language development (or linguistic development) is the development of communication skills. This includes verbal skills (talking) and **non-verbal communication** skills (gesture, eye contact, body movements), reading and writing. Early language development is mainly concerned with expressive language (spoken or signed). Written language and reading are

language development
The development of communication skills, which includes non-verbal communication, reading and writing skills, as well as spoken language; also called linguistic development

non-verbal communication
Non-spoken communication, for example, bodily movements, eye contact, gestures and facial expression; sometimes used to enhance or replace speech

later skills. Again, like all other skills, expressive language skills are acquired, practised and refined through use. As children play they use expressive language for many things:

- describing
- discussing
- reporting
- imagining
- predicting
- asking and answering questions
- practising new words
- forming and maintaining relationships.

To enable children to learn and practise their spoken language they need:

- good role models
- the opportunity to speak and to practise their speech
- adults who are sensitive to both their present level of development and the next stage.

Play provides the opportunity for children to interact with adults and other children to hear and see language, and to practise and develop their own skills. Interaction can occur during any activity or experience.

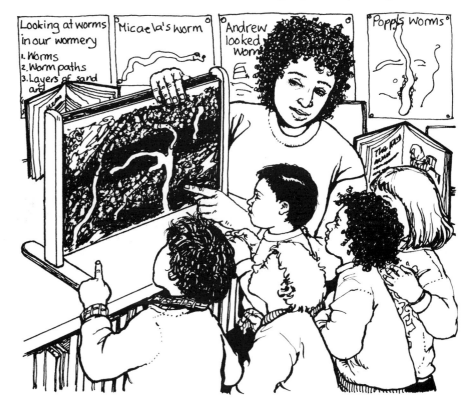

Talking with others is necessary for children to pick up language and to adjust and refine their language skills

Non-verbal communication

As well as verbal or expressive language, children acquire non-verbal communication skills through play. These are bodily movements, gestures, eye contact, facial expression, and so on. Non-verbal communication sometimes replaces speech, for example a finger on the lips indicating a command to be quiet. It also forms part of what we are saying when speaking, for example pointing to emphasis a point, facial expression reflecting what is being said. The meanings of these non-verbal signs are understood in the same way as spoken language. They have a powerful impact, and when the non-verbal clues are misunderstood, the meaning of what is being said can be misinterpreted. (It is important to realise that there are cultural differences in the meanings of some non-verbal signs. This can also lead to misinterpretation of what is being said or meant.)

Children's interaction with others in their play provides the opportunity to observe, learn and practise these non-verbal communication signs. For example, a child can become other people in a role-play and adopt their use of spoken language, tone of voice and non-verbal signs. They can observe the effect these have on others and adapt and change them as they wish. This is all done in the knowledge that the child can opt out of the play at any time if they begin to feel uncomfortable in the role.

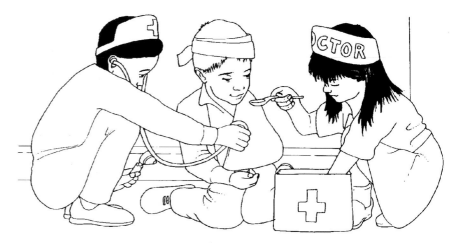

A child can become other people in a role-play, but opt out of the play at any time if they begin to feel uncomfortable

---

Think about it

1 What non-verbal signs can you identify, that either replace speech or form part of what is being said?
2 Are there situations that you can remember where there has been a mismatch between what is being said and the non-verbal messages given? What was the effect of this mismatch?

Case study: Using communication skills in imaginary play

Sarah and Christopher were playing in the imaginary play area which was a shop. Sarah was the shopkeeper and Christopher the customer.

Sarah   Can I help you?
Christopher Yes, some people are coming to my house for tea and I need to buy some food.

Sarah	We have got bread and beans. Do your friends like beans on toast?
Christopher	I think so. There are hundreds of my friends coming so I will need lots of food.
Sarah	OK. We have got huge tins in our shop. How many will you need?
Christopher	Twenty hundred.
Sarah	There you are. Fifteen pence please.

1 How did Sarah and Christopher use language in this interchange? (Refer to the list on page 69.)
2 Which non-verbal signs may they have used?
3 How may this activity helped their development?

Developing an understanding of reading and writing

Children also need opportunities to develop an understanding of reading and writing. Play provides this opportunity. For example, if notepads, pencils, menus, pricelists and notices are provided in an imaginative play area that is a cafe or restaurant, children have the opportunity to develop early reading and writing skills. By imitating what they have seen in cafes or restaurants, they may pretend to read the menus, make marks on the paper to represent writing when taking orders and refer to pricelists. This puts reading and writing into a realistic context where children can begin to understand the importance of these skills. Older children who have acquired some reading and writing skills can further develop them in similar play situations.

Do this!   *5.3*

1 Observe a group of children involved in an activity.
   a) Identify the ways in which they use language. Use the list in the paragraph *Language development* on page 69.
   b) What was the adult role in the talking?
   c) How did the activity contribute to the children's use and/or development of language?

2 Suggest reasons why play is a good way for children to learn and develop their language skills.

Emotional development

Emotional development includes the development of the healthy control and expression of feelings and emotions. These are learned skills and are often culturally defined. Emotional development is also concerned with the development of feelings about self (self-esteem).

Feelings exist and cannot be changed. It is the behaviour that results from the feelings that can be modified. Through play, children have the opportunity to explore feelings that they have. They have the opportunity to experiment with responses to their feelings. Play enables children to express positive feelings openly and begin to develop ways of expressing difficult feelings in acceptable ways.

Case study: Expressing and exploring emotions in imaginary play

Amelia's mummy had just had a new baby. Initially she was excited and spoke a lot about the baby and what she did to help look after her. Once this initial excitement had died down, the staff noticed how she would role-play being her mummy over and over again.

In the home corner, with a friend, Amelia would be the mummy and her friend became Amelia. They looked after the baby together. However, in role, Amelia would tell her friend that she was too tired to play and that they couldn't go to the park now because the baby needed to be fed. During this play, Amelia instructed her friend to cry when she was told that she couldn't do something that she wanted to do. Amelia responded by sighing a lot, putting her arm around her friend and kissing her, and sitting her on her knee to comfort her.

1 Why do you think Amelia wanted to play like this?
2 What are the benefits of this role-play?

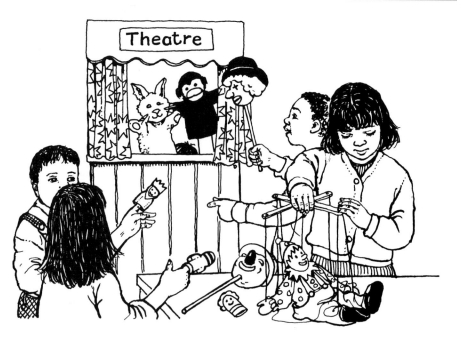

Imaginative play enables children to feel what it is like to be somebody or something else

self-concept (or self-image)
The picture we have of ourselves and the way we think other people see us

Play can also be a positive **self-concept** builder. The way that we feel about ourselves has a large impact on all aspects of our lives. It is therefore important that children develop a positive self-esteem. Play is familiar and natural to them and so is not a threatening experience – play cannot be wrong. Children play at their own level and so the risk of constant failure is minimised. This familiar positive environment gives them the opportunity to develop a positive sense of their achievements and to begin to feel good about themselves. This in turn affects their later development.

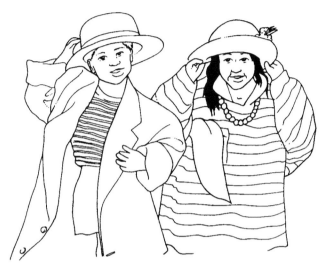

Play is also a positive self-concept builder

Do this! 5.4

1 a) List the ways in which you can enhance a child's self-concept.

  b) Link each of these suggestions to a play activity.

2 Suggest why play is a good way of developing a child's self-concept.

Social development

social development
The growth of the ability to relate to others appropriately and become independent, within a social framework

Social development is concerned with the development of skills that enable children to get on successfully with other people. Social skills enable a child to become a reasonable, acceptable and effective member of a community. These skills are learned through interaction with other people. It is a life-long process. Young children need to begin to acquire skills such as:

■ sharing
■ taking turns
■ co-operating
■ making and maintaining friendships
■ responding to people in an appropriate way.

Play acts as a bridge to social skills and relationships. It provides children with the opportunity to interact with others, both adults and children, at an appropriate level. This in itself helps children acquire the necessary skills for getting on with others and becoming part of a group. Through play, children are also given the opportunity to practise and perfect social skills in situations that are not permanent. The activity, game or experience will finish but the social skills used will eventually be remembered. In this way the child is not made to feel inadequate as new skills are acquired.

The development of social play

How children play within the group follows a developmental pattern. Progress through the stages of development depends upon having the opportunity to play with other children. As children learn and develop social skills these are taken into account in their play. The pattern is summarised in the diagram below.

Solitary play
A child plays alone.

Parallel play
A child plays side-by-side with another child, but without interacting; their play activities remain separate.

Associative play
Play begins with other children; children make intermittent interactions and/or are involved in the same activity although their play may remain personal.

Co-operative play
Children are able to play together co-operatively; they are able to adopt a role within the group and to take account of others' needs and actions.

The development of social play

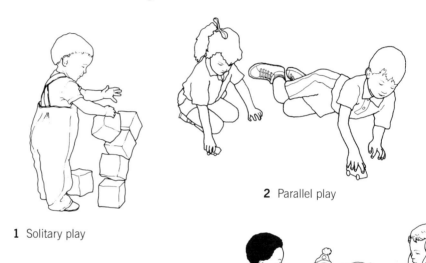

1 Solitary play

2 Parallel play

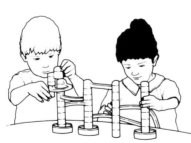

3 Associative play

4 Co-operative play

Do this! 5.5

a) List some of the social skills that a child needs to function well within society.
b) Link these skills to activities that give the child the opportunity to develop them.
c) What is your role in promoting social skills during these activities?

Progress check

1 How does play contribute to the development of fine and gross motor skills?
2 a) Why is outdoor play beneficial to children?
  b) What needs to be considered when planning outdoor play?
3 a) What is intellectual development?
  b) How can play contribute to the development of intellectual skills?
4 a) What is language development?
  b) How can play help language development?
5 What are:
  a) verbal skills?
  b) non-verbal skills?
6 List the ways in which children may use language when playing.
7 a) What is emotional development?
  b) List some ways in which play can contribute positively to a child's emotional development.
8 What is self-image (or self-concept) and why is it important?
9 a) What are social skills?
  b) Why are they important?
10 a) How are social skills acquired?
  b) Why is play a good way for children to develop these skills?

The adult's role in play

Adults have an important role in children's play to ensure that the maximum benefit is gained from it. The adult needs to plan and prepare the activities carefully. They also need to interact with the children during the activity and monitor what is happening through observation. The adult's role in play is summarised in the diagram on page 76.

Think about it

Study the diagram on page 76.
1 Why is it important to plan for children's play?
2 Why should activities be attractively presented?
3 Describe some specific instances where you have seen an adult interacting with a child during play.
4 Suggest some ways that an adult could extend a child's play.
5 Suggest some ways that an adult could observe and monitor children's development during play.

What are the children's developmental levels?
What are the special needs of children within the group?
Which skills do the children need to develop?
How much space is available?
How much time is available?
What are the staffing levels and expertise?
Is there a current theme or topic?
Does the planning reflect cultural diversity?
What activities do the children enjoy?
Are there any safety issues to be considered?

The children:
■ Does the play provided meet their needs?
■ Who is playing with which activity? Is this significant?
■ What interaction with the child/children is appropriate?
■ How can the children's play be extended?

The activity:
■ Is the activity appropriate for the group of children?
■ Is it attractively presented?
■ Is all the necessary equipment available so that the children can be as independent as possible?
■ Was there enough time and space for the children to play with the activity successfully?
■ Was the adult's time and expertise made full use of?

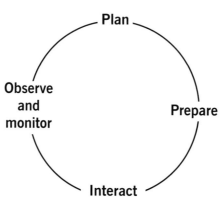

The activity needs to be attractive and easily accessible to the children.
Is all the necessary equipment available?
Is the activity presented in an inviting way? This may include beginning the activity to suggest ways of doing it to the children.
Is there enough space, time and adult help available to enable the child to be successful at the activity?
Is the area safe?

Ways of interacting with the children include:
■ joining in the children's play
■ playing alongside the children
■ providing a commentary on the play
■ suggesting new or different ideas for the play
■ introducing different equipment to extend the play
■ discussing the activity prior to or after the play.
Observe the play without direct intervention allowing the child/children to develop their own ideas.

The role of the adult in children's play

Do this!   5.6

Observe an adult who works with children.
a) Make a note of how they plan for the children's play, how activities are set up and how they interact with the children during play.
b) Ask the adult what they look for when observing children informally during their play.
c) Suggest reasons for their actions.
d) Where possible compare your findings with others. What are the similarities and differences?
e) What conclusions can you draw from the fact that there are similarities and differences?

The play environment

There are some important considerations in developing a positive play environment.

- Repetition is an important part of learning; children need some consistency in what is provided for them so that they can improve their skills.
- There should be a variety of activities provided at any one time to ensure that all necessary skills can be developed.
- There should be a balance between play where the children develop their own themes and ideas independently (sometimes called *free play*) and play where the adult guides the play towards the next stage of development (sometimes called *structured play*).
- Safety should be an important consideration at all times; this includes the maintenance of safe equipment.
- The best starting points for a positive play environment are the children's backgrounds, interests and knowledge. These can be extended and built upon and used to develop other necessary skills.

Think about it

1 How could you provide free play?
2 How could you provide structured play?
3 How can you ensure that the play environment is safe?
4 Think of some possible starting points for developing a play environment.

✓ *Progress check*

1 Why is the adult important in children's play?
2 What should be taken into account when planning children's play?
3 What is important about the presentation of an activity?
4 List the ways in which adults can interact with children during play.
5 Why is it important to observe and monitor children?
6 What should an adult be looking for when observing and monitoring an activity?
7 Why is it important for children to repeat activities?
8 How can the variety of activities contribute to a child's all-round development?
9 What is the best starting point for a play environment?

Key terms

You need to know what these words and phrases mean. Go back through the chapter and find out.

associative play
co-operative play
cognitive development
emotional development
fine motor skills
gross motor skills
language development
non-verbal communication
parallel play
physical development
self-concept (or self-image)
self-esteem
social development
solitary play

Now try these questions

1 Why is play a good way of meeting young children's needs?

2 Describe the range of skills and concepts that a child can develop through play.

3 What is the role of the adult in children's play?

4 What should be considered when planning a play environment?

6 *Philosophy and approaches*

This chapter includes:

- **Approaches to the curriculum**
- **Curriculum models**
- **Curriculum frameworks**
- **Curriculum planning and organisation**
- **Equal opportunities and the 'hidden' curriculum**

This chapter looks at various approaches to the early years curriculum and considers how these approaches are informed by what is known about the way in which children learn. It looks at statutory requirements concerning the content of the curriculum and at some aspects of curriculum planning and organisation. Finally, it examines the issue of equal opportunities and the curriculum.

You may find it helpful to read this chapter in conjunction with:

▶ **Book 1, Chapter 7** An introduction to language and cognitive development
▶ **Book 2, Chapter 5** Play
▶ **Book 2, Chapter 7** Curriculum components

Approaches to the curriculum

> **curriculum**
> The content and methods that comprise a course of study

A 'course of study' is the simple dictionary definition of **curriculum**. But in the early years, the term curriculum carries more than this simple academic definition implies. The curriculum also transmits the values of the setting and those who work within it. Through it, children learn about themselves and their place in the world.

In the past

Look in history books and see if you can find drawings or photographs of schools in the early 1900s. You might see very large classes of children, sitting in rows facing a stern-looking teacher, who might be pointing to a list of words on a blackboard with a long stick. There might be a chart or a map on the walls and probably a list of rules, but not much else. The windows would be placed high on the walls so that children could not be distracted by what was going on outside the schoolroom. The only sounds heard would be the voice of the teacher or children chanting their multiplication tables in unison. Children were expected to learn facts by heart, to listen passively and to absorb knowledge from adults. They were not encouraged to take any responsibility for their own learning, to contribute their ideas or to follow up their own interests. Education was not expected to be enjoyable. (*Hard Times* by Charles Dickens and *Cider with Rosie* by Laurie Lee both give vivid accounts of bygone schooldays.)

Current practice

Studies of the way that children learn, and Piaget's work in particular, indicate that concepts are best understood through actual experiences, in effect, that children *learn by doing*. These theories have had a significant influence on the way that we organise early years provision and have led to an approach to learning that takes into account the child's individual capabilities and interests (**child-centred**) and which is achieved through experience (**experiential**).

child-centred
With the child at the centre, taking into account the perspective of the child

experiential
Achieving through experience

Case study: Making a rainhat for teddy

An activity was set up for the 5-year-olds in the class to work at in groups. Children were provided with a range of different fabrics, a bowl of water and a water squirter. They were asked to examine all the fabrics carefully and decide which would be most suitable to use to make a rainhat for teddy. The nursery nurse worked with the children at the table getting them to talk about what a rainhat was required to do and also encouraging them to use the equipment provided to test out their choices.

After some time spent squirting water on each of the fabric samples, they were able to eliminate most of the samples as no good for keeping teddy dry and then were able to decide on a 'best choice' from those that were left. Later on that day they were able to test out the rainhat that they had made by taking teddy out during a heavy shower. By the end of the session they had gained a considerable understanding of the concept of absorbency and were beginning to develop their own methods of scientific enquiry. They also experienced a sense of achievement and satisfaction at being able to follow the task all the way through to completion.

1 Why was this a successful activity for the children?
2 What do you think the children learned from this?
3 How did the adult support children's learning here?
4 An adult could tell children about absorbency and the properties of fabrics. Would this enable them to understand this concept?

In most settings the environment is carefully organised so that children have the maximum opportunity for hands-on experience. Equipment will be accessible so that they can make choices and follow up interests, fostering a responsibility for their own learning. A number of activities will be available at any one time and the atmosphere buzzes with busy noise. Children will be involved in planning and working collaboratively, both with adults and with each other, and will be encouraged to contribute

Think about it

Do you remember your early years at nursery or in school? How was your day organised? Can you recall anything that you particularly enjoyed? Anything you hated? Would you describe your experience as child-centred?

their own ideas. Staff monitor progress, interact with children and plan and provide for the next learning activity.

This current approach to the curriculum assumes that if children engage with and enjoy what they are doing, then their learning will be both effective and meaningful.

> ### ✓ *Progress check*
>
> 1 What do you understand by the term 'curriculum'?
> 2 How does our current approach to the early years curriculum differ from that of the past?
> 3 What is experiential learning?
> 4 How has Piaget's work influenced the way that we provide for young children's learning?

Curriculum models

The curriculum models of Montessori, Steiner and Highscope examined below have much in common. All three are based on an understanding that children learn through active involvement with their environment and that this is often best achieved through the medium of play. They all acknowledge that childhood is a sensitive learning time and that children are highly receptive to all experiences. Where they differ is in the emphasis placed on the various elements of the curriculum and on the methods used.

The influence of these approaches is not limited to the relatively small number of centres that have adopted them in their entirety: some elements of all of these approaches can be recognised in much of what is considered 'mainstream' provision.

Montessori education

Montessori education is named after its founder, Maria Montessori, who devised an approach to learning based on her observations of children she worked with. The child is at the centre of the Montessori method. She believed that children learn best through their own spontaneous activity and that they have a natural inquisitiveness and eagerness to learn. The role of the adult is to provide a planned environment that will allow the child the opportunity to develop skills and concepts.

Montessori classrooms follow a similar pattern. Furniture is child-sized, including long, low cupboards so that children can select their own materials. There are rugs so that children can sit on the floor and the classroom is bright and light with pictures on the wall and plants and flowers around the room.

Central to the Montessori method are the didactic (teaching) materials. These consist of blocks, beads, cylinders and rods provided for the children to play with. Experimentation with these materials allows the children to discover and understand basic concepts for themselves. There is no time limit to this exploration; the children continue until satisfied. To achieve this, the materials are:

■ simple – though not easy – so that the child can understand them and the observant adult can decide when to become involved
■ inherently interesting
■ self-checking, so that the child knows whether they have succeeded without the need for adult intervention.

Children's exploration of the didactic materials remains an important part of the Montessori curriculum although this is usually presented alongside a broader range of experiences.

In a Montessori classroom, the adult's role is considered to be that of 'director', that is to keep children's interest through guiding, but also to withdraw so that the children do things for themselves and develop a sense of independence and self-confidence. The director observes the individual children and notes the stage achieved on records that relate to the didactic materials. The director will then determine what activities are suitable for the next steps in each child's learning and guide the child toward them.

Steiner education (the Waldorf schools)

Steiner education is based on the educational philosophy of Rudolf Steiner. He did not believe that the purpose and focus of education should be a narrow teaching of skills that are required for society's economic growth, but rather that the true purpose of education was to allow the individual's impulses and talents to unfold. Steiner felt that as children learn from what happens all around them, the environment had the most significant influence on the child and that this included experiences and interactions with other people as well as the physical environment. Steiner believed strongly in the need for children to develop their own inner world, valuing creativity and self-expression most highly. The Steiner method encourages these qualities through activities such as drawing, dancing, music, movement and all kinds of fantasy and pretend play. Eurhythmy – whole body rhythmical movement – is also valued as an important means of creative self-expression.

A Steiner kindergarten will have many or all of the following features:

■ items made from natural materials, wherever possible
■ toys and articles that can be used in an open-ended, imaginative way
■ a room that is pleasing to the child with factors such as light and use of colour considered
■ plenty of paper, pens and modelling clay provided
■ large boxes, pieces of carpet and lengths of fabric for children to develop their own role play themes
■ a garden where children can come into contact with the natural cycle of planting, tending and harvesting.

The adult's role in the Steiner system is that of provider and guide. The adult should not initiate play but become involved where appropriate. Steiner believed that children learn through imitation and interaction. Therefore, the good behaviour of adults towards one another and towards children serves as a powerful role model to influence children's own standards of behaviour.

Although Steiner's approach may appear unconventional in the current educational climate, it should be noted that education in the Steiner system does not preclude children from achieving conventional educational targets, such as success in public examinations, alongside the Steiner aims of developing individual talents.

Highscope

Highscope is an approach to the early years curriculum that was developed in the United States in the 1960s as part of the Headstart **compensatory education** programme. It has been shown to have good results, particularly in terms of developing in children a sense of responsibility for their own learning and actions. Follow-up research, which has tracked those children involved in the original Highscope project for 30 years, has shown that this type of pre-school experience has had a positive effect on the participants well into their adult lives, which is indicated by their social and economic well-being. The Highscope approach has been adopted by number of centres in the UK, not necessarily as part of a compensatory programme but because its principles are recognised as developmentally appropriate for young children.

> **compensatory education**
> A programme or initiative that is offered to those who might be likely to experience disadvantage in the education system

Highscope is characterised by:

- *The daily routine* This comprises the Plan–Do–Review approach, where children are required to indicate to an adult what they are going to do during a session (plan), to carry out this plan during the 'worktime' part of the session (do) and then to recall what they have done (review). This recall time will often include some kind of representation such as a drawing, or showing the work, or describing what's been done. Recall may be incorporated into 'small group time' when children are involved in structured, adult-led activities. Also incorporated into the daily schedule will be sessions of outside time – usually focused on vigorous activity – and circle time, when the whole group get together to sing, discuss or play games.
- *Room and equipment organisation* The room is arranged for particular activities in distinct work areas, usually with a book area, a construction area, a home area and an art area. All equipment and materials are stored and clearly labelled so that children have independent access to them.
- *Key terms, concepts and experiences* The curriculum is designed to develop a range of key experiences and cognitive skills and the child's progress is reviewed with reference to these. Key experiences provide the focus for adult–child interaction. These may be specifically planned for small group time or arise incidentally during a worktime. It is the adult's

responsibility to guide play and talk in such a way as to draw these key experiences into focus.

■ *The role of the adult* The role of the adult in the Highscope curriculum is to encourage, demonstrate and to assist but not to dominate. The adult creates a framework for learning that values and acts upon the children's initiatives and interests.

This approach actively involves children in decisions about their learning and fosters responsibility and independence. (To find out more about Highscope, contact the Highscope Institute 190–2 Maple Road, Penge, London SE20 8HT)

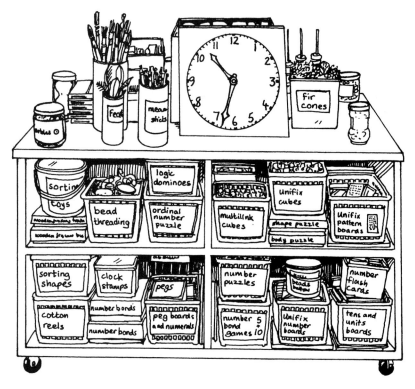

Children have independent access to clearly labelled equipment

---

Do this! 6.1

Re-read the section on curriculum models. Compile a chart with sections on aims, environment and role of the adult and complete each section with reference to the Montessori, Steiner and Highscope approaches.

✓ Progress check

1 Outline the curriculum models described in this section.
2 What similarities are there in the various approaches?
3 What is compensatory education?
4 What are the features of the Highscope approach? How does this approach develop responsibility?

Curriculum frameworks

This section summarises the statutory (laid down by law) curriculum requirements in the UK for state schools and for nurseries and other settings who are in receipt of government grant for the provision of education.

The National Curriculum

> **National Curriculum**
> A course of study, laid down by government, that all children between 5 and 16 in state schools in the UK must follow

The **National Curriculum** was introduced in England and Wales as part of the of the 1988 Education Reform Act (a similar act relates to Scotland). The main points of relevance to the early years can be summarised as follows.

- The National Curriculum is compulsory for all children between the ages of 5 and 16 in all state schools (this includes special schools).
- The curriculum comprises the three core subjects of English, maths and science (plus Welsh in Welsh-speaking schools) and seven foundation subjects – technology, history, geography, art, music, physical education, with a modern foreign language introduced at 11. Priority is to be given to the three core subjects. In addition, teaching in religious education must be provided.

> **attainment targets**
> Different elements of a curriculum area. For example, the attainment targets for English are speaking, reading and writing

- Subjects are divided into **attainment targets**, each with a programme of study.
- Schooling is divided into four key stages. Children between 5 and 7 years are at Key Stage 1.
- At the end of each key stage, children's progress in the core subjects is assessed by Standard Assessment Tasks (SATs) and, at Key Stage 1, by teacher assessment. The child's progress is then reported back to parents. Schools' results are aggregated and published in league tables. Information about the performance of individual children is not made public.

The effect of the National Curriculum and its implications for child-care workers

- Though its format and compulsory nature were new, most of the content of the National Curriculum was already part of good early years programmes.
- The importance of science and technology in the early years has been highlighted by the National Curriculum. In-service training and investment in equipment have given staff the opportunity to plan and deliver these subjects with increased confidence.
- Planning a programme to meet the requirements of the National Curriculum has encouraged staff to work collaboratively. Nursery nurses and classroom assistants have much to contribute here.
- Evidence needs to be gathered to support teacher assessment. This may mean observations of the children as well as actual pieces of work. Everyone who works with the children will have a part to play in collecting this.

> **baseline assessment**
> An assessment of a child's capabilities on entry to school at 5 years

- **Baseline assessment** for all children at 5 years, at the beginning of Key Stage 1, has been introduced. This provides staff with a profile of the child's capabilities on entry to school which will inform planning and the setting of targets for individuals and groups. Baseline assessment also allows schools to measure the progress made by individual children during Key Stage 1.

- Children (and parents) may become anxious at the prospect of formal assessment at 7. Child-care workers must take time to reassure both parents and children and avoid putting pressure on children.

- Young children learn most effectively through child-centred and experiential methods. These have been shown to be the most appropriate methods for delivering the National Curriculum too, although research has also demonstrated the effectiveness of some whole-group teaching.

- The content and structure of the National Curriculum has been changed a great deal in a relatively short space of time. Concerns have been raised that the curriculum for Key Stage 1 is overloaded and that inadequate time is available to devote to developing the key skills of literacy and numeracy. There is a renewed emphasis on improving literacy standards with the introduction in September 1998 of a daily Literacy Hour and the setting of annual literacy targets for schools. A daily Numeracy Hour is also planned.

The Desirable Outcomes Curriculum

> **Desirable Outcomes Curriculum**
> The curriculum that must be provided by all centres receiving government funding for the education of 4-year-olds

The **Desirable Outcomes Curriculum** was introduced in 1996 as part of government initiatives to expand the provision of nursery education. It is a requirement that any establishment receiving government funding for the education of 4-year-olds provides a programme that will allow children to achieve the specified outcomes for learning by the time they reach compulsory school age at 5. No distinction is made between the types of setting: private day nurseries, playgroups, family centres and nursery classes in primary schools are all required to provide the full curriculum. Although this is essentially a curriculum for 4-year-olds, many settings base their 3 to 5 curriculum on a programme that works towards developing children's skills and concepts towards achieving these outcomes by 5. The curriculum is divided into six areas of learning:

- Personal and social development
- Language and literacy
- Mathematics
- Knowledge and understanding of the world
- Physical development
- Creative development.

As with the National Curriculum, these requirements were derived from what was considered to be good early years practice for this age group. For each area of learning, there is a statement that defines the skills and concepts young children need to develop (see the diagram opposite). There is no formal assessment requirement for this age group but

Personal and social development

Children are confident, show appropriate self-respect and are able to establish effective relationships with other children and with adults. They work as part of a group and independently, are able to concentrate and persevere in their learning and to seek help where needed. They are eager to explore new learning, and show the ability to initiate ideas and to solve simple, practical problems. They demonstrate independence in selecting an activity or resources and in dressing and personal hygiene.

Children are sensitive to the needs and feelings of others and show respect for people of other cultures and beliefs. They take turns and share fairly. They express their feelings and behave in appropriate ways, developing an understanding of what is right, what is wrong and why. They treat living things, property and their environment with care and concern. They respond to relevant cultural and religious events and show a range of feelings, such as wonder, joy or sorrow, in response to their experiences of the world.

Language and literacy

In small and large groups, children listen attentively and talk about their experiences. They use a growing vocabulary with increasing fluency to express thoughts and convey meanings to the listener. They listen and respond to stories, songs, nursery rhymes and poems. They make up their own stories and take part in role-play with confidence.

Children enjoy books and handle them carefully, understanding how they are organised. They know that words and pictures carry meaning and that, in English, print is read from left to right and from top to bottom. They begin to associate sounds with patterns in rhymes, with syllables, and with words and letters. They recognise their own names and some familiar words. They recognise letters of the alphabet by shape and sound. In their writing they use pictures, symbols, familiar words and letters, to communicate meaning, showing awareness of some of the different purposes of writing. They write their names with appropriate use of upper and lower case letters.

Knowledge and understanding of the world

Children talk about where they live, their environment, their families and past and present events in their own lives. They explore and recognise features of living things, objects and events in the natural and made world and look closely at similarities and differences, patterns and change.

They show an awareness of the purposes of some features of the area in which they live. They talk about their observations, sometimes recording them and ask questions to gain information about why things happen and how things work. They explore and select materials and equipment and use skills such as cutting, joining, folding and building for a variety of purposes. They use technology, where appropriate, to support their learning.

Desirable outcomes for children's learning

Mathematics

Children use mathematical language, such as circle, in front of, bigger than and more, to describe shape, position, size and quantity. They recognise and recreate patterns. They are familiar with number rhymes, songs, stories, counting games and activities. They compare, sort, match, order sequence and count using everyday objects. They recognise and use numbers to ten and are familiar with larger numbers from their everyday lives. They begin to use their developing mathematical understanding to solve practical problems. Through practical activities children understand and record numbers, begin to show awareness of number operations, such as addition and subtraction, and begin to use the language involved.

Physical development

Children move confidently and imaginatively with increasing control and co-ordination and an awareness of space and others. They use a range of small and large equipment and balancing and climbing apparatus, with increasing skill. They handle appropriate tools, objects, construction and malleable materials safely and with increasing control.

Creative development

Children explore sound and colour, texture, shape, form and space in two and three dimensions. They respond in a variety of ways to what they see, hear, smell, touch and feel. Through art, music, dance, stories and imaginative play, they show an increasing ability to use their imagination, to listen and to observe. They use a widening range of materials, suitable tools, instruments and other resources to express ideas and to communicate their feelings.

The skills and concepts young children need to develop for each area of the Desirable Outcomes for Children's Learning (DfEE with SCAA, 1996) establishments are expected to assess individual children as part of their provision. These assessments may be used to contribute towards baseline assessment at 5.

✔ *Progress check*

1 What does the term 'statutory' mean with regard to the curriculum?
2 a) Who does the National Curriculum apply to?
   b) Who does the Desirable Outcomes Curriculum apply to?
3 What are the six areas of learning in the Desirable Outcomes Curriculum?
4 What subjects are studied by children between 5 and 7?
5 When are children assessed by SATs? What happens to their scores?
6 Which pre-school establishments are required to provide the Desirable Outcomes Curriculum?

Curriculum planning and organisation

Planning for the long, medium and short term

Effective curriculum delivery is organised around long-, medium- and short-term planning. At every stage of planning, specific learning objectives for the children should be identified in terms of:

- knowledge to be gained
- concepts to be developed
- skills to be practised.

The activities and experiences presented will provide the means through which children can achieve this learning.

The needs of all children should be considered as part of the planning process. This will include provision for children who have identified special educational needs but will also include **differentiation** of some activities and experiences so that children across the range of ability can gain maximum benefit from them.

> **differentiation**
> The matching of provision to the individual needs and developmental level of the child

Long-term planning

Long-term planning looks at the overall curriculum aims and philosophy of the centre and the methods that will be used to achieve these. Long-term plans indicate how statutory and other curriculum requirements will be fulfilled over a period of time. These plans will also need to consider attendance patterns within the group, for example around transfer to school. There may be implications for resources, the organisation of the learning environment and training to consider at this stage of planning.

Medium-term planning

Medium-term planning will cover a period of weeks, say a term or half-term. This may involve planning around a theme that is used to promote learning through a range of linked activities and experiences (see *Themes and topics* below). It is important at this stage of planning to identify the particular *learning outcomes* that are to be targeted during this period of time and consider how to provide a *balanced curriculum*, that is, one that gives appropriate emphasis to the different areas of learning.

Short-term planning

This deals with the day-to-day or week-to-week implementation of the programme. It will link staff and resources to activities and experiences, identifying *learning objectives* for groups or individual children. Again, these plans will need to consider the balance of activities provided for children over the session, day or week.

Recording planning

Planning needs to be recorded for reference, so that staff, parents and children know what is going on, and for accountability, so that centres can show what they intend to do alongside what they have already done. There is no one way of doing this and centres develop ways of recording planning that meet their own needs.

Evaluating planning

Evaluation is an essential feature of the planning process. It is through observation of children's responses and progress that staff can assess whether their planning and delivery is meeting the developmental and curriculum needs of children. Evaluation of the current programme will enable staff to plan most effectively for the next steps in learning.

Themes and topics

Many early years settings plan using themes or topics as a vehicle for integrating different areas of the curriculum. The requirements of the Desirable Outcomes for Children's Learning and the National Curriculum can be successfully incorporated into a thematically planned programme (see the topic planner on page 91). There are several advantages here.

- Children can contribute to the development of the theme with their own interests and experiences.
- Involvement in the theme will promote and sustain children's interest.
- Themes and topics can promote useful links between home and the setting.
- Parents and families can contribute and become involved.
- The theme can provide a unifying focus, linking the different areas of the centre and providing staff with an opportunity to plan collaboratively.

The curriculum for the early years needs to be both broad and balanced. Planning will need to provide for a range of activities and experiences that will fulfil children's developmental as well as learning needs. Often these activities will be integrated into a theme or topic that will be developed over a period of time.

Case study: Working through a theme

As part of the of the half-term's theme on 'Travel', the nursery staff included the following activities.

- The imaginative play area is presented as a transport cafe. Children are 'reading' menus, 'writing' orders and serving customers.
- On the carpet, a road playmat has been set out and small cars are being steered around it.
- At the painting easels some children are painting pictures of journeys.
- A group of children are making models of vehicles from junk.
- A road with traffic signs has been chalked on the outside play area and children are negotiating the 'road' on the wheeled toys.
- Children are looking at catalogues, selecting and cutting out pictures for a transport collage.
- At carpet time, the children sing songs and listen to stories about travelling and journeys.
- A walk to the nearby station and a trip on a train is planned.
- The school's crossing warden is coming in to talk to the children about her job.
- Children have brought in postcards, tickets and pictures, all linked to travel and these have been displayed on an interest table, providing a focus for conversation.
- Children have recorded how they travel to nursery and this is presented in graph form.

1 Why do you think that using the theme approach is successful here?
2 How might parents be involved in this theme?
3 Refer to the Desirable Outcomes chart (page 87) and suggest how other learning outcomes could be developed through this theme.

When planning, it is important to bear in mind that it will often not be possible for all important aspects of the curriculum to receive appropriate and adequate attention through a theme. These areas must be planned for and covered through a range of activities and experiences that may not be linked to the current theme.

The integrated day

Much early years provision is organised as an integrated day. A number of activities and tasks are provided and the children either make a choice as to what to do (often the case in nursery) or are directed towards a sequence of tasks that need to be completed. Children can work at their own pace and at a level appropriate to their stage of development. This is especially important given the range of ages and abilities provided for in settings. Most nursery classes will have children between the ages of 3 and 5 years, and the practice of vertical or family grouping, where classes are comprised of children from more than one year group, is common in primary schools.

Language and literacy

- Describing themselves – extend vocabulary for body parts.
- Talking about families and family roles.
- Listening to each other – news and special occasions.
- Stories and rhymes about ourselves include 'head, shoulders, knees and toes' and 'I am sitting, I am sitting'. Also stories about family life and different types of families, e.g. *Alex's Bed, Janine and the Baby, Alfie* stories.
- Recognising own names and writing them.
- Making 'passports' – write in name, address and age.
- Recognising names of other family members.
- Imaginative play – family play in home corner; baby clinic; and role-play celebration with wedding.
- Also family play in small world.

Personal and social development

- Talking about feelings – describing happy, sad, angry and excited (link to stories).
- Different family styles (link to stories).
- Talk about similarities and differences between ourselves and others.
- Holding a baby – watching a new baby have a bath. (Get Mrs M. to come in.)
- Celebrations – get Rukshana to show us photographs and bring in wedding dress and talk about weddings in Pakistan (link to imaginative play).

Physical development

- Moving on particular parts of the body e.g. crawling through barrels; creeping on tip-toes.
- 'Simon says' emphasising body parts.
- Setting individual challenges in outdoor play e.g. Can you hop five times? Can you catch a bean-bag? Can you pedal the tricycle?

All About Me

Knowledge and understanding of the world

Science
- Exploration of senses – what we can see, taste, touch, hear and smell.
- Looking after living things – ourselves, our pets and plants.
- Parts of the body – joints and making models (linked to technology).

Geography
- Exploring the immediate locality – shops, houses, what else?
- Looking at photographs of local places – can you recognise them?
- Look at different types of buildings and open spaces.

History
- Photo-display of babies – 'look how you've grown!'
- Talking around – 'when I was little, I . . .'.
- Sorting and sequencing photographs of babies, children, adults and old people.
- Looking at old photographs of the locality – what's different?

Technology
- Follow up work on joints by making jointed figures using split pins, hinges and thread.
- Recording own voices (use cassette recorder) – can you recognize the voice?
- Computer programmes – making faces; also, getting dressed.

Mathematics

- Classifying – boys, girls, men and women. Use Logi-people.
- Making sets – brown hair, curly hair, blue eyes, etc.
- Using mathematical language to describe – smaller than, taller than, smallest and tallest.
- Counting up to ten fingers and toes.
- Talking about pairs – of hands, feet, arms and legs. Also socks, shoes and gloves.
- Measuring in handspans and footsteps – making cut-outs of hands and feet and comparing.
- Birthday display – 3s, 4s and 5s in birthday train.
- Recognise own birthday numeral and also house number.

Creative development

- Painting and collage of faces (mix paint for skin tones)
- Full-size paintings of tallest and smallest.
- Songs and rhymes, including action songs.
- Children to choose favourite music at circle time.
- Moving to music – angry music, happy music (linked to PSD on feelings).
- Making music using body sounds – clapping, stamping, tapping and clicking.
- Making models of own house.

An example of a topic planned around the theme 'All about me'

With an integrated approach, space and equipment can be used fully. Adults can spend time with small groups of children at activities that require close supervision or direction, for example reading practice, or introducing a new skill, while other groups of children are given some responsibility for their own learning as they work at activities that they manage themselves. There will naturally be times when the whole group of children come together, for example, at story time, for PE or assembly or to examine a particular concept. Research has shown that periods of whole-group teaching can be very effective in focusing children's concentration and attention. Good early years provision operates using a variety of teaching methods in order to meet the developmental and curriculum needs of children.

To operate effectively, the integrated day takes much careful preparation and organisation. Accurate records need to be kept for each child to ensure that progress is achieved and maintained.

Think about it

How is the children's day is organised in your workplace?
- Is there a routine that they follow?
- How do children move from one activity to another?
- What kind of records are kept?
- Do children have any responsibility for recording what they do?
- Are there any times when children come together as a whole group?

Do this! 6.2

a) Make a 'snapshot' observation of your workplace. Draw a plan of the room and indicate what activities are available in each area. Choose a time and record, at that moment, the position of the children on the diagram. Show where the adults are and what they are doing.

b) What does your diagram tell you about the way that the space is organised? Are the adults fully involved in supporting children's learning?

✓ Progress check

1 Why is planning an important aspect of the early years curriculum?
2 Why do centres need to plan for the long, medium and short term?
3 How can the curriculum be delivered through themes and topics? Why is this approach appropriate for the early years?
4 What do you understand by the term 'a balanced curriculum'?
5 What are the benefits of an integrated approach to organising children's learning?
6 Why is evaluation an important aspect of the planning process?

Equal opportunities and the curriculum

equal opportunities
All people participating in society to the best of their abilities, regardless of race, religion, disability, gender or social background

The curriculum can be a powerful tool in promoting **equal opportunities**. Child-care workers have a responsibility to present the curriculum in a way that includes and enables all children and that reflects the experiences of all sections of society. The planning and delivery of the curriculum must provide for equality of opportunity, irrespective of race and culture, gender, socio-economic background or disability. It must also consider how best to develop the potential of children who are more timid or aggressive or more confident than might be expected of the group. Treating all children the same will not provide for equality of opportunity. We need to recognise that some children in our society are more likely to experience disadvantage than others and that some **positive action** might be necessary to enable them to succeed. This is an important consideration when planning the curriculum.

positive action
Taking steps to ensure that a particular individual or group has an equal chance to succeed

The curriculum transmits not just skills and knowledge, but attitudes and values too. The early years are crucial in the formation of children's attitudes about themselves and about the world that they live in. A curriculum that promotes equality of opportunity will enable children to feel positively about themselves and their achievements, to avoid the limitations of **stereotyping** and to value diversity.

Promoting equal opportunities through the curriculum

stereotyping
When people think that all the members of a group have the same characteristics as each other; often applied on the basis of race, gender or disability

This section suggests some practical pointers to promoting equal opportunities through the curriculum. It is important to understand that resources in themselves do not promote equal opportunities. It is up to staff to make an equal opportunities perspective integral to curriculum planning and to present activities and resources in a way that develops children's awareness of the issues.

In the visual environment

positive images
The representation of a cross-section of a whole variety of roles and everyday situations, to challenge stereotypes and to extend and increase expectations

- Display **positive images** in the setting. Black people, women, and people with disabilities are under-represented in the wider visual environment. Choose images that challenge stereotypes, for example a black barrister, a disabled doctor, a woman police officer.
- Give children the opportunity to represent themselves accurately. Provide mirrors and paints and crayons that enable children to match their own skin tones.
- Look at the illustrations in books and posters that you provide. Do they convey a positive image or do you see line drawings of white children shaded to represent black races, girls always in the background taking a supporting role, disabled people portrayed as helpless and reliant on others?
- Visitors in the setting can challenge stereotypes – a father with his new baby, a black dentist, a female electrician.

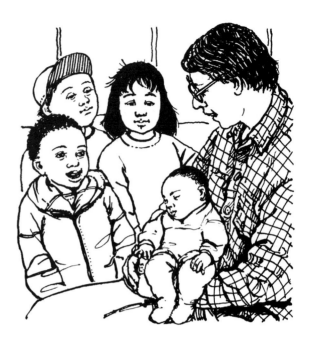

Visitors to the centre can challenge stereotypes

Choosing toys and planning activities

■ Look at jigsaws, games, play figures, musical instruments and their packaging too. Do they reflect cultural diversity? Do they encourage both boys and girls to play? Are children with disabilities represented?

■ Provide dolls that represent different racial groups. Do not buy black dolls that have white facial features or hair. Monitor the way that the dolls are played with. Think of the message conveyed when the white dolls are tucked up in prams and the black dolls thrown into a box. Encourage boys to show that they can cuddle and care for 'babies'.

■ Home corner play can be a secure and comforting play space. Make sure that your provision of cooking equipment and play food reflects a variety cultural styles and traditions. If you introduce some new or unfamiliar equipment, such as chopsticks, make sure that the children know how to use it properly.

■ Dressing-up clothes give children an opportunity to elaborate their role play. Avoid identifying items as 'for boys' or 'for girls' and encourage children to try out everything. Provide everyday clothes from a range of cultures but do not over generalise – Pakistani children are as likely to wear tracksuits or jeans as they are shalwar-kameez!

■ Mark a range of festivals. Children who celebrate these festivals at home will feel valued: others can gain an insight and understanding of unfamiliar traditions. Care needs to be taken in this area to avoid a **tokenistic** approach which emphasises the 'exotic' aspects of cultural difference. Festival celebrations need to be researched carefully if they are to have any real educational significance. Enlist help from community groups or parents. (Think about the message that you are sending about the relative worth of festivals if you spend six weeks building up to Christmas and an afternoon on Diwali.)

tokenistic
A superficial representation of minority or disadvantaged groups, for example including a single black child in a school brochure, a single woman on a board of directors

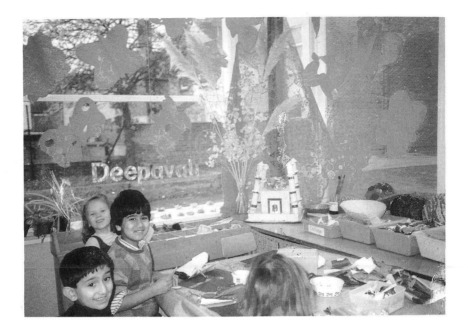

Mark a range of festivals

- Cooking sessions can present an opportunity to try different recipes and taste a range of foods. They can also provide children with a chance to confront any stereotypical ideas about whose job it is to cook. Again, when talking about cultural preferences in diet avoid over-generalisations. Children from Caribbean families may like to eat rice and peas, but they will also eat pizza and visit McDonalds.
- Make sure that activities are not dominated by one group of children to the exclusion of others. It may be necessary to exclude one group for a while so that others can have a chance to gain confidence and skills.
- Provision for creative activities should reflect cultural diversity. Introduce children to a range of artistic traditions and styles and provide a range of materials for them to work with. Play all kinds of music, provide instruments and this will influence the children's own music-making.
- Make sure that all children can participate in the range of activities, including those with disabilities. This may involve an adjustment to the physical environment, such as moving a construction activity to a table-top so that a child in a wheelchair can reach it or it may mean providing appropriate equipment, such as tactile dominoes so that a child with a visual impairment can be included in the game.

Case study: Valuing diversity

Karen felt the children in the small, all-white, rural playgroup which she ran had a very limited experience of a cultures other than their own. As part of their regular listening to music sessions, she played some Indian music to the children. Karen had planned the session carefully and had borrowed a box of Indian instruments from a nearby resource centre. After playing the tape a couple of times, she showed the children the instruments and demonstrated the sounds that they made, passing them round so that the children could try them out for themselves. As she played the tape through again, the children were able to recognise some of the instruments as they appeared in the piece. Once the children had become familiar with the instruments and had been shown how to use them, they were placed alongside the other equipment in the music corner so that they could use them in their own play. Indian music was introduced as part of the playgroup's regular dance sessions and later on that term, Karen was able to organise a visit to the playgroup by a group of Indian dancers, based at a nearby Community Arts Group.

1 Why was this a valuable experience for the children?
2 How did ensure that this activity would be successful?
3 Think of other, meaningful ways in which this group's experience of cultural diversity could be extended.

Recognising the power of language

- Value language diversity. Encourage children to listen to languages other than their own. Teach greetings and rhymes and share dual-language books with children.
- Choose books and tell stories that challenge stereotypes and provide positive role models.
- Introduce stories and rhymes from many literary traditions.

The hidden curriculum

Perhaps even more important than the 'official' curriculum in promoting equal opportunities are the attitudes and values of those who work with children and deliver the curriculum. This is sometimes known as the **hidden curriculum** and is communicated to children in the way that we talk to them and in the expectations that we have of them.

Here are some examples of ways in which the hidden curriculum can operate against equal opportunities:

- an expectation and acceptance that boys' play is rougher than girls'
- adults giving more time to boys (many studies show this to be true)
- having low expectations of the behaviour and achievement of children from minority groups
- regarding particular games and activities as sex-appropriate
- overprotecting children with disabilities
- comments such as: 'Boys don't cry'; 'Here's a picture of a wedding. The girls will like this'; 'Find me two strong boys to move this table'; 'The girls can wash the cups'; 'It's not ladylike to fight'.

Children absorb these messages and they can affect their view of themselves. The attitudes and values of the staff as well as the content of the curriculum need to address the issues of equal opportunities.

hidden curriculum
Messages, often unintended, that are communicated to children as a consequence of the attitudes and values of the adults who deliver the curriculum

Child-care workers are very influential in the formation of children's attitudes and values – children will take their cue from adult responses and reactions. Because of their powerful role, it is important that staff take issues of equality seriously and do not skate over them.

✅ *Progress check*

1 Why is equal opportunities an important aspect of the curriculum?
2 How can equal opportunities be promoted through the curriculum?
3 What is stereotyping and why should we challenge stereotypes?
4 Why is the promotion of equal opportunities an issue for all settings?
5 How can staff show that they are committed to promoting equal opportunities?

Key terms

You need to know what these words and phrases mean. Go back through the chapter and find out.

attainment targets
baseline assessment
child-centred
compensatory education
curriculum
Desirable Outcomes Curriculum
differentiation
equal opportunities
experiential
hidden curriculum
National Curriculum
positive action
positive images
stereotyping
tokenistic

Now try these questions

1 Explain why a child-centred approach to children's learning is appropriate for the early years.

2 How does the Highscope approach to curriculum delivery promote children's independence?

3 Describe how planning contributes to effective curriculum delivery.

4 How can a child-care centre demonstrate its commitment to promoting equal opportunities?

5 Why is the consideration of equality of opportunity an important issue when implementing the curriculum?

7 *Curriculum components*

This chapter includes:

- **Early literacy**
- **Children's books**
- **Developing maths**
- **Science and technology**
- **History and geography**
- **Creativity**
- **Physical activities**

This chapter looks at the elements that go together to make up the curriculum for the early years and suggest some ways in which the child-care worker can support children's learning in these areas. These subjects will not be taught in isolation but will be presented as part of an integrated and balanced programme of learning.

You may find it helpful to read this chapter in conjunction with:

- **Book 2, Chapter 5**   Play
- **Book 2, Chapter 6**   Philosophy and approaches

Early literacy

literacy
The aspects of language concerned with reading and writing

Think about it

Why is so much emphasis placed on children learning to read and write?

We live in a literate world, in a society that values reading and writing (**literacy**). Consequently, a great deal of emphasis is placed on becoming competent in these areas. Children begin to notice and respond to this literate world long before they begin the formal process of learning to read and write. Their environment contains many examples of writing, from the signs in the supermarket and on the bus ticket, to the postcard from Granny and the bedtime story book. Through their everyday experiences, children become familiar with the product of writing. When they see someone take a telephone message or write a cheque, they become aware of the process of writing too. These experiences have an impact; once children realise that writing carries meaning, they have taken their first step towards becoming literate.

Do this!   7.1

List as many examples as you can of where and how children meet the written word in their everyday environment. Compare your list with a colleague. How many of these involved the process of writing too?

Learning to read and write

Learning to read and write is a long and complex process for most children. They will need to learn skills and rules and have plenty of practice to consolidate them. If children have already begun to enjoy books, then it is likely that this will spur them on and give them a reason to persevere. (See *Children's books*, page 104.)

By the age of 5, many children will have a sight vocabulary of a number of words. Most will recognise their own name; many will be able to write it. Formal instruction in reading and writing will often begin in a pre-school environment alongside other, less formal, experiences and activities that contribute to the development of reading and writing skills. These include activities that involve any or all of the following:

- *hand–eye co-ordination and fine motor skills* – you need to control a pencil to write
- *visual discrimination* – it is important to be able to distinguish one word or letter from another
- *sequencing* – the order of the letters or words affects the meaning
- *auditory discrimination* – hearing the difference between sounds and combinations of sounds helps reading
- *use of symbols* – reading and writing are representational forms in which one thing – a combination of letters – stands for something else.

Also very important at this stage is using reading and writing as a meaningful part of play, for example, 'reading' the menu in the cafe, 'writing' a telephone message in the home corner.

Remember that reading and writing are essential tools for later learning. They are used and practised in every area of the curriculum.

Do this! 7.2

a) List the activities that might be available during a typical nursery session.

b) Look at the list of reading and writing skills given above. Link the activities that you thought of with the skills.

c) Write down any other experiences and activities you can think of that will promote reading and writing skills.

---

look and say
An approach to reading that relies on recognition of the shape or pattern of a word

phonics
An approach to reading that is based on recognition of sounds

Reading

There are basically two approaches used in the teaching of reading:

- **look and say**
- **phonics**.

There is some debate over which is the most effective method, with a combination of both usually being applied.

Look and say involves the recognition of whole words by their shape. Words are often written on flashcards and children will attempt to memorise them, often practising at home. Children can then read simple stories comprised of the words that they have learned. They recognise words from their shapes, from the look of them. The shortcoming of this approach is that early readers will have no way of recognising words that they have not yet learned.

Phonics breaks down words into sounds and encourages the sounding out of words. Children are encouraged to pick out patterns in the sounds of words, noticing rhymes and rhythms. This disadvantage with this method is that English is not phonically regular – a letter may make one sound in one word and a completely different sound in another. It is not very rewarding for the early reader to be limited to phonically regular words that can be sounded out. On the other hand, a knowledge of phonics will give children a good strategy for attempting unfamiliar words.

Reading schemes or 'real books'?

Reading schemes are carefully structured and graded. A limited number of words is introduced in each book and there is much repetition of these words. The same characters usually appear in a number of books so children have the opportunity to become familiar with them.

Critics of reading schemes say that the stories are contrived and that the language of the books is stilted. They advocate the use of 'real books' for readers, that is picture books and story books that represent good children's literature. They maintain that interesting books make children want to read and that this motivation brings success. Critics of the 'real books' approach say that children miss the step-by-step structure and may choose books that are beyond their capabilities.

Most settings use a mixture of both reading schemes and 'real books', adjusting their approach to what best suits the individual child alongside the preference of the teacher.

> **Think about it**
>
> Look at how reading is approached in you workplace. Do they use phonic methods, a look and say approach, or a mixture of both? Try to remember the methods that were used when you learned to read.

> **Do this!**   **7.3**
>
> a) Compare some books from a reading scheme with some picture books. Look at the following:
> - the characters: do they hold your interest?
> - the language: sentence structure and vocabulary
> - the story itself: is it interesting, exciting?
> - the illustrations.
> b) Prepare for a 5-minute talk to your colleagues describing your findings. Summarise these on a word-processed handout for the group.

How can you help?

Early readers need lots of practice. When you listen to children read you can help them by:

- giving them your attention
- finding a place with minimal distractions
- giving the child thinking time
- helping when necessary – sometimes a bit of encouragement or a clue, for example 'What's that sound?', can help the child move on
- talking about the book and getting them to talk to you – the child may lose the sense of a story when reading it word by word
- monitoring and recording their progress – you may notice that a child is not doing very well on a particular book, so suggest something else, different approaches suit different children
- alerting them to patterns in words and sounds
- being positive about their achievements.

You might also be involved in making special individual books for children. These usually consist of photographs of the child with simple text about themselves, their family and so on, mounted on card and bound in some way. These are very popular and are often the first books that children get to read.

Remember that reading is a complex skill that may take years to achieve. As with all skills, some children will grasp it easily and progress quickly, while others find it more difficult.

Case study: A book for Nathan

Nathan, at $5\frac{1}{2}$, was showing himself to be a very reluctant reader. Whilst most of the other children in his class were making progress with the early levels of the reading scheme, he seemed uninterested. When Maria, the nursery nurse, tried to interest him in the books, he replied that they were boring and just for babies. She decided to involve him in making a special book, just for him. They spent some time together talking about him and what he liked to do and his favourite things. Maria took some photographs of Nathan and found other illustrations from magazines and she made a book using these pictures and simple text that was all about Nathan and presented it to him. Nathan was very pleased with his book and worked hard with Maria to read the text. Maria followed this up with another book, this time about Nathan's pets. After a few weeks, he began to express an interest in the other reading books around the classroom.

1 Why do you think Nathan rejected the reading books?
2 Why was Maria's approach successful?
3 Why is important to encourage reluctant readers early on?
4 What could you learn from this case study?

Writing

Children begin writing by making marks. To adults this may appear to be meaningless scribble, but to the child it is a telephone message, a letter to Santa, their name. During their early years in school, children need to learn the rules and conventions of writing. It becomes an important tool that they use to communicate with themselves and with the outside world.

The conventions of writing

- *Letter formation* Children need to know how to form letters correctly and consistently. This means where you start and where you finish and requires a great deal of practice. Children also learn to recognise the feel of a letter when they write it. Tracing in the air and in sand helps to reinforce this.
- *Orientation* In English (and many other languages) this means writing (and reading) from left to right and from top to bottom. Bilingual children may have experienced a written language, Urdu or Hebrew for example, that is oriented differently.
- *Spacing* Groups of letters go together to form words and spaces separate these words. Spacing words correctly needs practice.
- *Spelling* Children need to learn that there is a standard way of spelling words. However, excessive concentration on this at the very early stages will limit and inhibit children's writing.
- *Punctuation* This is a skill acquired later, but children notice punctuation early on in their reading and begin to introduce it into their writing. It also includes the appropriate use of upper and lower case letters.

Children's writing is not just about the technical skills listed above, it is about content too. Sometimes children become overwhelmed by these technical skills and this affects the content of their writing. A child who is limited to the words that they can spell correctly or who is afraid to make a mistake will not become involved in or enjoy writing. It will become a task to be completed because an adult demands it. A sensitive adult will watch the child's progress and introduce the need for correct spelling at the right stage, ensuring that child retains confidence in their writing abilities.

Teaching writing

Writing is taught in a variety of different ways. All approaches will ensure that children learn to form letters correctly and develop fluency in their handwriting style. Some schools favour an approach where the child writes completely on their own and then reads the writing back to an adult who may then identify something with the child that can be discussed. This approach is known as **emergent writing** (or developmental writing). It enables children to get on with what they want to write without waiting for an adult to show them the correct way to write a word. Critics say that technical accuracy takes longer to establish with this method. Other schools place an earlier emphasis on accuracy, with children relying on adults for correct spelling at an early stage with independent writing coming later. Critics of this approach say that children become over-dependent on adults and may not have the confidence to make their own attempts. Of course, there are merits in both approaches and most schools

emergent writing
An approach to writing that encourages children to write independently

Think about it

How might the content of children's writing be affected by their lack of technical skills?

will strike a balance with the aim of producing children's writing that shows both independence and accuracy.

Case study: Emergent writing

The reception class had been working on a topic about minibeasts which had involved searching for wildlife in the school garden and examining the animals closely. The school encouraged independent writing by valuing children's emergent writing. After the session in the garden with the microscopes and bug-boxes, the children were encouraged to write about their investigations. Katy was engrossed and spent a long time over her writing. When she had finished, she took it to her teacher and read out her writing to her.

Katy's emergent writing

This is what she read: 'The snail's teeth is on its tongue and I am going to a party tomorrow and the snail's tongue works like a cheese grater.'

1 What purpose was Katy using her writing for?
2 What did she gain from this exercise?
3 What was the teacher's role here?
4 Refer back to the section on the conventions of writing. Which of the conventions of writing has Katy grasped?

Do this! 7.4

Investigate the methods used in your workplace to get children writing. Evaluate both approaches to writing. Note down strengths and weaknesses.

How can you help?

- Sit with children and help them form letters correctly. Left-handed children may need extra help.
- Be a good role model. Let children watch you making notes for your file, filling in a register and so on, so they see that writing is a part of everyday life.

- When you write for children, make sure that your writing is clear, legible and accurate. If children are going to copy your writing, make sure that it is large enough.
- Talk to children about their writing, use it in displays. Let them know that you value it.
- Present children with a variety of writing tasks, not just stories. Get them to make shopping lists, record experiments, write letters and invitations.
- Show children that writing can be found in many different places. Collect examples – involve children in this – and make a display of comics, cereal boxes, bus tickets, labels, and so on.
- Help children to present their writing in different ways, such as making books, using a word processor.

> ### ✓ Progress check
>
> 1 What does the term literacy mean? Why is it important that children become literate?
> 2 Why is it important that children have an understanding of the purposes of reading and writing?
> 3 What are the differences between the phonic method and the look and say approach to teaching reading?
> 4 Why is it important that children learn the conventions of writing?
> 5 What is emergent writing?

Children's books

Books are an important and integral part of the early years curriculum. They are provided in all nurseries and classrooms. Reading and story time are part of each day. Some children also have books at home and read with parents and carers. This early experience of books is very important in establishing positive attitudes to books and to reading.

Why are books important?

Books and stories are an important part of children's development. Outlined below are some of the main skills that can be developed and nurtured. Books and stories can be introduced to very young children. Although the child may not fully understand the story, a quiet intimate time reading with a parent or carer forms a positive association for the child. This in turn helps to establish a habit of reading and listening to stories that has many benefits for the child.

Language development

Language is learned: the more exposure a child has to different patterns in language, the richer their own language is likely to be. Initially this will be expressive (spoken) language, later read and written language. Listening to stories and talking about books enables young children to listen and respond to the sound and rhythm of spoken language. This is important to speech development at all levels. Initially children need to recognise the sounds and rhythms that occur in their language; once this has been established they need to practise and refine their use of spoken language.

Listening to stories can also extend a child's vocabulary. As long as most of the language in the text is familiar to the child new, imaginative language can be introduced. The child will begin to understand these new words by their context, that is, how they are used and linked with the story line and the pictures.

Experience with books and story telling is also an important part of a child's early understanding of symbols. A child who has contact with books begins to understand that the squiggles on the page represent speech. This is a vital skill in the development of reading and writing.

Emotional development

Books and stories are enjoyable. They give children the opportunity to express a whole range of positive emotions. They provide a rich imaginative world that can be a source of great pleasure to the child, and through identification with the characters and the storyline children can develop and practise their own responses to events and experience situations and feelings that are beyond their own life experiences. This can be done in a safe environment where the child has an element of control over events.

Cognitive development

Books, if carefully chosen, can provide a rich source of imagination for a child. They can stimulate interesting and exciting thoughts and ideas. The development of imagination is an important part of being creative. Creative thoughts and ideas are an important part of the quality of life and necessary to the development of society.

Books can also introduce children to a wide range of concepts. Repetition and context enable children to develop their understanding of the world that they live in. Listening to stories, recalling and sequencing the events are also positive ways of extending young children's concentration span and memory.

Social development

Books and stories are more than just the presentation of a sequence of events; they carry in them a whole range of messages about how a society functions. This includes acceptable patterns of behaviour, expectations of groups within the society and moral codes of right and wrong. Children pick up these messages. It is therefore vital that books for young children portray a positive view of society and the people within that society. This positive view of the world contributes towards young children developing a balanced and constructive outlook on life.

Group story time and sharing books contribute to the development of social skills of sharing, turn taking and co-operating with others. Children begin to learn that they have to take other people's needs and wishes into account. Story time can also provide children and adults with the opportunity to build and maintain relationships. If a cosy and comfortable environment is provided it offers a sense of closeness and intimacy for the children and adults involved.

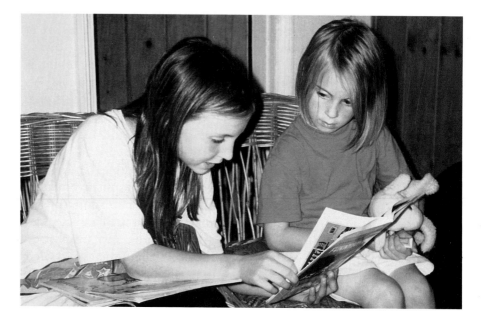

Sharing books contributes to the development of social skills

Think about it

Why is it important to choose a book or story appropriate to the audience? Why are different books appropriate to children of different ages?

Choosing children's books

It is important that children's books are chosen carefully. Children have different needs and interests at different stages of their development. The maximum benefit can be gained if the book chosen meets the child's needs. All children are individual and will have different needs, likes and dislikes. This needs to be taken into account. There are, however, are some general points to consider when choosing a book for a young child and these are listed in the table opposite.

Do this!   7.5

a) Draw up a checklist for choosing appropriate books within each age range. Make sure that they meet the criteria listed in the table opposite, including the need to reflect positive images of all sections of society in the books we present to children.

b) Using your checklist, choose a selection of books for each age range.

Guidelines for choosing books for young children

Books are a powerful way of influencing children's views about the society they live in. Books for children must, therefore, reflect positive images of all sections of society, in both the text and the illustrations.

0–3
- Picture books are appropriate for this age range, especially for children under 1 year.
- Where there is text, it needs to be limited, especially for children aged 0–1
- The pictures need to have bright colours and bold shapes.
- The pictures need little detail. They need to be simplified so that they are easily identified – the most obvious features stressed.
- Children enjoy familiar themes, for example families, animals.
- The complexity of pictures and text can be increased for children aged 2+.
- The context of the story time is as important as the book itself; the cosy, close and intimate time gives children a positive association with books and reading.

3–5
- Repetition is important – for language development and for the enjoyment of the sound and rhythm of language.
- Books need to be reasonably short, to match children's concentration span.
- Books need minimum language with plenty of pictures that relate to the text.
- Popular themes are still everyday objects and occurrences.

5–7
- A clearly identifiable story and setting are important.
- Children's wider interests, experiences and imagination should be reflected in themes.
- The characters can be developed through the story.
- Language can be richer – playing with rhyme and rhythm, the introduction of new vocabulary and the use of repetition for dramatic effect.

3–7
- Illustrations still need to be bold, bright and eye-catching, but can be more detailed and have more meaning than pure recognition.
- Sequenced stories become popular – with a beginning, middle and end.
- The storyline needs to be easy to follow with a limited number of characters.
- Repetition is important so that the reader or listener can become involved in the text.
- Animated objects are popular – children can enter into the fantasy.
- Children enjoy humour in stories, but it needs to be obvious humour, not puns or sarcasm.

Planning story time

Story time needs to be planned as carefully as any other activity for children. The following points should be considered for all story telling, whether on a one-to-one basis, or in a small or large group.

- The choice of an book should be appropriate to the child/children involved.
- Allow the child to see the pages as the story is being told.
- Point to the words as you read them, demonstrating left to right tracking and identifying individual words as you say them. This will help children to develop aural reading and writing skills.
- Tell of the story enthusiastically; show that you are enjoying it.
- Talk about the book after you have read it through.

When telling a story to a group of children you also need to think about:
- the area – it should be cosy, quiet, warm, comfortable
- the structure of the session – introduction, story, discussion topics and questions, rhymes or songs appropriate, where possible, to the story
- visual aids – storyboard, puppets, props

■ behaviour management – how will you manage the behaviour to minimise interruptions and to make sure that all children can be involved in the session?

Do this! 7.6

Plan three story sessions, one each for children aged 2, 4 and 7 years.
Think about:
■ choosing the book
■ the area
■ the structure of the session
■ appropriate visual aids
■ behaviour management
■ the size of the group.
Present your planning in an appropriate format.

✓ **Progress check**

1 Why is it important to introduce books and stories to young children?
2 How can books and story telling contribute to children's all-round development?
3 How can books and stories influence children's view of the society that they are growing up in?
4 What criteria should be used when selecting books to use with children?
5 Why should an area for telling a story be cosy, quiet, warm and comfortable?
6 What are the benefits of using visual aids in story telling?

Developing maths

Maths in the early years should be approached primarily through practical activities that children will be able to relate to and understand. Children who 'do' maths through first-hand experiences are most likely to develop confidence and understanding in the subject. Much of what children experience in activities will involve an element of maths. This may be something that is planned, for example measuring sunflowers to find out which is tallest, or it may arise incidentally, perhaps when a child is sharing out birthday sweets. The child-care worker needs to be aware of the mathematical potential of any situation and be prepared to extend and develop this through interactions with the children.

Remember that many adults feel nervous about maths, perhaps recalling negative experiences from their own schooldays. It is important that this negative attitude is not passed on to children.

What is maths?

Maths is all around us and children have many mathematical experiences in their everyday lives before they begin the formal study of maths.

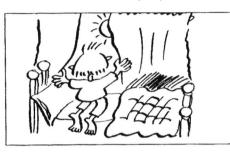

1. Getting up. Is it still dark? (Time; making logical deductions)

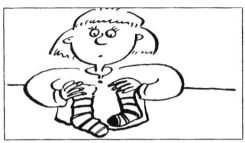

2. Getting dressed; putting clothes on in the right order. Are these socks a pair? (Sorting, sequencing, matching)

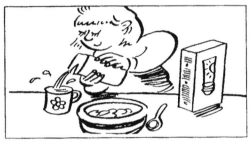

3. Having breakfast; pour cornflakes into a bowl and juice into a cup. Oops! Don't spill it! (Estimating quantity, volume)

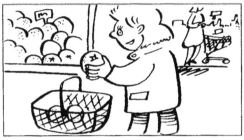

4. Going shopping. How many oranges? A large packet or a small packet? How much does it cost? (Counting, size, money)

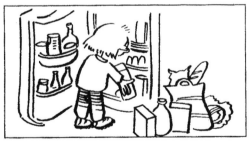

5. Unpacking the bags. Where will these boxes fit? What goes in the fridge? (Sorting, shape, size)

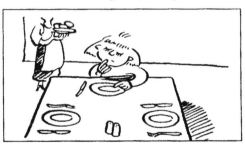

6. Laying the table. How many places? Are there enough plates? How long before we eat? (Matching, counting, time)

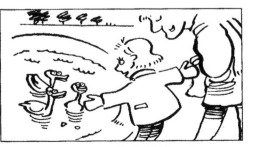

Mary's mathematical day, showing how maths is a part of children's everyday experiences

7. Out for a walk. How far is it? Have I seen more buses or more lorries? How many ducks on the pond? (Estimating, comparing, counting)

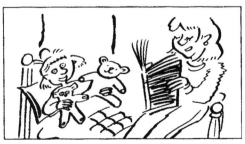

8. Bedtime. Can I have one more story? I'll have the big teddy and the little teddy. How long is it till morning? (Number, size, time)

> ### Do this!   7.7
>
> Using Mary's day on page 109 as a guide, draw a comic strip of your own mathematical day.

Maths is much more than figures and formulae.

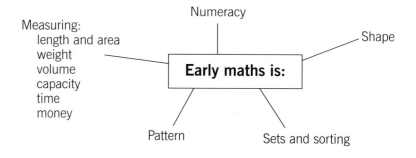

Below are some brief details about each of the areas of maths in the diagram and some examples of activities that are linked to them.

Shape

Children need to be able to recognise shapes in both two and three dimensions. They need to learn about the properties of shapes, for example that cylinders roll, cubes have right angles, how they fit together and the space that they occupy.

- *Activities:* identifying shapes in the environment; drawing around shapes; sorting junk and modelling with it; making shapes with playdough or clay; building with bricks.

Sets and sorting

Children need to be able to sort objects into sets and explain why they belong there. This contributes to the development of their logical abilities.

- *Activities:* sorting with structured sorting apparatus and with collections of shells, beads, etc.; sorting for colour, for shape, for more complex attributes, for example, making a set of animals that live on farms. Older children will begin to record their findings on diagrams and in other ways.

Pattern

Pattern occurs both in number and in shape. It is an important mathematical concept that lays the foundation for algebra. The essential features of a pattern are that it is regular and predictable.

- *Activities:* looking for pattern in the environment, for example in brick walls, on floor tiles, on fabrics and also in nature, in animal markings and in plant life; making patterns with beads bricks and other materials including painting, printing and collage; copying and continuing patterns with bricks, beads and peg boards and also using computer software.

Numeracy

Numeracy includes counting, estimating, recording numbers and the four rules of number – addition, subtraction, multiplication and division – and also simple fractions.

- *Activities:* taking every opportunity to count, for example children in the class, coats on the pegs, bottles in the crate; matching one thing to another, children to chairs, saucers to cups; linking number symbols to groups of objects; dividing apples into halves, quarters and sharing them out; using real objects to add to, take away, share. As they develop an understanding of number, children will begin to recognise numerals and use symbols to record their work.

Money

As for numeracy, but additionally children will become familiar with coins and understand about equivalence, that is that one coin may be worth the same as, say, ten other coins.

- *Activities:* making shops in the classroom and buying and selling; counting real money, for example milk or trip money; handling play money and sorting coins; making a collection of price tags, receipts, etc.

Time

Children need to understand that time can be measured and to be familiar with how we measure time. At about 7 years, we expect children to be able to read the time from both analogue and digital clock faces. They also need to be able to sort events into past, present and future.

- *Activities:* talking about daily routines; filling in daily calendars; using all kinds of timers to measure, for example, how many jumps in a minute, etc.; using movable clock faces. Stories such as *Sleeping Beauty* deal with the passing of time and can be helpful to children's understanding of this concept.

Weight

Children need to be able to use non-standard (a book weighs as much as three apples) and standard (grams and kilograms, pounds and ounces) measures. They need to be able to apply the concept of equivalence (equal weight) and be able to make comparisons based on weight.

- *Activities:* practical experience of holding things and talking about *heavy* and *light*, then *heavier than*, *lighter than*; cooking activities using non-standard (cups, spoons) or standard measures; using balance scales to weigh first with non-standard, then with standard measures (balance scales provide clear evidence of equivalence that the children can see); investigation of other types of scales.

Length and area

Children need to be able to estimate and measure length and area using non-standard as well as standard measures. They need to be able to select the most appropriate unit of measurement for the task.

- *Activities:* measuring with hand spans, strides, pencils, etc.; measuring using standard measures, rulers, tapes, trundle wheels; measuring and making charts of height – who is tallest?, who is smallest? – ordering: smallest to tallest, tallest to smallest; drawing around hands, feet, children on squared paper and counting the squares; covering box models with paper and estimating how much is needed.

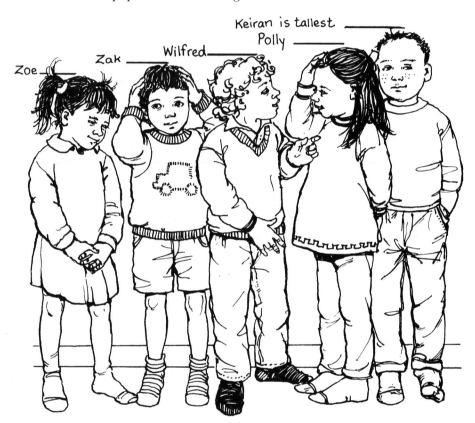

Make charts of children's heights

Case study: Measuring the playground

The children in the nursery had been talking about measuring. They had taken part in a number of different measuring activities, using handspans, strides, pencils, bricks and conkers. A group of the older children wanted to measure the playground. After some discussion, they settled on using pencils as their unit of measurement, placing a number of pencils end to end. The task proved too much for them and they soon gave up. At group time later that morning they talked about their difficulties and, together with the nursery nurse, decided on other ways of going about the task in the afternoon.

1 Why did this prove such a difficult task for the children?

2 What would you have suggested to help them?

3 What did the children learn from this unsuccessful attempt?

Capacity and volume

This is a difficult concept for young children to grasp. They need to understand that capacity and volume can be measured using non-standard as well as standard measures. They need to be able to compare containers of different sizes and shapes and to make comparisons about their capacity.

- *Activities:* filling buckets, beakers, containers with sand or water. Posing problems – how many cups to fill a bucket? Using standard measures to compare the capacity of other containers; 'real life' questions – how many beakers can you fill from a squash bottle?

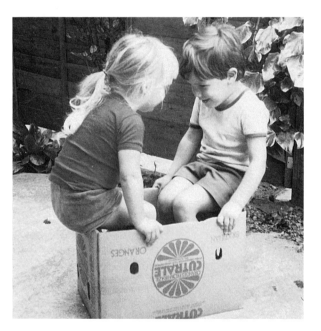

How can we fit into this box?

How can you help?

- Encourage and explain. Many children take a while to grasp new ideas.
- Talk to the children about their work. Introduce mathematical language, *more than*, *less than*, etc. Name shapes accurately.
- Use everyday experiences to reinforce mathematical learning, for example counting stairs, sharing biscuits, laying the table.
- Be aware of the mathematical potential of activities and experiences and develop children's understanding.
- Observe progress on an individual level and use this to plan the next step.

> ### Do this! 7.8
>
> Make a copy of the chart 'Early maths is' (page 110) and alongside each area, list any activities you have seen, or you can think of, that promote an understanding of the mathematical concept.

> ### ✓ Progress check
>
> 1 How should early maths be approached?
> 2 What are the elements of early maths?
> 3 Why is it vital to promote positive attitudes to maths in the early years?
> 4 Why is it important to give children practical experiences to develop their mathematical understanding?
> 5 How can the adult promote children's mathematical development?

Science and technology

Children are naturally curious about themselves and about the world they inhabit. Good early years provision will harness this curiosity, providing the foundation for children's scientific understanding. Science and technology are aspects of the 'Knowledge and understanding of the world' programme of learning in the Desirable Outcomes for Children's Learning and have separate programmes of study at Key Stage 1 of the National Curriculum.

What is science?

There are many situations in which the young child can be a scientist. Here are some examples:

- the natural world – caring for plants and animals, looking at the seasons, caring for the environment, life cycles, work on growth, ourselves
- natural materials – discovering the properties of water, wood, clay, sand, air, and so on
- creative materials – identifying the science in painting, collage, junk modelling, music
- the physical world – using magnets and batteries, investigating light and colour with lenses and mirrors, looking at movement and forces
- chemistry – combining substances, watching changes, cooking.

Science is not approached in isolation. In the pre-school years, it is an integral part of many of the activities provided routinely such as outdoor play, construction, sand, water, paint. In school, scientific themes will be developed through topic work.

How can you help?

The adult's role in promoting the growth of children's scientific understanding is crucial. Their role is to:

- provide a rich and stimulating environment for the children
- interact and question the children, encouraging them to think, to pose questions and to solve problems for themselves
- help children decide on ways to try out their ideas, including ways of designing a fair test
- help children to organise their understanding of what has happened, that is, to draw conclusions and to form concepts
- encourage children to record their findings using a variety of methods including talking, drawing, making tables, writing
- monitor children's progress and provide opportunities to extend learning.

Case study: Planting seeds

The Year 1 class were to plant some bean seeds as part of their work around the theme of growing. Sally, the nursery nurse, gathered a small group of children together to talk about what they were going to do. She wanted the children to understand that living things would only grow if they received the care that they needed.

They looked at the seeds carefully, examining them with magnifying glasses. The children were encouraged to describe them, commenting that they were hard and shiny. They talked about what they would do to make them grow. Some of the children had experience of growing things at home and were keen to make suggestions. They all agreed that the beans needed soil and water to grow but they couldn't decide on whether they needed a warm place or a cool place and whether it should be light or dark. Eventually they decided that they would try out a number of places. They would plant all the seeds in soil and keep them moist, but would put one pot in the fridge (cool and dark), one in the cupboard (warm and dark), another on the windowsill (warm and light) and the last outside (cool and light). They marked on the calendar when they'd planted them and examined them every week on the same day, recording their seed's progress by drawing it on the right pot on the weekly progress sheet.

After three weeks, Sally got the group together and asked them to look at the seeds in the pots and decide which had grown most successfully. They were then able to decide, from their experience, on what conditions were best for growing seeds. They recorded their decision on the final progress sheet and used the school camera to record the 'evidence'.

1 What did children learn about the principles of scientific investigation from this activity?
2 Why was it important that the children were able to follow through their own ideas about growing?
3 How were children's observational skills developed here?
4 How did the adult support the children's learning through this activity?
5 Think of some other activities that would encourage children to develop early science skills.

Technology

Technology for the early years is closely linked to science. It involves the use of tools and materials in practical projects. Children need opportunities to plan and design as well as to make. As their experience increases, their designs will become more complex. In this area of learning, the adult's role is to give the children access to a range of materials and to encourage them to complete and evaluate their projects. This will include the teaching and practising of techniques such as cutting, joining things and sewing, as well as encouraging the children in their projects.

Technology should be available for use by children's to support their learning across the curriculum. They will have access to a range of equipment, for example, cassette recorders, cameras, electronic keyboards, televisions and video recorders.

Information technology, involving the use of computers, is now very much a part of the early years curriculum. Children will become familiar with the operation of the equipment and work on software programs specially designed to meet their learning needs.

> ### ✓ Progress check
>
> 1 What kinds of activities will allow children to develop scientific understanding?
> 2 What is the role of the adult in promoting children's scientific understanding?
> 3 Why is it important that children be encouraged to ask questions? What is the adult's role in asking and answering questions?
> 4 In what ways can children record their investigations and findings?
> 5 What does early years technology consist of?
> 6 How can children use technology to support their learning across the curriculum? Give examples.

History and geography

History and geography will be included in any thematic approach to the early years curriculum. There are National Curriculum programmes of study for history and geography at Key Stage 1. In the Desirable Outcomes for Children's Learning, these subjects are part of the programme for 'Knowledge and understanding of the world'.

History

The concept of time is not an easy one for young children to grasp (see *Developing maths*, page 111). 'A long time ago' to a small child could equally be last week or when dinosaurs were about. However, there are some ways of making the notion of the past meaningful to children.

Skin rashes and blemishes

Measles

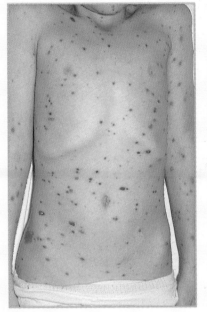

Chicken pox

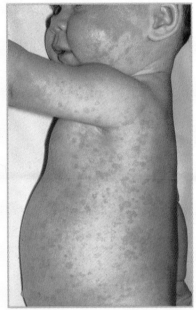

Rubella

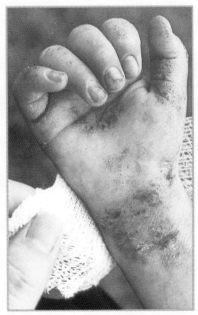

Eczema

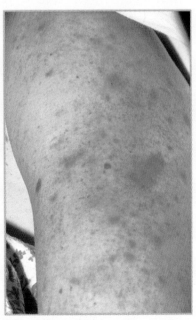

Meningococcal rash

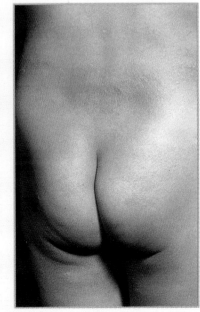

Mongolian blue spot

Developing manipulative skills: all in a day's work

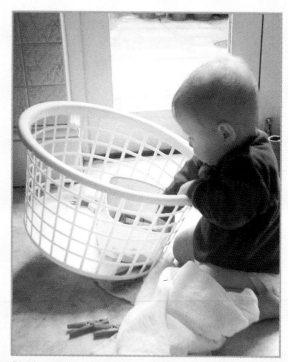

Picking up the pegs

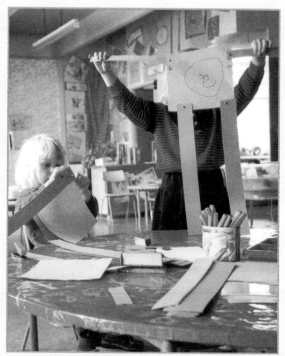

Cutting, joining and folding

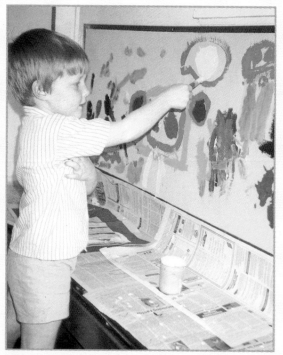

Young artist

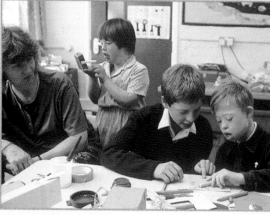

Designing and making

Role play: let's pretend

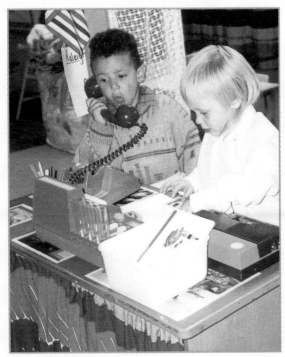

'I'm just putting you through'

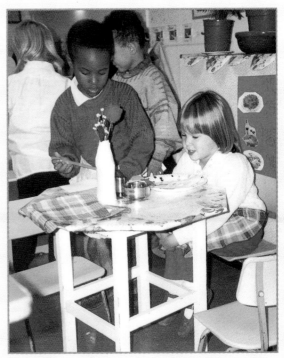

'Can I take your order?'

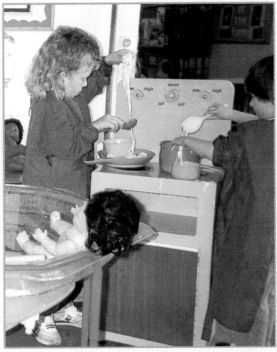

'It'll soon be ready'

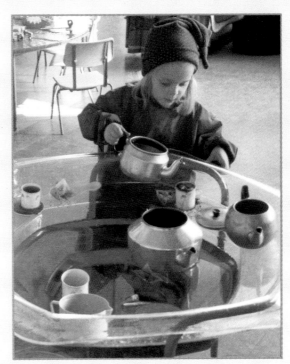

'Is there enough for another cup?'

A stimulating environment

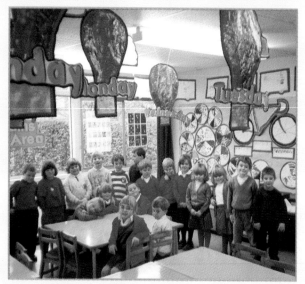

A bright and stimulating classroom

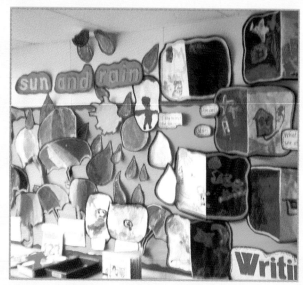

Displaying children's work effectively

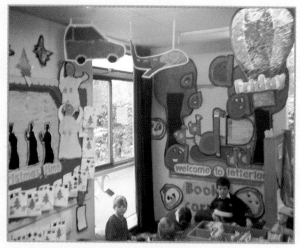

An attractive environment encourages children to participate

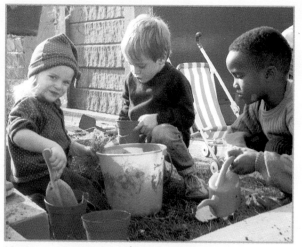

Making good use of the outdoor environment

- Ordering and sequencing events in their own lives, for example looking at photographs of themselves as babies and toddlers and comparing with the present day.
- Comparisons with 'then' and 'now' can be very successful, particularly if children have a chance to handle objects from the past and make a direct comparison with now, for example, comparing the dolly tub with an automatic washing machine.
- Many museums run excellent programmes that get children to experience, say, a Victorian schoolroom, complete with costumes and tasks.
- Getting older people to talk to children about the past can be helpful. Children can question their own parents and grandparents for insights about the recent past.
- Old newspapers and photographs can provide useful starting points. Children might search for clues and put them in chronological order.

Case study: Toys then and now

The nursery's topic for the term was 'Toys'. The children had been looking at their own toys and investigating what they were made of and what they could do with them. To develop the topic further, the nursery teacher brought in a selection her own toys from 20 years ago and asked the children's parents and grandparents if they had any toys that could be borrowed. They were all examined very thoroughly and the children commented on how different these toys were from their own. To further the investigation, the teacher was able to borrow a small collection of Victorian toys from a local museum. The children were fascinated when their teacher described how children would play in the street with whips and tops and would roll hoops along the gutter. When one child asked why the children hadn't been knocked over by cars whilst playing with their toys, the nursery teacher showed the children a photograph of the period so that they could judge the danger from traffic for themselves.

1 Why was this an appropriate starting point for historical investigation?
2 Why do you think it was important that the children had a chance to handle the toys?
3 What do think the children understand about the Victorian period as a result of this activity?

Geography

The geography curriculum encourages children to investigate the physical and human features of their immediate surroundings and, from this basis, to learn about the wider world. The following activities would contribute to this understanding:

- making simple maps, perhaps of home-to-school routes

- reading simple maps by following directions and identifying features
- looking at similarities and differences in locations, for example between a city school and a village school. Many schools 'twin' to achieve this
- providing opportunities to look carefully at the local environment, giving children a chance to recognise different uses of land and to notice changes. Children could also be asked to suggest how their environment could be improved
- noticing and recording the weather and acknowledging its importance and that of the seasonal cycle.

As children learn through direct experience with the world, much of this learning should be achieved by going out into the local environment. This may be to observe certain features, such as buildings or ponds, or to experience certain conditions, such as wind or snow. The adult's role here is to focus children's observation and to draw their attention to relevant features in the environment.

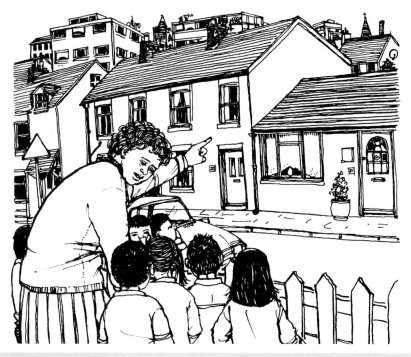

The adult can draw children's attention to relevant features in the environment

✓ Progress check

1 Why is the concept of history difficult for young children to grasp?
2 List some of the ways in which history can be made relevant to young children.
3 What does the early years geography curriculum consist of?
4 Why is it important that children should go out and observe their environment?
5 Suggest some experiences that would contribute to children's geographical understanding.

Creativity

creativity
The expression of ideas in a personal and unique way, using the imagination

Creativity involves the expression of ideas. Creative activities provide children with a means of communication with themselves and with the outside world. Creative activities are those which value the process as well as the product of any endeavour. Opportunities for children to be creative, to develop their own ideas through a variety of media, should be provided throughout the early years.

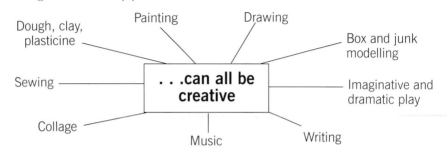

Providing for creativity

The way an activity is presented affects how much scope it offers for creativity. Consider the following activities.

1 Children have been asked to make a collage using natural materials they collected on an autumn walk. Paper and glue are available and the children are interpreting this brief in a number of ways.
2 Children are busy cutting around circles of paper. They are then sticking them onto an outline drawing of a clown on a piece of paper. They are matching the circles for size to spaces on the paper.

The first activity gives the children an opportunity to develop their own ideas, to be creative. The second activity, which is also a collage activity, is getting the children to practise the skill of cutting and is developing their concepts of size and shape. This activity provides an opportunity for children to develop valuable skills, but it does not allow them to be creative.

What we expect from children and what we provide for them in creative activities needs to be linked to their developmental stage. At the early stages they will explore and experiment with the materials, using them in a random manner. They finish quickly and then move on to something else. As they become more experienced, they build up a repertoire of skills and techniques that they can then apply creatively. They will work for a longer period at an activity and show more concern for the end product.

Good early years provision will ensure that all aspects of children's creative development are catered for. A stimulating environment will encourage children to take part in a wide range of experiences, giving them opportunities to explore and experiment.

Providing for drawing and painting

By the time they come to the child-care centre, children are likely to have widely varying experiences of drawing and painting. Most children will have had opportunities to use different types of drawing media and some will be familiar with paint. However, it is not helpful to assume that all children have had common experiences.

Drawing

A variety of drawing media will allow children to discover different properties and applications. The following would provide a range of effects.

- *Pencil* Offer thick and thin, carbon and coloured.
- *Charcoal* demonstrate the techniques associated with the medium.
- *Chalk* White and coloured chalks offer different effects and textures.
- *Wax crayons* Provide different thicknesses and textures.
- *Felt and fibre-tip pens* Provide a wide range, including those where the colours blend together.
- *Pastels* Oil and water pastels produce a wide range of effects, although they are expensive and fragile.

Painting

The way that painting is provided for will depend on the space available and, to some extent, on the budget. With this in mind, here are some general points.

- *Provide a variety of paints* Include powder paint, redimix paint in squeezy bottles and finger paints. Mix paint with glue or paste for different effects.
- *Provide a variety of brushes and tools* Include thick and thin brushes, decorators' brushes for large areas. Introduce tools that can be used with paint such as sponges, corks, old toothbrushes and straws and demonstrate these techniques.
- *Provide a variety of paper* Give children the chance to paint on different surfaces, rough, smooth, shiny, corrugated. Cut paper to different sizes and shapes and offer a range of colours.
- *Consider the space* Large-scale works will need some floor space. Try to offer easels as well as tables so that children can discover how paint behaves in a vertical plane.

Providing for collage

Collage involves sticking two- or three-dimensional materials such as fabrics, paper, twigs, feathers and introduces children to a variety of textures.

- *Supply the correct adhesive* Children will soon become frustrated trying to stick carpet with wallpaper paste!
- *Collect and store a stimulating range of materials* Get children and parents to help.
- *Organise storage so that materials are accessible to children* Vet all materials for safety.
- *Present materials that are themed*, for example natural materials or shiny things. Choosing from within a theme can provide a framework for children to work within.
- *Provide a variety of surfaces for children to stick onto* – card, board, fabric, etc.

■ *Teach children different tearing and cutting techniques*, and provide effective scissors.

Providing for box and junk modelling

Working in three dimensions presents another challenge to children's creativity as it provides them with more problems to solve.

■ Collect sufficient materials to allow the children maximum flexibility.
■ Store materials in an organised and accessible way.
■ Demonstrate and resource a variety of joining techniques. As well as glue, include sellotape, treasury tags, split pins, staples, cutting flaps and hinges.
■ Provide enough space and time for the activity.
■ Protect the models when they are at the fragile, wet stage.

Clay, dough and other malleable materials

Using these media provides another means of creative expression. Children will need time to familiarise themselves with the materials before they become aware of their potential. They will practise techniques of cutting and rolling and experiment with tools. These materials can be combined with others with contrasting textures such as pebbles, fir cones and shells. For some malleable materials, baking and firing will extend the activity further.

Music

The early years environment should provide children with opportunities to listen and respond to music and to make their own music. As well as fostering an appreciation of music, this will provide children with another channel for communication and self-expression.

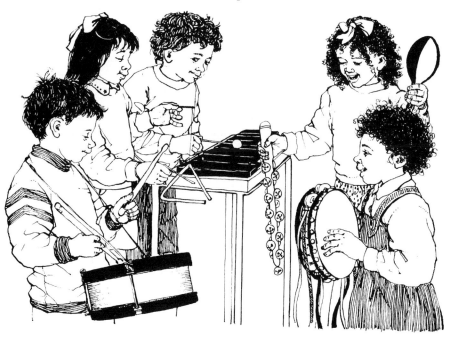

Give children an opportunity to make their own music

- *Provide opportunities for children to listen to music* Introduce a wide range of musical styles, classical, contemporary, electronic. Choose music that is culturally diverse. Alert the children to the characteristics of music – pitch, tone, pace – and listen for phrases that recur.
- *Teach children songs and rhymes* Include all sorts of rhymes – traditional, funny, number – and from all over the world. Alert children to rhythm in songs and rhymes. Introduce clapping and simple instrumental accompaniment.
- *Get children to move to music* Create a mood with music or use music to tell a story and get children to respond. Introduce children to different styles of dance and encourage children to respond to music with their bodies through dance.
- *Encourage children to make their own music* For maximum variety, provide commercially produced instruments alongside the children's home-made ones. Let children tape their own music to use in their play or to share with their parents.

Imaginative and dramatic play

Most settings will provide for a range of imaginative play opportunities. There is usually an area for domestic play and other provision for imaginative role-play such as a cafe or hospital. Children will be able to create their own scenarios in construction areas and with small world play. Dressing-up clothes are often available, either linked to a theme or as a separate activity. Sand and water and other messy activities may also provide a focus for children's imaginative play.

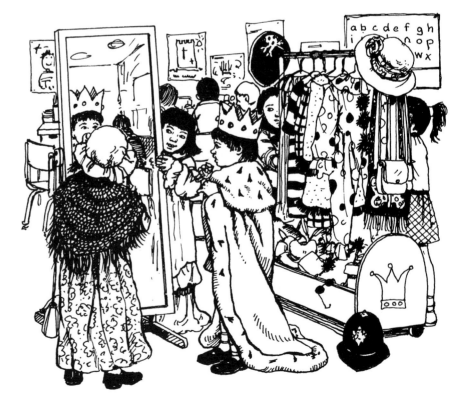

Children enjoy admiring themselves in a mirror

Imaginative play provides children with a means of communication with others and themselves. It can also give them another perspective on the world and their role in it.

To encourage imaginative play:

- Vary home corner provision, maintaining a balance between new and familiar equipment.
- Plan imaginative play areas to link with any theme that might be developed.
- Ensure dressing-up clothes are easy to put on. Provide hats, bags and other accessories and a mirror for children to admire themselves in.
- Provide for large brick play. This often involves collaboration and complex story lines.
- Show children that you value their imaginative play by talking to them about it and join in, if appropriate, and extend and challenge sensitively.
- Present small world play in varied ways, sometimes on playmats, sometimes in the sand, sometimes in with the bricks.
- Plan for imaginative play outside too. Tents can be made from blankets and drapes. Chalk markings on the playground can trigger all kinds of games.
- Give children the time and space to develop their own imaginative play. Encourage them to use resources in their own unique ways.

Do this!   7.9

For each of the aspects of creativity shown in the diagram on page 119, briefly describe an activity that you think is creative. Indicate the age group of the children you are planning for.

The role of the adult

Provision

- Select and present materials and equipment appropriate to the stage of development of the child, for example thick brushes for 3-year-olds, finer ones for 7-year-olds.
- Organise storage of materials so that they are accessible and easily maintained.
- Introduce new materials. They can act as a stimulus to children's ideas.
- Display children's work with care, showing that you value their own efforts.

Planning

- Give time and space to creative activities.
- Organise experiences that will act as a stimulus to creative activities.

Working alongside

- Encourage the child.

Think about it

Look at your workplace. How is children's creativity provided for? Is creativity valued? How can you tell?

- Do not judge by adult standards. Value the child's work for its own sake.
- Do not do it for the child. You will make him dissatisfied with his own efforts and dependent on you.
- Children may be affronted if you ask 'What is it?' – 'Could you tell me about it?' might be better!
- Teach children techniques. Children's creativity may be hindered if they lack the skills associated with the activity.

✓ Progress check

1 What is creativity?
2 What kinds of activities allow children to explore their creativity?
3 Why are creative activities important to children's development?
4 Make a list of the points that you should consider when providing for children's creativity?
5 How can adults support the development of children's creativity?

Physical activities

Physical activities are a vital part of the early years curriculum. They are important for the health and development of children and may also provide a starting point for leisure activities. All nurseries will provide regular opportunities for vigorous outside play. This kind of play is important for all areas of development, not just the physical (see Chapter 5, *Play*).

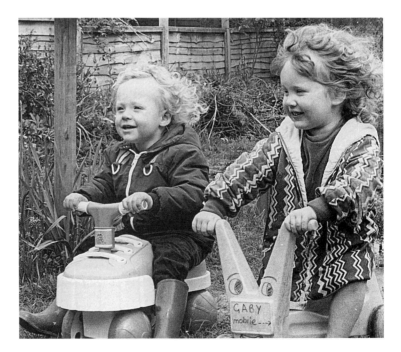

Vigorous outside play is important for all areas of development, not just the physical

Many centres will provide some or all of the following as part of the PE curriculum:

- gymnastics sessions that include floorwork as well as the use of large and small apparatus. Children often work with a theme in mind, for example moving on different parts of the body. They are encouraged to set targets for themselves. Some younger children might find the large apparatus daunting and adults should be sensitive to this and allow the child to stand by and watch until ready to join in. Children also have a part to play in the setting up and putting away of equipment; adequate supervision is vital here
- opportunities for dance to live or recorded music. Dance styles from a variety of cultures may be introduced, sometimes by demonstration
- games and games' skills will be introduced during the early school years. These could be indoor or outdoor sessions. Younger children may have difficulty remembering rules but can usually manage simple games. Large team games are not suitable at this stage as the children spend too much time waiting. Remember that there can be quite significant differences in children's physical co-ordination, balance and manual dexterity at this age and this range needs to be catered for in any skills sessions.

  Equipment is important too: a beanbag is easier to catch than a tennis ball; a full-size football is too big for a small child. Make sure that all children take part. They will not enjoy playing the game if they have not had a chance to learn the skills
- swimming may be offered in areas where facilities are available. Children who have not experienced swimming before may be frightened at the prospect and need reassurance. If staffing is adequate, an adult in the water will help too. Sessions need to be short but frequent and children should never be forced into situations if they feel unsure
- playtime will provide another opportunity for physical activities, often without the direction of an adult. Some children organise themselves in complicated games, others will enjoy just running around. Children new to the situation and used to the organisation and adult interaction of the nursery playground, may find the frenetic activity of the school playground frightening and will want to find a quiet place to observe until they feel more secure.

Remember to allow plenty of time for changing both before and after PE sessions, as many children will need help.

Case study: Learning to swim

Dominic's class were to have a regular trip to the swimming baths once a week for the summer term. Many of the 6 and 7-year-olds were regulars at the baths, but Dominic had never been before. The class teacher talked to the whole class about what they would be doing and reminded children to bring their swimsuits and towels for the session.

Although Dominic felt quite excited on the bus, when he got to the side of the pool he was too frightened to get in. Seeing the other children jumping in and splashing, obviously enjoying themselves made him feel worse. His teacher told him to wrap himself up in his towel and find a place where he could watch. He didn't need to worry about going into the pool today.

Before the next session, the teacher had a word with Gina, one of the nursery nurse students on placement at the school, and arranged for her to go swimming with the group and join them in the water. Dominic started off on the side of the pool as before but five minutes from the end of the session Gina managed to persuade him to sit with his legs dangling in the water, splashing and kicking.

Week by week, Dominic became more adventurous and, with Gina's help, by the end of the term he was spending the full time in the pool and asking his mum to take him swimming at the weekend.

1 Why was the class teacher right to respond to Dominic's fears in the way that she did?
2 What would have happened if Dominic had been forced into the water?
3 Why do you think Gina's approach was successful in calming Dominic's fears?

✅ *Progress check*

1 Why is vigorous play important for children's development?
2 What kinds of physical activities are provided in school?
3 Why is it important to teach games skills to children?
4 How should you deal with children who are reluctant to join in with some physical activities?

Key terms

You need to know what these words and phrases mean. Go back through the chapter and find out.
creativity
emergent writing
literacy
look and say
phonics

Now try these questions

1 How can the child-care worker promote the development of children's writing?

2 What mathematical concepts could be introduced to children as part of a biscuit-making activity?

3 What points would you bear in mind when selecting books for 3 to 5 year olds?

4 Describe how you would promote children's creativity in painting?

5 How can you present the concept of history to children in an accessible way?

Part 3: The Social and Legal Framework

The vast majority of children are brought up within their family. Child-care workers have differing amounts of contact with the parents of the children in their care, according to the setting in which they are working. A thorough knowledge of different types of child-care provision and support services available to families is valuable to their work.

All workers are required to recognise the prime importance of the parental role and to work in partnership with parents. In order to work effectively with parents, workers need a good understanding of the possible differences in family background of the children in their care. This will enable them to work without making assumptions about people that are based solely on their own experiences of life.

Child-care workers also need to have a good awareness of the different pressures that families may be experiencing and why parents respond differently to such pressures. This will help them to adopt a non-judgmental and professional approach in their work.

8 *Early years care and education*

This chapter includes:

- **The range of services**
- **The political structure for service provision in the UK**
- **Child-care and education services**
- **Personal social services**
- **Housing**
- **Social security**
- **Health**

There is a wide range of statutory, voluntary and private services that support children and their families in the UK today. The UK has a welfare state that provides statutory services. It was introduced by the government during the 1940s. The aim of the welfare state is to ensure that all citizens have adequate standards of income, housing, education and health services. The welfare state and the services provided by it have changed a great deal since they were introduced. Recent governments have supported the growth of private and voluntary provision to supplement state services.

You may find it helpful to read this chapter in conjunction with:

- ▶ **Book 2, Chapter 9**   The family
- ▶ **Book 2, Chapter 10** Social issues
- ▶ **Book 2, Chapter 14** Child protection procedures

The range of services

Care and education services for children and their families are provided either by

- the state – referred to as **statutory services**
- private individuals or companies – referred to as **private services**
- volunteers or voluntary groups – referred to as **voluntary services**.

statutory service
A service provided by the government after a law (or statute) has been passed in parliament

Statutory services

What are they?

A statutory service is one provided by the government after a law (or statute) has been passed in parliament. Such laws say that a service either:

- *must* be provided (i.e. there is a duty to provide it), for example, education for 5–16 year olds

or

- *can* be provided (i.e. there is a power to provide it, if an authority chooses), for example local authority day nurseries.

What do they provide?

Statutory services provide, amongst other things, education, health care, financial support, personal social services, housing, leisure services, public health. Government provision is sometimes referred to as 'the state sector'.

How are they financed?

Statutory services are financed by the state, which gets its money through taxation and National Insurance. There may be some fund-raising activities and charging for services (for example, through sponsorships, fairs and concerts in schools, and charges for school outings and prescription charges). There has been increasing pressure on state services to be more accountable financially and to be run more like private organisations, only with the government providing the funding. This philosophy has affected the way that both state hospitals and state schools are funded.

How are they staffed?

Most people working in statutory organisations are trained and paid for their work, but volunteers may carry out some tasks (for example, parent-helpers in schools, WRVS workers in hospitals).

Voluntary services

> **voluntary services**
> Services provided by voluntary organisations which are founded by people who want to help certain groups of people they believe are in need of support

What are they?

Organisations are referred to as voluntary when they are founded by people who want to help certain groups of people who they believe are in need of support (i.e. they are formed *voluntarily*, like Barnados and the NSPCC). The basic difference between voluntary and statutory organisations is that no legislation needs to be passed in order for voluntary organisations to be set up. The government is very positive about some services being provided by 'the voluntary sector', but it does pass laws that require certain of them to register, so that the services they provide can be inspected by government officers in order to protect the people who use them (for example, playgroups and childminders under the Children Act 1989).

What do they provide?

There is a long and varied tradition of voluntary work in the UK, and as a result there is a wide variety of voluntary organisations. In some European countries, the church has been the only source of voluntary activity. Voluntary organisations have a number of different functions. Some organisations combine more than one of these functions. They:

- act as information and campaigning bodies (for example, Shelter and the Pre-School Learning Alliance or PLA)

- provide money to help people in particular circumstances; these are sometimes called benevolent funds or charities (for example, the Family Welfare Association)
- help and support some people who have health conditions or impairments (for example, Scope, RNIB)
- support and care for families and children, and other individuals (for example, Barnados and NCH day centres and family centres, Mencap, Relate).

How are they financed?

Money for voluntary organisations comes from a variety of sources that include donations, fund-raising, grants from central or local government, lottery grants and fees for the services they provide.

How are they staffed?

Some people work without pay and have no qualifications (for example, in self-help groups), and this is the reason that most people think they are called 'voluntary'. In contrast, many people who work for voluntary organisations are professionally trained and qualified and receive a salary (for example, inspectors in the NSPCC, workers in NCH family centres). Some voluntary organisations may employ one person who then organises volunteers (for example, Homestart), or pay several people a small amount (for example, playgroup leaders). They may be run by a voluntary management committee, as is the case for many playgroups and community groups.

Private services

private services
Services provided by individuals, groups of people, or companies to meet a demand, provide a service, and make a financial profit

What are they?

Private services are provided by individuals, groups of people, or companies to meet a demand, provide a service, and make a financial profit. As with voluntary organisations, the government is also positive about certain services being provided by 'the private sector'. The law requires some of them to register, so that the services they provide can be inspected by government officials in order to protect the people who use them (for example, childminders and private day nurseries, under the Children Act 1989).

What do they provide?

Private services aim both to provide a service *and* make a financial profit for their owners. They therefore need to be what is called 'financially viable', i.e. not run at a loss. They provide, amongst other things, nursery care, education, health care, counselling services, housing and leisure services. Nannies and childminders are part of the private sector.

How are they financed?

The financing of private services comes both from private investment by people wishing to make a return on their investment, and from the fees that they charge for their use. In some cases, the state may pay the fees for someone to use a private service, usually because, although it has a duty to provide a service for a particular client, there is a lack of provision within the state sector in a particular area (for example, day care for a child who is considered to be 'in need' under the Children Act 1989).

How are they staffed?

Private services are staffed according to the need of the organisation. This may mean employing professionally qualified staff, both if the state demands it (for example, there must be 50 per cent professionally qualified staff in a private day nursery) and if users want it (for example, qualified nannies).

✅ **Progress check**

1 Define 'statutory organisations' and give an example.
2 Define 'voluntary organisations' and give an example.
3 Define 'private organisations' and give an example.
4 Which Act of Parliament covers the procedures for registering and inspecting private and voluntary organisations that care for children?

The political structure for service provision in the UK

Statutory, voluntary and private services for children and their families are provided within the political structure of a country. Political structures vary between countries and there are therefore differences between the UK and other European countries in their provision. In the UK, although some service provision is administered centrally, other provision depends on the choices made by politicians in a local authority. Services may therefore vary from one area to another. Political parties change and services may be modified as a result.

Political attitudes and the level of service provision

Differences in levels of service provision, like that of state-run day nurseries, may reflect the political beliefs of the party in power in a local area or centrally in a country. A simple way of understanding why this is so is to look at the basic ideas behind opposing political beliefs. These basic ideas may be described as either 'right-wing' or 'left-wing'.

Right-wing beliefs

Right-wing beliefs include ideas such as:

■ People should be responsible for themselves and their own families.
■ The money the state collects in taxes should be kept to a minimum.

- Spending by the state on services should be kept to a minimum.
- People should pay little tax and be free to keep and spend their money on which services they choose.
- It is better if services are provided by private or voluntary bodies to meet a demand by people who can pay for them.

Left-wing beliefs

Left-wing beliefs include ideas that:

- The state has responsibilities for the welfare of all its citizens.
- Sufficient money should be collected in taxes, and more should be collected from those who have the highest incomes.
- The government should spend taxpayers' money to provide services.
- The state should provide services free for everyone who needs them, regardless of whether they have contributed towards them through taxes or insurance.

Do this! 8.1

Make a study of the area that you live in. Find out how many state-run nursery classes and day nurseries there are, and if there is any private or voluntary provision. Summarise the information you have obtained and present it as an information leaflet.

Statutory services: Central government provision

Some statutory services are provided by central government, through many different departments. The *political process* that leads to this provision involves the following.

- In a general election, citizens elect politicians, called Members of Parliament (MPs). MPs make policy decisions about the services they want to provide, based on their political beliefs. They then pass laws (statutes) to say which services should be provided.
- MPs employ officers to put their policies into practice. These officers are called civil servants and are paid out of taxes. These officers work both in central and regional offices throughout the country.

The Departments of Health, the Inland Revenue, and the Department of Social Security are all organised as central government departments with regional offices.

Statutory services: Local government provision

Some statutory services are provided by local government, through a local authority. The organisation of local authorities in the UK is varied and complicated. The two main differences are as follows.

- Some areas of the country have two tiers (or layers) of local government, both of which have elected councils, which are:

     – a district council, which may represent a borough, city or district
     – a county council, which will contain several districts.
    In such areas the provision of services is divided between the two authorities.

■ Others areas have just one tier (or layer) of local government and only one elected council. These are called *unitary authorities*, because one body provides all local services.

The *political process* that leads to the provision of services involves the following.

■ Citizens vote for and elect councillors in district and county council elections. These councillors then form the local council. The party that has the greatest number of councillors takes charge (this is called the democratic process). The powers of local councils are given to them by Acts of Parliament and through passing local by-laws.

■ Councillors appoint officers to put their policies into practice and to organise and provide services in that area. These are called local government officers and they are paid out of local and central taxation. These officers work both in town halls, civic centres and other offices in the area.

Some schools and other education services, social services, leisure services and housing are all provided in this way by local government departments.

Do this!   8.2

a) Carry out some research to find out the structure of local government in your area and the cost of services.
    Find out what services are provided and who is responsible for each. This information is usually enclosed with a council tax bill, but it can also be obtained from the headquarters of your local council(s), which may be at a county hall, a civic centre or a town hall. There are also books that give a general description of the structure of local government.

b) Make a graph to show the relative cost of different services in your local authority.

Private and voluntary services

The extent to which the state encourages private or voluntary provision depends on its political outlook. Conservative governments have traditionally been associated with support for the private sector. However, it is a fact that recent governments, of both political persuasions, have increasingly encouraged the provision of private and voluntary services. In order to protect the people who use them, the state passes laws requiring these services to reach certain standards, to register and to be inspected by government officials (for example, childminders and private day nurseries, under the Children Act 1989).

Apart from this, private services can charge the amount that people will pay for a service. They meet the demands of 'the market place'. Voluntary providers are usually controlled by some form of committee that decides who should be helped by their service. This may mean that people have to subscribe to a certain belief, or be seen as 'deserving'. This is in contrast to state provision which is available as a right to citizens.

✓ Progress check

1 Why may levels of service provision differ according the political party that is or has been in power?
2 What is a right-wing political belief?
3 What is a left-wing political belief?
4 Who is voted for in a general election?
5 Who are civil servants appointed by and what do they do?
6 Who are local government officers appointed by and what do they do?
7 What are unitary authorities?

Child-care and education services

Statutory provision

statutory school age
The ages at which a child legally has to receive education: from the beginning of the term after their fifth birthday, until the end of the school year in which they have their sixteenth birthday

The state is required by law to ensure that all children, including those with disabilities, receive education if they are of **statutory school age**. This means from the beginning of the term after their fifth birthday, until the end of the school year in which they have their sixteenth birthday.

Primary education

The structure of primary school provision varies from one area to another. Primary education may be provided for children in:

- one primary school until the age of 11
- an infant school until the age of 7, then a junior school until the age of 11
- a first school until the age of 8, followed by a middle school from 9–13 years.

Grant-maintained status

grant-maintained status
Schools which receive their money (grant) directly from the government, not from their local authority

All state schools were under the control of their local education authority (LEA), until the Education Reform Act 1988 was passed by the Conservative government. In passing this law, the government hoped to encourage schools to 'opt out' of local authority control and have **grant-maintained status (GMS)**. This means that they receive their money (grant) directly from the government, not from their local authority. This money is then used by the school to buy the staff and services they need. A small proportion of schools have chosen to do this, and they tend to be grouped in certain areas, or counties. In January 1996, there were only 453 primary grant-maintained schools in England and Wales. Schools have been less likely to opt out in areas where the local education is seen as supportive and a good provider of resources to schools. The Labour government elected in 1997 has allowed schools to keep their grant-maintained status, but is not actively encouraging others to take this status.

Local management of schools

Local education authorities now give a large proportion of their education budget directly to schools. The head teacher and the governors of a school decide how to spend this money and how to staff the school. They are responsible for the financial and overall management of their school. This system is called the **local management of schools (LMS)**. Most people in education view this as a successful a policy that has given power and discretion to schools to manage their own budgets.

The National Curriculum

All state schools are now required by law to follow a national curriculum. This is to ensure that all children follow a broad-based and balanced curriculum and study the same subjects. The content of the National Curriculum and arrangements for testing it have been amended several times, which has been stressful to those working in education. (See Chapter 6, *Philosophy and approaches*.)

Nursery schools and classes

Think about it

What are the advantages and disadvantages of LMS and GMS? Discuss this with a teacher or head teacher if you are able to.

Local authorities have had the power to provide pre-school education for many years, but they have not used this power uniformly either across the country, or within their own areas. Nationally, state provision of nursery schools and classes is therefore varied, both because of this lack of compulsion and because provision is expensive. Some councils provide separate nursery schools, others provide nursery units attached to a primary school, others provide very little. Education in these is usually part-time, either every morning or afternoon.

The government has now undertaken to fund pre-school education for all 4-year-olds, and intends to extend this to all 3-year-olds. This funding is provided for children in both state, private and voluntary establishments. They have to be inspected and judged to be offering provision that will satisfactorily promote the desirable outcomes for children's learning by the time they are 5 (see Chapter 6, page 86). There is still a strong emphasis on play and exploration in these schools. Where there is no state nursery provision, many schools are taking rising-5s (children older than 4) into primary schools. Nursery schools are most often found in areas of highest social need.

Most European countries have more nursery education than the UK, but statutory school age is usually older. For example, in France and Germany there is a legal entitlement to a place in a kindergarten for every child from 3 to 6 years old. In Italy, 92 per cent of children attend pre-primary education as part of the state system from 3 to 6 years; this figure is 95 per cent in Belgium. In Sweden, all parents who work or study are entitled to a place for their children in a publicly-funded centre from the age of 1.

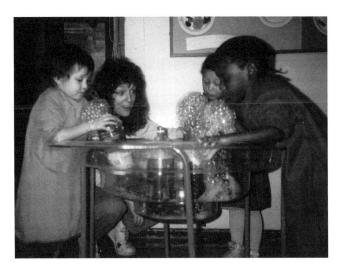

There is a strong emphasis on play and exploration in nursery education

Day nurseries and family centres

The social services department (SSD) of a local authority has the power to provide day care for children in day nurseries and family centres, and a duty under the Children Act 1989 to provide for **children in need** in its area (see *Children in need*, page 141). Many of these powers in England have now been transferred to the Department for Education and Employment (DfEE), who have done much of the work in developing policies for Early Years Development Plans and Partnerships and for setting up the first Early Years Excellence Centres.

> **children in need**
> A child is 'in need' if they are unlikely to achieve or maintain a reasonable standard of health or development without the provision of services, or if they are disabled

The National Childcare Strategy

The development by the Labour government of a **National Childcare Strategy** is also taking place in the DfEE. In May 1998 the government unveiled its plans to spend more than £300 million on funding child-care places over the following five years. Its aim is to ensure good quality, accessible and affordable child care for children aged up to 14 in every neighbourhood in England. Its strategy includes measures to make child care more affordable, including new tax credits for working families, and more accessible, by increasing places and encouraging diversity in provision that will satisfy the preferences of parents. A similar strategy is in place for Wales.

> **National Childcare Strategy**
> A strategy introduced by the UK government in May 1998 to ensure good quality, accessible, affordable child care for children aged up to 14

Do this!	8.3

1 a) Investigate how primary education is provided in your area. Information will be available from your LEA.
   b) Find out how and where the education of 4-year-olds is provided.
   c) Collate and present your information.
2 Find out about the current requirements of the National Curriculum and the arrangements for testing it (referred to as SATs – what does this stand for?).

Voluntary sector provision

Playgroups

The playgroup movement in the UK began in the 1960s with the formation of one group by a parent. It then rapidly spread throughout the country. Over the years it has filled a much needed gap in pre-school provision, but recent changes in funding, and rises in provision by other sectors has led to a fall in the number of playgroups nationally.

To form a playgroup, local people usually come together, rent premises and form a committee that organises and appoints workers. Parents sometimes help at sessions on a rota basis. There are usually a limited number of part-time sessions available a week and a charge is made for each child. Pre-school playgroups have traditionally provided play facilities and social contact, but now, if they take funded 4-year-old children, they must show that their programme can enable children to achieve the desirable outcomes for children's learning by the time they are 5 (see Chapter 6, page 86). The Ofsted inspection process has been very demanding for some pre-school playgroups, as staff are often low-paid and lacking in professional qualifications. Playgroups also have to register with and be inspected by the social services department.

Parent and toddler groups sometimes use the same facilities as playgroups. At these, carers bring children from babies upwards, but remain with them while they play.

The Pre-School Learning Alliance (PLA) is a national educational charity with many years' experience in the field of pre-school education and care. It offers a national training programme for parents and pre-school staff, and publishes educational materials and advice for pre-school playgroups.

Children and family centres

Children and family centres are sometimes provided in areas of high social need by voluntary organisations which were once more traditionally involved in providing residential care. Now that there is less demand for such care, organisations including Barnados and NCH Action for Children have diverted resources and research into providing day care and family support in their own communities for families who are experiencing difficulties.

Private sector provision

Childminders

Childminders are people who look after other people's children in their own homes. They have a legal duty to register, previously with the SSD, but now with the DfEE, and must conform to standards in the guidance to the Children Act 1989. They must be of good health and character and have non-discriminatory attitudes. The Act lays down standards for safety, floor space and for child–minder ratios according to the different ages. Childminders are free to fix their own charges. They are sometimes paid by the SSD to care for children in need.

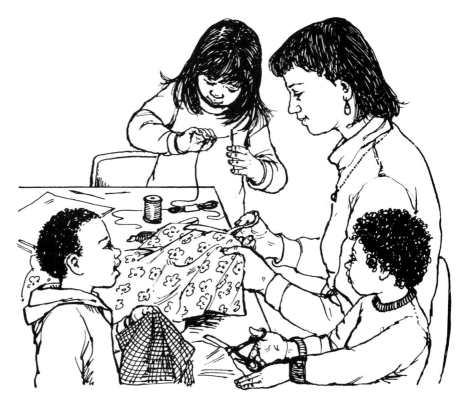

Childminders are people who look after other people's children in their own homes

Private day nurseries

Private day nursery provision more than trebled over the period from 1987 to 1997, when there were an estimated 6,100 day nurseries in England providing 194,000 places. Private day nurseries occupy many types of premises and vary in size. They all have to register and conform to standards in the same way as childminders, and there are regulations about qualified staffing levels. They provide full- or part-time care and education for children under school age, and many provide for babies. Some also provide before and after-school care, and care during the school holidays, especially for children who previously attended. Charges vary, and to some extent they reflect what people in an area are able to pay for child care.

Out-of-school clubs

Out-of-school clubs are provided in school, nursery or other premises and have had considerable financial backing from government in recent years. They provide invaluable support for the children of working parents in the periods between working hours and school hours. In 1997, the number of clubs was 2,600, providing places for 79,000 children from 5 to 7 years – a rise of 13 per cent over the previous year. These numbers are set to rise still further.

Private nursery schools

Private nursery schools exist to meet a demand from parents who want their children to be educated in the private sector. They are often part of a private school for children up to the age of 11 years. These schools provide full- and part-time education for children usually from 3 years old during school hours, and may also provide before- and after-school care. Their fees vary. Small class sizes are a key feature of this provision. Schools have to register with the DfEE and meet certain standards. If they are providing nursery education for funded children, they have to be inspected by Ofsted nursery inspectors.

Nannies

Nannies are privately employed to look after children in the child's family home. They may live in or out of the home. They negotiate their contract, which includes hours, pay and duties, with their employer. They do not have to be qualified or registered, unless they are looking after the children of three or more families at the same time. There has been a call for nannies to be registered under a national system. This raises numerous problems, and some experts believe that registration would be unworkable and in any case not serve to protect children. A set of guidelines has been published by the Federation of Recruitment and Employment Services (FRES) for anyone looking to employ a nanny. It provides a ten-point list for prospective employers to help them to choose the right nanny.

Workplace nurseries

Provision of day care at places of work is fairly uncommon. In 1998, only 25 of 500 top companies provided a workplace nursery. Ten companies had reserved places at nurseries and 15 had after-school clubs. When asked, 88 per cent of the companies said they did not think that working mothers were less reliable staff members than employees in general, and 65 per cent agreed they should do more to help working parents. They may do this if they recognise a strong business case for investing in child care, with increasing numbers of mothers with young children returning to work.

Case study: Child care and education for children of working parents

Rose, Anne, Stephanie and Aisha are four friends who met at antenatal classes. They have remained in touch as their babies have grown older and sometimes discuss their concerns about making the right decisions about child care and education for their children. They all live with working partners, but agree that although they have made joint decisions, they are the ones who feel most responsible for arranging child care for their children. None of them has any close relatives living nearby. They all agree on the need for a flexible system that enables them to fulfil their work commitments, but gives their children good care in a suitably stimulating environment.

- Rose has a child of 18 months. She works from home and has some flexibility in her hours, but nevertheless most days she aims to complete six hours work a day in her office.
- Anne has a baby of 6 months and one of 20 months. She has just returned to work part-time for one whole day and three half days a week in a departmental store.
- Stephanie has a 19-month-old and a $3\frac{1}{2}$-year-old, and works full-time as a nursery nurse in a primary school.
- Aisha has three children of 18 months, 4 and 7. She works as a clerk in a busy solicitors office.

1 Outline what you think would be the most suitable, practical child-care arrangements for each of these families.
2 Give an acceptable alternative for each family.
3 Give reasons for your choices in each case.

✅ Progress check

1 What child-care and education services are provided by the state sector?
2 What child-care and education services are provided in the voluntary sector?
3 What child-care and education services are provided by the private sector?

Personal social services

Statutory provision

Children in need

Local authorities provide personal social services through their social services departments (SSD). The Children Act 1989 gave them a duty to provide services for children in need in their area to help them to stay with their families and be brought up by them.

A child is defined as 'in need' if:

- the child is unlikely to achieve or maintain, or to have the opportunity of achieving or maintaining, a reasonable standard of health or development without the provision of services
- the child's health or development is likely to be significantly impaired, or further impaired, without the provision of such services
- the child is disabled.

The SSD tries to keep families together by offering them support in the community. It may provide social work support and counselling, practical support in the home, family centres, short periods of relief care, help with providing essential household needs and welfare rights advice.

Children at risk

The SSD has a duty to investigate the circumstances of any child believed to be at risk of harm and take action on their behalf to protect them using child protection procedures. It also provides care in residential or foster homes for children who are made the subject of care orders by a court.

Provision of accommodation

The SSD provides accommodation for children who, with the agreement of their parents, need a period of care away from their family. Children will often be looked after by foster carers whom the department approves and pays. It also provides community homes for some children. All SSDs provide an adoption service.

Special needs

There is also a range of services that are provided for children with disabilities alongside those provided by the health and education authorities.

The National Health Service and Community Care Act (1990) placed on local authorities the responsibility for assessing the needs of individual clients who, for a variety of reasons, need help to enable them to continue to live in the community.

Case study: Children 'in need'

Jeanette was 17 when her first child was born. The child's father was not named on the birth certificate. She subsequently had two more children by different fathers, the last of whom lived with her but he was sometimes violent towards her and little involved with the children. Jeanette found it very difficult to manage. Her partner gave her little money and the children were sometimes unfed and poorly cared for. The health visitor called but never seemed to find them in. A neighbour referred them to the local social services office because she considered the children were being neglected.

After an enquiry and a case conference, the children's names were put on the child protection register because of the neglect and the presence of a potentially violent male in the household. The protection plan included recommending nursery centre places for her 2- and 3-year-old. These were provided on a part-time basis, but this was on condition that Jeanette stayed with them for two mornings each week to learn about play and physical care. The 5-year-old had a place in a local primary school. This school had a partnership with social services to provide before-school care, including breakfasts, for some referred children. A social worker visited Jeanette and befriended her, helping her with advice and guidance. She also discussed her taking up a place with a local training agency to undertake some training for work.

A year later Jeanette had matured into a much more confident and mature young woman. She told her partner to leave, took control of her finances and embarked on a part-time course. Her children were thriving and noticeably more happy.

1 Why was Jeanette referred to the local social services?
2 Why could her children be defined as being 'in need' in terms of the Children Act 1989?
3 What help did social services give when the children were registered?
4 Why do you think that a year later her children were thriving and noticeably more happy?
5 Why is this called preventive work?

Do this!   8.4

Find out about your local social services department. Where are its offices? These will be listed in the telephone directory or your local library. The SSD will have some leaflets to inform the public about their services. Try to obtain these.

Voluntary provision

There is a wide range of voluntary organisations that help to support families and children; some of these are shown in the table on pages 144–5. These organisations supplement the work of the social services department. Addresses and further information can be obtained from *The Charities Digest*, published by The Family Welfare Association and available in public libraries.

National voluntary organisations

Organisation	Provision
African-Caribbean, Indian, Pakistani community centres	Exist in areas where there are numbers of people of Caribbean and Asian origin. They offer a range of advice and support services for local people. There are also a wide range of local organisations that aim to meet the needs of other minority communities. Some of these provide nurseries.
Barnados	Works with children and their families to help to relieve the effects of disadvantage and disability. It runs many community projects, including day centres where young children who are at risk can be cared for and their families supported. It also provides residential accommodation for children with special needs. It carries out research into areas of need and publishes the results of research.
ChildLine	Provides a national telephone counselling helpline for children in trouble or danger. It listens, comforts and protects. Its freephone number is 0800 1111.
The Children's Society	Offers child-care services to children and families in need. It aims to help children to grow up in their own families and communities.
National Association of Citizens' Advice Bureau	Provides free, impartial (not biased), confidential advice and help to anyone. It has over a thousand local offices that provide information, advice and legal guidance on many subjects. These include social security, housing, money, family and personal matters.
Contact-a-Family	Promotes mutual support between families caring for disabled children. It has community-based projects that assist parents' self-help groups, and runs a national helpline.
Family Service Units	Provide a range of social and community work services and support to disadvantaged families and communities with the aim of preventing family breakdown.
Family Welfare Association	Offers services for families, children and people with disabilities. It provides financial help for families in exceptional need, social work support and drop-in centres.
Gingerbread	Provides emotional support, practical help and social activities for lone parents and their children.
Jewish Care	Provides help and support for people of the Jewish faith and their families. Among other facilities, it runs day centres and provides social work teams and domiciliary (home) assistance.
Mencap	Aims to increase public awareness of the problems faced by people with mental disabilities and their families. It supports day centres and other facilities.
MIND	Is concerned with improving services for people with mental disorders and promoting mental health and better services.
NCH Action for children (previously the National Children's Homes)	Provides support for children who are disadvantaged and their families. It runs many schemes, including family centres, foster care and aid and support to families. It also carries out and publishes the results of research.
National Deaf Children's Society	A national charity working specially for deaf children and their families. It gives information, advice and support directly to families with deaf children. It helps them to identify local help and support.
National Society for the Prevention for Cruelty to Children (NSPCC)	Has a network of child protection teams throughout England and Wales. The RSSPCC works similarly in Scotland. Central to the NSPCC's services is the free 24-hour Child Protection Helpline – 0800 800500 – which provides counselling, information and advice to anyone concerned about a child at risk. It investigates referrals and also offers support in family care centres. It is very involved in research and publication, and provides information and training for other professionals. It also campaigns to change attitudes towards children and their care.
Parentline	Offers a telephone support helpline for parents who are having any kind of problem with their children – 01702 559900.

continued

National voluntary organisations *continued*

Organisation	Provision
Playmatters: The National Toy Libraries Association	Exists to promote awareness of the importance of play for the developing child. Libraries are organised locally, loaning good quality toys to all families with young children.
Relate (formerly the National Marriage Guidance Council)	Trains and provides counsellors to work with people who are experiencing difficulty in their relationships. This service may be free, or people may make a contribution.
The Samaritans	Provides confidential and emotional support to people in crisis and at risk of suicide. The Samaritans is available 24 hours a day. Local branches can be found in the phone book under S, or phone 0345 909090.

Local voluntary organisations

In most areas there are local voluntary organisations that have grown up to meet the needs of the local population. They are often listed and co-ordinated by a local Council for Voluntary Service (CVS). They are also listed under 'Voluntary organisations' in *Yellow Pages* telephone directories. There is a wide range of these organisations. Some are self-help groups. Others meet the needs of people from a variety of ethnic and national backgrounds. They may provide specific information services, advice and support.

Do this!   8.5

1   Find out about and list any locally based organisations in your area. You may be able to obtain some leaflets about them.

2   Make a leaflet for parent and carers of children at a local school about the local and national voluntary services that are available in their area.

Private provision

Some support services can be purchased privately, for example personal and family therapy, different forms of counselling, domestic and care assistance. These services tend to be expensive and financially impossible for many people, but they can provide a very useful service for many people in need of personal support.

✅ Progress check

1   Which Act of Parliament gave the local authority a duty to provide services for children in need in their area?
2   Who is a 'child in need'? Try to put the definition in your own words.
3   Which Act gave local authorities the responsibility for assessing the individual needs of clients?
4   What do the NSPCC, NCH and Barnados provide?
5   Which voluntary societies provide telephone helplines for the public?
6   Which private personal services can people purchase themselves?

Housing

State provision

Local authorities act as enablers in the provision of housing and are expected to take a strategic approach encompassing all housing issues in their area. They encourage new house building by others in the private and voluntary sector, and have a duty to ensure that families in their area are not homeless. They first provided council housing at the beginning of the twentieth century, but the demand for council housing has always been greater than the supply, and has always therefore been limited to certain categories of people. There was a massive slum clearance and rebuilding programme after the Second World War, and local authorities continue to have a duty to rehouse certain families displaced by slum clearance or redevelopment schemes.

Local authorities are expected to maintain the condition of their existing housing stock, but the amount of council housing is constantly declining since the Conservative government introduced the 'right to buy' policy in the early 1980s. People have been encouraged to buy their council houses, but councils were not allowed by law to build new houses with the money gained from sales. As a result, there are fewer houses available for families. The sale of council houses has, in part, contributed to the rise in homelessness.

> **Think about it**
>
> What are the advantages and disadvantages both to the individual and to the state of the right for occupiers to buy their council homes?

Homelessness

Local authorities have a duty to house homeless families but, as they have insufficient accommodation, they often have to place homeless families in hostels, of which there are few, or in bed and breakfast accommodation, which is a very expensive and unsuitable, especially when there are young children.

Housing Benefit is paid by local councils to people who need help to pay their rent.

Voluntary provision

Housing associations

Large charitable trusts, such as the Guinness Trust and the Peabody Trust, have a long history of providing housing in some cities. More recently, other voluntary bodies have formed **housing associations**. The government has supported this movement, encouraging the growth of housing associations and providing money for them through the Housing Corporation, which is based in London.

Housing associations provide an alternative to council housing. They exist to provide homes for people in need of housing from a variety of social and cultural backgrounds; they are non-profit-making. They provide homes by building new units or by improving or converting older property.

> **housing associations**
> Non-profit-making organisations that exist to provide homes for people in need of housing from a variety of social and cultural backgrounds

Women's refuges

The local authorities help to finance refuges for women and their children, who are the victims of violent male partners. These refuges often act as half-way houses until they can re-accommodate the women.

Do this! 8.6

a) Find out about the housing associations in your area from your local CVS or from the Housing Corporation.
b) Make a list of those that provide housing for families with dependent children.

Private provision

Ownership

About 65 per cent of housing in the UK is owner-occupied. There has been an enormous growth in owner-occupation during the twentieth century. It is difficult for people on a low income to buy their own home, both because of the deposit required and the high cost of mortgage repayments.

Rental

The number of properties available for private rental has declined enormously during the twentieth century. This is especially so at the cheaper end of the market, where for a variety of reasons it is no longer very attractive to owners to let their properties to families. Nevertheless, nearly 10 per cent of all households live in privately rented accommodation. People with these tenancies are protected by law from sudden eviction.

✓ Progress check

1 Who does the state have a duty to provide accommodation for?
2 Why has there been a fall in the number of council houses available for renting?
3 Where might a homeless family be accommodated if there are no council houses available?
4 What is a housing association?
5 Where might a woman and her children go if they are the victims of violence?
6 How many households live in privately rented accommodation?
7 In what way are private tenants protected?

Social security

Statutory social security

The aim of statutory social security is to make sure that all adults have a basic income when they are unable to earn enough to keep themselves and their dependents. There is a range of financial benefits and allowances payable by the Department of Social Security (DSS) (central government) through its local Benefits Agency to people in a range of different circumstances. The Social Security Act (1986) set out the main changes, which were introduced in April 1988.

Changes to the system since 1998

In the spring of 1998 the Labour government announced major changes to the ways that state benefits are to be paid. This is part of its New Deal Welfare-to-Work programme. Its aim is to help and encourage people to work where they are capable of doing so, to support families and children, tackle child poverty, and to establish a flexible and efficient welfare system which is easier for people to use.

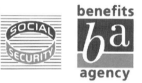

Logos of Social Security and the Benefits Agency

Types of benefits

Contributory benefits
Contributory benefits include sickness, unemployment, disability, old age, maternity and widowhood benefits. These are paid to people in particular categories providing they have previously made a contribution (National Insurance contributions are deducted from a person's pay).

Non-contributory benefits
To receive non-contributory benefits a person has to be in a particular financial group or category, but does not have to have made a contribution beforehand. Non-contributory benefits fall into two groups:
- *universal benefits* – given to all people in a certain category who claim them, whatever their income. These include Child Benefit, payable to all mothers, and Disability Living Allowance (Some politicians think that these benefits should be means-tested like those below.)
- *means-tested benefits* – only given to people in a certain category providing their income and savings are below a certain level. To claim, these people must fill in lengthy forms (tests) about their income (means), hence the phrase **means test**. This can put people off claiming them.

---

means test
An assessment of a person's income and savings, made by completing a form (test) about their income (means) to determine whether they are eligible to receive certain benefits

Major benefits for families

Child Benefit

This is seen as the cornerstone of the government's support for the family (it was formally called Family Allowance). It is considered to be the fairest, most efficient and most cost-effective way of recognising the extra costs and responsibilities borne by all parents. Rises in the amount of benefits paid are accompanied by the suggestion that taxation of high-paid families who receive this benefit is likely. The one-parent benefit that was previously paid has been abolished.

Income Support

Income Support is one of the main benefits in this group; it is payable to people who are not in paid employment, or who are employed part-time, according to the DSS definition, and whose income falls below a certain level. Any income, whether from wages, or from Child or Unemployment Benefit, is deducted from Income Support. The amount of money given in Income Support includes allowances for members of the family and for different needs. The level at which payments are is set is a political decision. The government has for many years fixed this at the *poverty line*. This means that below this level of income people are accepted as living in relative poverty. This benefit is believed by some to be inadequate because those who live on Income Support for a long time are effectively living in poverty.

New initiatives to help unemployed claimants

The Labour government is continuing the movement by the previous Conservative government to encourage people to work if they are able. It aims to rebuild the welfare state on the 'work ethic', and now calls benefits for those who are registered as unemployed the **Job Seekers' Allowance**. Its work-or-training scheme for 18–24-year-olds, which became effective in April 1998, has been extended in many directions. In June 1998, the 225,000 people over 25, who had been receiving benefits for two years or more, received a £75-a-week subsidy for employers to take them on, described by the government as a 'passport to work'. The New Deal also includes rights for up to 250,000 partners of unemployed claimants, 95 per cent of them women, who had previously been denied access to unemployment programmes. Lone parents looking for work have also been targeted for support.

Job Seekers' Allowance
Benefits paid to people who are registered as unemployed

Family Credit

Until October 1999, Family Credit is a payment to families where a parent is in full-time work, but their income is below a certain level. The government advertises this benefit, but many people who are eligible do not claim it. The claim form is long, and completing can be difficult for some people who may need assistance. It also acts as a disincentive for people to earn more, because at a certain point they loose their Family Credit and may be worse off. This has prompted new initiatives with the aim of giving self-respect and dignity back to low-paid workers by allowing them to keep more of their earnings.

New initiatives to help working families who are low paid

In the March 1998 Budget, effective from October 1999, hundreds of thousands of low-paid families are guaranteed a minimum income of £180 a week through the introduction of an American-style Working Family Tax Credit (WFTC), which replaces Family Credit. It is designed to lift the 'ceiling on the aspirations of men and women wanting to work their way up'. This reverses the situation where low-paid workers are sometimes forced to exist on state benefits because high rates of taxation make it uneconomic to work.

Under the WFTC, low-paid workers keep more of what they earn. Low-income families can also claim a tax credit which provides a maximum of 70 per cent of their child-care costs up to a ceiling of £150 a week; this, together with other initiatives, aims to ensure that 'all work pays'. Families are able to choose which partner receives the tax credit, which is either paid through the wage packet or directly to a non-working parent. Claimants must work a minimum of 16 hours a week, but those working more than 30 hours receive extra credit

Social Fund

The Social Fund is a fund out of which payments are made to meet special needs not covered by Income Support. Most of this money is given in the

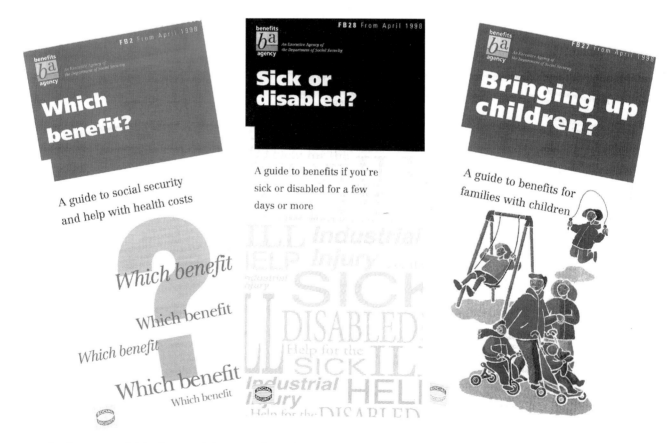

Leaflets are available about a whole range of benefits

form of loans to meet crisis and special household expenses. The criticisms of this benefit are that:

- it is discretionary (officers can chose whether to give it or not)
- it requires repayments by claimants who already have a low income
- there is a limited amount of money in the fund each year.

Do this! 8.7

Obtain current information about the whole range of social security benefits, and how much is payable. Leaflets are available at post offices and local social security offices (addresses in the telephone directory). Using the information:

a) Calculate the amount of Income Support that might be paid to a lone mother who has two children aged 3 and 5 and who does not work.

b) Find out what is regarded as full-time and part-time work by the government for benefit purposes. Then make some calculations of your own about the amount of money which would be given in Income Support to some imaginary families of different sizes and structures.

c) Work out how much some families of different sizes can earn and still be eligible for Family Credit up to October 1999 or WFTC after that.

Voluntary provision

Charities

There are many charities that give financial assistance to people in need in different situations. People need first to be aware of these and then to put in an application stating their case. Gaining awareness and making applications can both be difficult and people may need help with this. A further difficulty is that since the social security changes in 1988, the pressure on charities has been greatly increased and demand for their funds far exceeds money available. *The Charities Digest* gives the names of some charities with funds to help children and families.

Private services

People are at liberty to borrow money from private sources. Those who are already financially secure, with a job and a house, are more likely to be able to borrow from sources like banks and building societies, and to have credit cards.

Those who are less secure have to go to less reputable sources if they need extra money, these include private companies and individuals (sometimes referred to as 'loan sharks'). People borrowing in this way may be charged higher interest rates and thus be put at a further disadvantage, and slide deeper into debt.

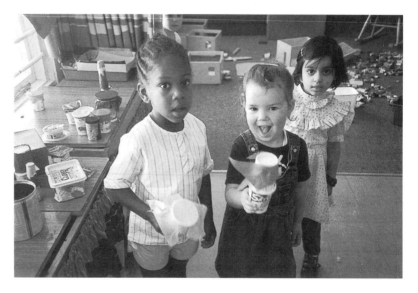

The National Childcare Strategy aims to ensure good quality, accessible, affordable child care for all children

Health

Statutory provision

The National Health Service (NHS) was created in 1948 to give free health care to the entire population of the UK. Since it was founded:

■ the general health of both children and adults has improved
■ the demand for services has continued to increase, despite improvements in general health
■ more expensive technology and treatments has meant that the cost of the service has increased enormously and is continuing to do so.

This increase in cost has resulted in a series of reforms over the years aimed at achieving greater efficiency, and to what some regard as a decline in standards, for example the increase in hospital waiting lists and the introduction and gradual increase in prescription charges.

District Health Authorities

The Department of Health (central government) is in overall charge of policy and planning for the health service and social care. It gives power and money to the 192 district health authorities (DHAs) in Britain.

The role of each district health authority is to:

- determine the full range of health needs of the local population, from vaccinations, to mending fractures to treating cancer
- plan the shape of the services required, including the services of dentists, pharmacists and opticians
- purchase the services required to meet local health needs
- review their effectiveness and make any necessary changes.

The National Health Service and Community Care Act 1990 led to a series of reforms. This Act aimed to bring the 'market place' into the health service. This means that within the service there is a health authority that *purchases* services in a planned way from different trusts (hospitals and other services) that *provide* health care to patients.

NHS trusts

More recently the concept of a 'market' for health care has been modified, with health authorities co-ordinating groups of primary health care teams (GPs and community nurses) to commission the services that their patients need from NHS trusts. These are both:

- community trusts, providing community services such as health visitors, midwives and clinics at health centres
- hospital trusts, providing a range of out- and in-patient services.

The work of the NHS trusts includes emergency and acute services, as well as meeting longer term needs in mental health and disability.

Voluntary provision

There is a long history of health care and provision through the voluntary sector in the UK. Many hospitals with voluntary status however, including famous ones like such as St Bartholomew's in London, became a part of the NHS when it was formed in 1948. Prior to this, people had to pay to see a GP, and if they could not afford this they sometimes went to a charitable hospital instead.

There are many voluntary organisations and self-help groups covering a very wide range of medical conditions and impairments that aim to help and support people, and to fund research.

The Sick Children's Trust is a national charity providing accommodation for the families of sick children at centres of specialist paediatric care. The trust owns houses in different cities in which it aims to provide homely accommodation to families at times of great stress.

Private provision

There has been a large growth in private sector provision since 1979. Increasingly, people who are able to, and wish to, pay into private insurance schemes and then receive their treatment privately. This usually means that they do not have to wait for treatment, and the physical standards in private hospitals is usually better. However, not all services are provided in the private sector, including accident and emergency services.

Some people believe that the presence of the private sector contributes to the growth of a two-tier health service, where those who can, pay for a good service, and those who cannot, make do with a poorer service by the NHS (similar to the effect of having private and state schools).

Think about it

1 It has been found that the people who most need services are often the least likely to use them. This is especially true, for example, in the use of antenatal and postnatal care. Why do you think this is?
2 Do you think that the presence of the private sector contributes to the growth of a two-tier health and education service?

Progress check

1 When and why was the NHS created?
2 What do District Health Authorities do?
3 What does the work of NHS trusts include?
4 What do self-help groups do?
5 Why do some people choose to pay for private health care?

Key terms

You need to know what these words and phrases mean. Go back through the chapter and find out.

children in need
grant-maintained status (GMS)
housing associations
Job Seekers' Allowance
local management of schools (LMS)
means test
National Childcare Strategy
private services
statutory school age
statutory services
voluntary services

Now try these questions

1 What are the main differences between a statutory, a voluntary and a private organisation.

2 How might differing political approaches affect the level of service provision in an area?

3 In what ways does the voluntary sector supplement the work of the state in providing services for children and their families?

4 What major new initiatives have there been in the area of social security provision for families?

5 How does the 'market place' affect the provision of health services?

9 The family

This chapter includes:

- **Care and protection: the alternatives**
- **The family**
- **The structure of the family**
- **Partnership arrangements**
- **Family size and family roles**
- **Alternative forms of child care in the UK**
- **Working with children and their families**

Children are totally dependent at birth. They move from dependence towards independence throughout childhood. In order to survive and develop during this period of dependency, they need care, security, protection, stimulation and social contact. In most societies, and at most times throughout history, children have most commonly been nurtured and cared for within families. The family is therefore of greatest significance to a child's development. However, people have different ideas about the groupings of people that can be defined as constituting 'a family'. Whatever the definition, it is clear that families have many functions in common, but many differences in their formation and how they carry out their tasks.

You may find it helpful to read this chapter in conjunction with:

▶ **Book 1, Chapter 10** An introduction to social and emotional development
▶ **Book 2, Chapter 8** Early years care and education
▶ **Book 2, Chapter 10** Social issues

Care and protection: the alternatives

The family, both in the past and present, is by far the most common environment for bringing up children, both in the UK and in other countries. The family is probably the most common arrangement for child care because it the most practical way to meet both children's and parents' needs. However, there are circumstances and places where alternatives to family life have been either necessary or thought to be preferable.

The most significant alternatives to family life are children's homes, communes and kibbutzim.

Children's homes

Large children's homes, sometimes called orphanages, used to exist in the UK. Children whose parents were either dead or unable to care for them were cared for in large groups. This type of institutional children's home is no longer provided for this purpose in the UK. Where there is a need, children are mainly cared for in foster homes or small residential units. Some large children's homes have been redesigned to provide respite care in small units for children with special needs. Large institutions do, however, still exist in some parts of Europe, especially in some former communist countries, where, as formerly happened in the UK, some children of very poor parents, children with disabilities and orphans are left in state care.

Communes

Occasionally people live together in communes. Adults share tasks and bring up their children collectively. This arrangement was popular among a small minority of people in the 1960s and 1970s in the USA and the UK.

Kibbutzim

Think about it

What are the advantages and disadvantages of the different types of alternative child-care arrangement described above?

Some people in Israel live on kibbutzim. A kibbutz is a place where people live and work together for the economic benefit of the whole community. Children are cared for together, in units separate from their parents, leaving parents free to use their time and energy for work. This system still exists but the separation of children and parents is now often modified. (See also Book 1, page 280.)

> ### ✓ Progress check
>
> 1 Why is the family the most common environment for child care?
> 2 What are the main reasons that children have been and still are cared for in institutions?
> 3 Where do large institutions still exist?
> 4 What is a kibbutz?

The family

What is a family?

It is surprisingly difficult to define what a family is, but it can be said that:
- all families have things in common
- all families are different.

One very general definition is:

'a group of related people who support each other in a variety of ways, emotionally, socially and/or economically'.

Case study: Different families

In a busy nursery class the teacher is aware of the personal details of some the children who attend. Anna lives with her grandmother, her mother is dead and her father is unknown. Royston lives with his mother, who is unmarried, and his half sister. Jamil lives with his grandparents, parents, uncle, aunt and cousins. Jasmin lives with her mother and her mother's female partner. Tom lives with his father, his father's new partner and her older daughter.

1 According to the definition above, which of these children are living in a 'family'?
2 Are there any reasons that some people might say that any of these children are not living in a family?

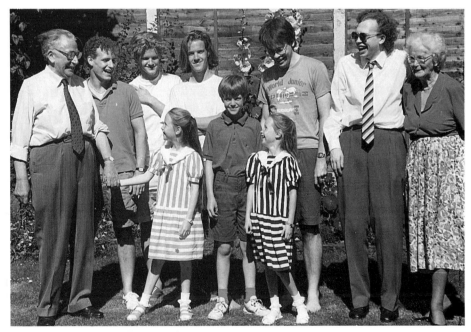

An extended family (see page 161) enables children to develop a variety of caring relationships

Why study the family?

Family life, in some form, is basic to the experience of most children. The family has a strong influence on every aspect of a child's life and development. For this reason, child-care workers need to:

- understand the importance of the family to children's development
- know the particular family background of the children in their care
- understand the possible influences and effects of different family circumstances on children.

The functions of the family and the similarities between families

The **functions of the family** are the things the family does for its members. Families all perform similar functions to a lesser or greater extent. These functions are:

- socialisation
- practical care and protection
- emotional, social support
- economic support.

Families do however have different traditions, customs and ways of carrying out these functions.

> **functions of the family**
> The things the family does for its members

Socialisation

Families provide the basic and most important environment in which children learn the **culture** of the society of which they are a part. The family consciously and unconsciously teaches children the main aspects of any culture. These are shared **values**, **norms** and a language.

The peer group, schools and the media have a strong influence as children grow older, but children learn the foundations of culture within the family

> **culture**
> The way of life, the language and the behaviour that is acceptable and appropriate to the society in which a person lives

Practical care and protection

The family is very effective in providing practical day-to-day care for its dependent members – children, those who are sick or have disabling conditions and those who are old. Caring for people outside the family is much more expensive, and often less effective.

> **values**
> Beliefs that certain things are important and to be valued, for example a person's right to their own belongings

Emotional and social support

Families perform a very important role. They give a baby a name and initial position in society. (When we hear of an abandoned baby, we immediately wonder who the child is and where the child comes from.) The family gives us an identity, a sense of belonging and a feeling of being valued.

A child's family is able to provide a positive feeling of worth that is fundamental (basic and very important) to healthy emotional development. It meets the basic need for love and affection, company and security. In a busy and crowded life, people are less likely to find this support outside their family where contacts are more impersonal. Foster care, or adoption (that is, a substitute family), is now the usual provision in the UK for children who lose their families. This is because the experience of family life is regarded as very important for emotional and social well-being.

> **norms**
> The rules and guidelines that turn values into action

Economic support

The extent of economic support that families provide varies between cultures. The family is still an economic unit in many ways. However, in the UK and other European countries, family members are no longer totally dependent on each other for survival. The state now provides an economic safety net, through for example social security benefits, which prevents the starvation and destitution that people experienced in the past when they were dependent on their families.

✓ **Progress check**

1 What is:
   a) a value?
   b) a norm?
2 What are the main functions of the family?

The structure of the family

Although there are many similarities between families, there are many variations in their structure and size. These differences can significantly affect the way families carry out their functions and, therefore, the lives of children.

The nuclear family with two parents

nuclear family
A family grouping where parents live with their children and form a small group with no other family members living near to them

family of origin
The family a child is born into

The **nuclear family** is a family grouping where parents live with their children and form a small group. They have no other relatives living with them or close by. This type of family has become increasingly common in modern societies like the UK, where many people move for work or education and leave their **family of origin** (that is, the one a person is born into).

In countries where there is an agricultural economy and people work on the land, they are much more likely to remain near their family of origin.

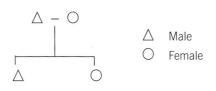

△ Male
○ Female

An example of a nuclear family

socio-economic group
Grouping of people according to their status in society, based on their occupation, which is closely related to their wealth/income; another way of referring to someone's social class

Social and cultural variations in nuclear families

Nuclear families are more common in higher **socio-economic groups** (see Chapter 10, page 177), that is among those employed in managerial, administrative and professional jobs (such as running businesses, teaching or the law). These families are more likely to move around for education and employment. The fact that they will earn higher incomes make this possible and worth doing. In some nuclear families, parents have developed a system of sharing family responsibilities. This is called a *democratic system*, because partners share earning money, child care and domestic jobs.

Life in a nuclear family

Children who grow up in a small nuclear family may:
■ experience close relationships within the family
■ receive a lot of individual attention
■ have more space and privacy.
They may, however:
■ feel a sense of isolation
■ experience intensity of attention from parents
■ have fewer people to turn to at times of stress
■ suffer if their parents have no support system to care for them at times of illness or need.

The nuclear family with one parent

The terms 'one-parent family' or 'lone-parent family' are used to describe families with dependent children that are headed by a lone parent. Of these, roughly 10 per cent are headed by men, 90 per cent by women. Of the women, about 60 per cent are divorced or separated, 23 per cent are single and 7 per cent widowed

Social and cultural variations in one-parent families

An increasing number of children in the UK (one in every eight) is born to women who are not married. The incomes of most lone parents are lower than those of most two-parent families. Many receive state benefits and their lifestyle is affected as there is little spare money for luxuries. Both they and their children are also vulnerable at times of difficulty, such as illness, if they do not have an extended family (see opposite) nearby to support them. The publicity given to the Child Support Agency has focused attention on the government's attempts to make fathers more financially responsible for their families following separation.

Only a small minority of lone parents are well off economically and receive incomes that enable them to work and to afford day care for their younger children. Most lone mothers are less likely to work, as their income would not enable them to pay for child care. However, the government now has a clear policy to support them with their child-care costs, and to encourage them not to be dependent on welfare benefits. Most lone parents are divorced or separated, a smaller number are single parents. A high proportion are in the lower socio-economic groups.

Although there are many married couples in the African-Caribbean community, there is also a tradition of single parenthood. This was one of the outcomes of slavery in the Caribbean, where the nurturing of children by their fathers was forbidden. Subsequent high unemployment rates both in the West Indies and in the UK have perpetuated this tradition of low involvement by fathers. Many African-Caribbean families, therefore, tend to be **matriarchal**, where women are important and dominant.

matriarchal family
A family in which women are important and dominant

Life in a one-parent family

Children who grow up in a one-parent family:

■ may establish a close, mutually supportive relationship with the parent they live with

■ may maintain a close relationship with their other parent and his or her family.

However, they may:

■ have experienced a period of grief and loss when their parents separated

■ lose contact with their other parent

■ experience lower material standards than children in a two-parent family

■ have less adult attention at times when their parent is coping with practical and emotional difficulties.

The extended family

> **extended family**
> A family grouping which includes other family members who live either together or very close to each other and are in frequent contact with each other

An **extended family** extends beyond parent(s) and children to include other family members, for example grandparents, uncles and aunts. A family is usually referred to as extended when its members:

■ live either together or very close to each other

■ are in frequent contact with each other.

Many people who live at a distance from their relatives gain a great deal of emotional support from them, but distance makes the practical support offered by a close extended family difficult. When an extended family who live together includes only two generations of relatives such as uncles, aunts and cousins, it is referred to as a *joint family*.

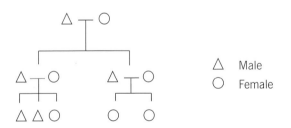

An example of an extended family

Social and cultural variations in extended families

People in lower socio-economic groups involved in semi-skilled or manual jobs are less likely to move from their locality for work or education. This means that they are more likely to be part of a long-established extended family system. In white, working-class families, there is a tradition of women staying close to their mothers. A matriarchal system is common. Roles within the family are likely to be divided, with men traditionally the bread-winners and women in charge domestically, although they may also work outside the home.

Families who came originally from India, Pakistan and Bangladesh have maintained a tradition of living in close extended families. Many came from rural areas where this was traditional. Their cultural and religious background also places a strong emphasis on the duty and responsibility to care for all generations of the family. These extended families are usually **patriarchal**, where men are dominant and make the important decisions. On marriage, a woman becomes a part of her husband's family and usually lives with or near them.

> **patriarchal family**
> A family in which men are dominant and make the important decisions

Families whose origins are in Mediterranean countries, such as Cyprus and Italy, also tend to have a strong extended family tradition. Family members frequently meet together for celebrations. Daughters tend to stay close to their mothers on marriage, but the man has considerable authority in the family.

Life in an extended family

Children who experience life within an extended family:
- have the opportunity to develop and experience a wide variety of caring relationships
- are surrounded by a network of practical and emotional support.

However, they may:
- have little personal space or privacy
- feel they are being observed by and have to please a large number of people
- have less opportunity to use individual initiative and action.

The reconstituted family

> **reconstituted family**
> A family grouping in which the adults and children who have previously been part of a different family

The **reconstituted family**, or reorganised family, is an increasingly common family system now that an increasing number of parents divorce and remarry. A reconstituted family contains adults and children who have previously been part of a different family. The children of the original partnership usually live with one parent and become the step-children of the new partner and step-siblings of the new partner's children. Children born to the new partnership become half-siblings. Such families vary in their size and structure, and may be quite complicated!

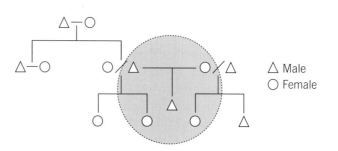

△ Male
○ Female

An example of a reconstituted family

Social and cultural variations in reconstituted families

Reconstituted families are more common among people who accept divorce. This could include people who have no religious beliefs, and Protestant Christians. Muslims do not forbid divorce, but are committed to family life and divorce is less common.

Reconstituted families are less common amongst people who have a strong belief in the family and who disapprove of divorce, usually because their religious doctrines are against it. These include Hindus, Sikhs and Roman Catholics to whom marriage is sacred and should not be dissolved.

Life in a reconstituted family

This can be a positive experience for a child because:
- their parent may be happier, more secure and have greater financial resources
- the child gains a parent and possibly an extended family.

However, they may:
- have difficulty relating to a step-parent and step-brothers and sisters
- have to compete for attention with children of their own age
- feel a loss of attention because they have to share their parent
- have to accept the birth of children of their parent's new relationship.

Do this!   **_9.1_**

Draw a diagram of your own family tree and show whether it is nuclear, extended or reconstituted.

✓ **_Progress check_**

1 What is a nuclear family?
2 What is an extended family?
3 What is a reconstituted family?
4 Why are there an increasing number of reconstituted families?

Partnership arrangements

Adults have a wide variety of arrangements for the way they form partnerships. These provide different care environments for children.

Partnership arrangements include:
- *monogamy* – the marriage between heterosexual partners (one partner of each gender); this is still popular in the UK, although the rate of marriage has declined since the 1960s
- *polygamy* – the marriage of a person of one gender (usually a man) to a number of others (usually women) at the same time; it is illegal to enter into this arrangement in the UK, where it is called *bigamy*. It has been very common in other countries, especially those with Muslim cultures

cohabitation
A relationship in which partners live together without being married

■ *serial monogamy* – a term used to describe one person of either gender having one partner followed by another over a period of time, each followed by separation or divorce

■ *cohabitation* – partners live together without the legal tie of marriage; this is increasingly common in the UK, where about 30 per cent of partners cohabit; although many later marry their partner, especially after they have children. This arrangement is now acceptable among many social groups who would have previously seen it as a disgrace; some people, including Asian families, continue to believe it is wrong and unacceptable

■ *homosexual partnerships* – especially between women, are increasingly viewed as an acceptable base for the rearing of children. As recently as the early 1980s, women who left their husbands to live with a woman often lost the custody of their children; such an arrangement was thought unsuitable. In June 1994, two women from Manchester became the first lesbian couple to be made the joint legal parents of the child of one of them. This was made possible by the Children Act (1989) because it enables parental responsibility to be shared by a range of people. All the research carried out since the 1960s shows no differences in the social and emotional development of children of lesbian and heterosexual partnerships, or to their gender orientation.

Think about it

In what ways do you think that the different partnership arrangements outlined above make any fundamental difference to a child's happiness and development?

Case study: Family life

Mr and Mrs Jameson were married 26 years ago. They have three children, Sylvia, Roy and Belinda. Sylvia divorced her husband and now lives with her new partner in a house in the same road as her parents and sees them frequently. She has two daughters and he has a son, all of whom live with them. Sylvia's ex-husband has remarried and now has a baby son. Roy is also married, to a woman who has a child but was never married; they have one son, but live many miles away. Belinda lives locally with her female partner and their two daughters each from previous relationships that have ended in divorce. Her parents baby-sit regularly while they work.

1 Which family members are monogamously married?
2 What proportion of all the people in this scenario's original marriages ended in divorce?
3 Which people are living as part of an extended family?
4 Are any people in this case study not living in a family?
5 Draw a family tree and try to include all these people!

Family breakdown: divorce and separation

Marriage is a legal contract between two people. It places on partners certain duties to behave reasonably and to support each other. It also gives certain rights to both partners, including the right to live in the marital home and to have equal parental responsibility for their children.

The sole grounds for divorce following the Divorce Reform Act (1969) is the 'irretrievable breakdown' of a marriage. The evidence that can be used to prove breakdown is:

- adultery
- unreasonable behaviour
- desertion for two years
- partners living separately for two years and each agreeing to a divorce
- partners living separately for five years.

The breakdown of the partnership between parents is usually experienced as stressful by children, whether their parents are legally married or not. Children can feel a deep sense of loss, and even blame themselves.

An unmarried father has no legal rights over his children following separation, unless he has acquired parental responsibility.

When a partnership breaks down, there can be disagreements between parents about where a child should live and how often each parent should see the child. In such a dispute, parents can apply to the court for orders under the Children Act 1989. This Act replaced orders that previously concerned custody and access with four new orders known as **Section 8 Orders**, which together with a *Family Assistance Order*, determine with whom a child should live, who they can have contact with, and some of the steps and decisions adults can take.

| **Section 8 Orders** |
| Passed by a court when there is a dispute about whom a child should live with, who they can have contact with, and some of the steps and decisions adults can take about them |

Section 8 Orders

The four Orders are:

- a *Residence Order*, stating who the child is to live with; it can be made in favour of more than one person and state how much time the child should spend with each person
- a *Contact Order*, requiring the person with whom the child lives to allow the child to have contact with the person named on the Order; parents, grandparents and other family members may apply for this if they are being denied contact with a child
- a *Prohibited Steps Order*, applied for if someone objects to something that a parent is doing concerning a child; the order aims to restrict the way that a person exercises their parental responsibility, for example, whether they can take a child abroad
- a *Specific Issues Order*, aiming to settle disputes about a child's care and upbringing; it can make a specific order, for example concerning education or medical treatment.

The Family Assistance Order aims to provide short-term help to a family who cannot overcome their disagreements concerning their children following separation.

| **Think about it** |
| Why is it important that child-care workers know of any court orders that relate to the children in their care? |

| ***Do this!***   **9.2** |
| Research the statistics about the rise in the rate of divorce in the past 150 years. Present your findings graphically and explore the reasons for the rise in divorce. |

> ✅ **Progress check**
>
> 1 What is:
>   a) monogamy?
>   b) polygamy?
>   c) cohabitation?
> 2 What are the sole grounds for divorce?
> 3 What are the four main Section 8 Orders?
> 4 What does a Family Assistance Order aim to provide?

Family size and family roles

Family size

The average number of dependent children per family in the UK is now a little less than two children This has gradually fallen since the middle of the last century when it was about six. The most significant reasons for this change are:

- the increased availability of contraception and legal abortion
- a rise in the standard of living, together with the fact that children are costly to support and they start work later than in the past
- changes in women's roles, attitudes and expectations; many women regard child-rearing as only a part of their lives and want to do other things as well.

Although the average family has two children, there are of course larger families. Children from large families have some differences in their life experiences. Research shows that on average their life chances are not as good as children from small families.

Many children grow up in families where they are the only child. These children are more successful, but there are possible social disadvantages for them.

Do this!	**9.3**
Carry out some research of your own: by writing a questionnaire and talking to people who are members of a large family, and people who are only children. Record the positive and negative aspects of their experiences and your own opinion, and present your results as a report	

Changing roles within the family

Domestic roles

There is evidence that, in families across a range of social and cultural groups in the UK, the traditional role of male as provider and bread-winner, and female as carer and homemaker, have changed. Men are increasingly involved in the care of their young children, and women are more likely to work outside the home. Research shows, however, that women still have the major responsibility for either doing or organising domestic work, whatever their social or cultural background.

Women and work

Nearly half the workforce in the UK is female. Although an increasing number of women with dependent children work outside the home, the younger their children are, the less likely they are to work either full or part-time. The growth of affordable child-care provision for young children is leading to an ever-increasing number of working mothers, and the government is encouraging this trend by supporting the expansion of child care. In some European countries, there is a much higher level of provision and a much higher proportion of mothers working outside the home.

Do this! 9.4

Find out some facts and figures about female employment and child-care facilities in the UK and other European countries. Interpret and present the data you collect.

Working parents

When both parents of young children work outside the home, they have to make some arrangement for the care of their children. An increasing choice of day care alternatives is available. Research shows that children's needs can be met if they are provided with good day care.

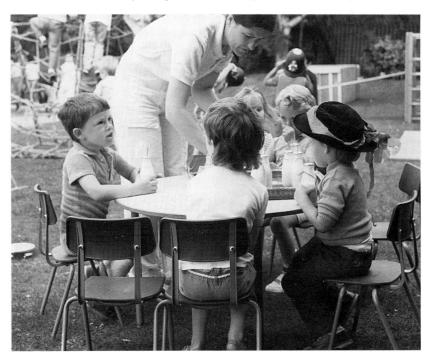

Research shows that children's needs can be met if they are provided with good day care

Case study: Changing roles

Wendy is married to John and they have a baby, Chloe, who is 9 months old. Chloe has attended a day nursery for five days a week since she was 6 months old, when her mother returned to work full-time as a pharmacist. Wendy and John share all the household tasks, including looking after Chloe, shopping and cooking. John's mother, Mary, sometimes visits and helps them out, but she has worked full-time for the past ten years so gets little spare time even for her own household tasks, though she does have a cleaner. She is a little concerned about her son and daughter-in-law's lifestyle, and often reminds them of how different it was when they were children. Wendy gets a bit annoyed when Mary reminds them of how she gave up work when her children were young and only returned part-time when they went to school. Wendy's grandfather, however, expresses very strong feelings about his grand-daughter's lifestyle. He remembers the time when his wife gave up work and became a housewife as soon as they were married. When Wendy, in her annoyance, once said to him 'What for?', he replied 'To look after me, that's what for. I went out early and she needed to be there to cook my breakfast'. Wendy decided not to respond to this.

1 What are the major changes in child-care practice that can be seen over these three generations?
2 How do the generations reveal the changing role of women in the world of work?
3 What changes can you see in men's and women's domestic roles?
4 Why do you think Wendy decided not to respond to her grandfather's statement?

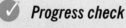 **Progress check**

1 What is the average number of dependent children per family in the UK?
2 What are the most significant reasons for the reduction in family size?
3 Why do an increasing number of mothers work?

Alternative forms of child care in the UK

Under the Children Act 1989, local authorities have a responsibility to provide a range of services to safeguard and provide welfare for 'children in need' in their area.

They can do this by providing advice, assistance and services to families, including day care. They may also look after children by providing accommodation for them on a full-time basis, in foster homes or community homes.

Local authority care

Provision of accommodation

Sometimes the most appropriate help a local authority can give a family is to provide accommodation for a child under a voluntary arrangement with the child's parents. This might be offered:

- to give parents respite (a break) from looking after a child who is difficult to care for. This can be a particularly valuable service for families with a child who has disabilities
- when a family situation makes it very difficult for parents to meet the needs of a child, through illness or severe family problems.

Parents may take their children home at any time under this voluntary arrangement, and they are encouraged to have regular contact with them.

Children in care

Local authorities aim to keep children and parents together, and to promote the care of children within their own families. There are, however, situations when a child's welfare can only be protected by removing them from their family. To do this, the local authority must obtain a court order. These orders are described in Chapter 14, *Child protection procedures*.

These orders include:

- an Emergency Protection Order
- a Child Assessment Order
- a Care Order.

Alternatively, the authority may be given the power to supervise a child compulsorily while they remain at home. To do this, the local authority needs:

- a Supervision Order

or

- an Education Supervision Order which places a school-age child under the supervision of the local authority if the court decides that the child is not attending school properly.

Types of substitute care

A local authority will provide the type of care for a child that is most appropriate to the child's needs. The type of care is not necessarily linked to whether the child is being looked after by being provided with accommodation under a voluntary agreement, or is the subject of a court order. Children may be placed in a foster home, a residential children's home or, in some circumstances, with adopters.

Foster care

Foster parents are people from all backgrounds who are recruited by a local authority to take children into their homes for short or longer periods of time. They can be single or married couples. They are interviewed at length concerning their suitability to look after children;

they need a range of qualities to meet the demands of looking after children whose behaviour may be disturbed by their life experiences. They may also have contact with the children's parents.

Once the foster parents are approved, they are paid a weekly allowance for children placed with them. Foster care is now considered the most appropriate form of substitute care for children who cannot be with their families. Local authority social services departments usually produce leaflets for the public to encourage them to apply to become foster parents or adopters.

Residential care

Residential care is the term used to describe children's homes, often referred to as *community homes*. They usually consist of small units, often ordinary houses within the community. They are staffed by residential social workers. They are generally considered to be unsuitable for the care of young children, except in special circumstances, such as emergencies or if their behaviour is initially very difficult to manage. They are more likely to be used to accommodate older children, larger families, or to assess children's developmental needs.

Adoption

Adoption is a legal process whereby the parental rights and responsibilities for a child are given up by one set of parents and taken on by another. Adoption must be arranged through a recognised adoption agency and an order made in court. All local authorities must provide an adoption service. Adopters go through a similar interview and selection process as foster parents. In recent years, the number of babies placed for adoption has declined enormously, from 2,649 in 1979 to 895 in 1991. Many adoptions now involve older children. Children have a right to make their wishes known at an adoption hearing. The current trend is towards open adoption, where some form of contact between a child and their birth parents or relatives is maintained. Attention is also given to the need to place children in families of the same ethnic origin.

Think about it
What qualities do you think foster parents or adopters need?

✓ Progress check

1 When might a child be provided with accommodation by a local authority?
2 How can a child be removed from home compulsorily?
3 Why is foster care considered to be the most suitable form of substitute care for young children?
4 Who is residential accommodation most likely to be provided for?
5 What does adoption do and in what circumstances may adoption be more suitable for a child than long-term foster care?

Working with children and their families

Good practice for child-care workers

There are some important points for anyone working with children and their families to remember.

- The family forms a central part of any child's life.
- Children come from a variety of family types and structures.
- Each child's family is important and meaningful to that individual child.
- Some children may be looked after in substitute families or establishments.
- We tend to be very self-centred in our view of families, seeing our own family as 'normal'.

Improving working practice

- Try to increase your awareness and understanding of different family patterns. You can do this by observing people around you, talking to them, reading books and articles, watching programmes on the television, films and videos. It is important to be open and willing to learn.
- Be aware of the alternative provisions for the care of children in the community.
- Inform yourself, when appropriate, of the family circumstances of each child in your care. Remember that confidentiality is essential, both in what you say to others and how you keep records.
- Assess the individual needs of each child. This is the only way that you can ensure equality of opportunity for each child. People who say that they 'treat all children the same' are denying children equality by not recognising and providing for their differences and particular needs.
- Plan the best way to meet children's individual needs and provide appropriate attention, care and stimulation.

✓ Progress check

1 Why does our view of families tend to be self-centred?
2 How can a worker increase their understanding of different types of families?
3 What is the best way a worker can meet children's individual needs?

Key terms

You need to know what these words and phrases mean. Go back through the chapter and find out.

cohabitation
culture
extended family
family of origin
functions of the family
matriarchal family
norms
nuclear family
patriarchal family
reconstituted family
Section 8 Orders
socio-economic group
values

Now try these questions

1 What are the most significant differences between the experience of life for a child in a nuclear, extended or reconstituted family?

2 Why have changes in women's roles, attitudes and expectations been one of the reasons for a fall in the number of children in the average family?

3 What might be the particular needs of only children and children from large families when they start at nursery?

4 What are the differences between the tasks that men and women do now compared to those in the past?

5 What should good substitute day care provide in order to meet the all-round developmental needs of young children?

10 Social issues

This chapter includes:

- **What is society?**
- **The individual and society**
- **Social action**
- **Social mobility**
- **Social pressures and social disadvantage**
- **People's differing responses to pressures and problems**

There are many things that affect the way that individuals and families live and experience life. Some of these are personal issues concerning their health, intelligence and personality, but others are social issues influenced by their experience of life, their education, wealth and position in society. Everyone experiences pressures in their life, but people have different practical, emotional and social resources to deal with these pressures. This can explain in part why people respond differently to problems and why some people are able to provide a good environment for their children despite considerable pressures, whilst others find it more difficult.

You may find it helpful to read this chapter in conjunction with:

- **Book 1, Chapter 12** Socialisation and social development
- **Book 2, Chapter 8** Early years care and education
- **Book 2, Chapter 9** The family

What is society?

What is society? One view is contained in the statement made in 1987 by Margaret Thatcher, the then Prime Minister of the UK: 'There is no such thing as Society. There are individual men and women, and there are families.' This statement has since been commented on by many people.

In contrast to this, many people believe that society does exist. They perceive that individuals and families do not live in isolation, but are both a part of a society and are strongly affected by their social and legal environment.

Society can be described as people living together within a framework of shared laws and customs that have been created over a period of time. Society provides the social, cultural, economic and physical environment for people's lives.

A multicultural society

All societies include different social groups. Many societies, including the UK, also include different cultural groups. A **multicultural society** is one that includes a variety of cultural groups who may have some differing social customs and rules. This can provide a varied and positive social environment. Sometimes the customs of one group become known and adopted by another group. In this way, people's lives are enriched. A simple example of this in the UK is the enjoyment by many people of the traditional foods of different cultural groups, for example Asian, Chinese and Italian.

For a multicultural society to work positively and be of benefit to all its members, it is essential that:

- certain laws are shared and respected by all
- there is mutual acceptance and tolerance of differences in customs
- no group has, or is thought to have, more power, status and resources than another.

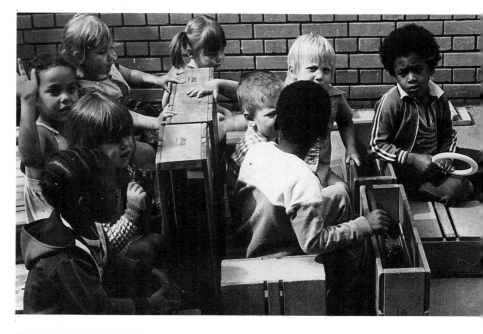

A multicultural society can provide a varied and positive social environment

Do this! 10.1

Discuss Margaret Thatcher's statement and decide what you think it means. Do you believe that something called 'society' exists in addition to individuals and families?

✔ Progress check

1 What is a society?
2 What is a multicultural society?
3 How can everyone benefit from living in a multicultural society?

The individual and society

The legal framework

The UK, like every democratic society, has a set of laws. These laws have been passed in parliament by elected representatives and apply to everyone. They form a framework of rules that cover the rights of citizens to be treated fairly and equally.

Laws include an outline of all citizens':

- rights to certain services
- right to protection from harm
- duties to behave in certain ways

and the penalties and punishments an individual will incur if they break the law.

Socially deviant behaviour

socially deviant behaviour
Behaviour that is socially different and does not follow the rules of the dominant group in a society

Socially deviant behaviour is behaviour that is socially different. Behaviour comes to be regarded as deviant by some people if it does not follow the rules of the dominant group in that society, or if it is unpredictable or undesirable to them.

There are two main types of deviant behaviour:

- *illegal* – this behaviour is criminal and carries legal sanctions to punish and prevent it; it includes violence, vandalism, theft and drug dealing
- *legal* – this behaviour may either be disapproved of or tolerated; it includes dressing and behaving differently, having no fixed abode, living and travelling in vehicles, prostitution.

The media can have a powerful influence on opinion if it labels certain groups as deviant, and then goes on to suggest that they are responsible for society's problems. The way that young people are sometimes portrayed is an example of this. Deviance does not necessarily result in poor parenting. Some parents whose behaviour is socially different, for example old style 'hippies', can meet the needs of their children very well. However, some lifestyles, including those involving drugs or alcohol abuse and criminal behaviour, may leave children more vulnerable to neglect.

Think about it

Why does deviant behaviour occur? Try to think of some explanations.

Do this! 10.2

a) List some common behaviour that is illegal but nevertheless regarded by many people as acceptable (breaking the speed limit, drinking and driving, using materials at work for your own purposes, etc.).

b) Devise a survey/questionnaire and ask a number of people whether they have ever done these things. Record their answers.

c) Collate your results and make a graph to illustrate them.

✅ **Progress check**

1 What makes up the legal framework of a democratic country like the UK?
2 What is socially deviant behaviour?
3 What may strongly influence people's attitudes to deviant behaviour?

Social action

Individual members of any society can significantly affect the society in which they live. They can do this by taking social action directed at other people in society in a variety of ways. Such behaviour can have both positive and negative effects.

Positive social action

- Throughout history individual politicians, social reformers, those in business, industry and the media have brought about positive changes to society and people's lives.
- On a smaller scale, some people work hard in their local communities. They give time and energy through different organisations, and contribute to the lives of the people around them. Others contribute to the richness of society by participating in everyday events within their local schools and community groups.
- Some members of society use their energy simply and positively to cope with their own lives and with their families.
- Sometimes people perceive that they have a worse position in society than others, but they do not accept their situation passively. They want to achieve a better position. They sometimes join together to fight what they see as an unfair system. The trade union movement, for example, grew out of this perception. People may use legal means to achieve this (like marches and strikes), or they may feel justified in taking illegal action (suffragettes who were trying to win the vote did this).

Negative social action

Think about it

Think of other examples of positive and negative social action.

In many societies there are people who believe, rightly or wrongly, that the system is against them achieving success or equality. They believe they are discriminated against and denied access to the things that are valued by society as a whole. They do not believe that they can achieve anything either by positive group action or legal means. They take destructive action either against themselves, for example through drug addiction, or against individuals or groups, for example through crime, or against society as a whole, for example by terrorist acts.

Social mobility

A person's socio-economic status or position is often referred to as their social class. It is determined by the structure of the society that they live in. In the UK, a person's social status is usually decided by the type of work they do, which is also closely related to their wealth. For example, manual work is of lower status and is usually paid less than non-manual work. **Social mobility** refers to the movement of people from one social class to another.

social mobility
The movement of a person from one social group (class) to another

Society and socio-economic status

The UK government uses six socio-economic categories for people according to the occupation of the head of their household, as shown in the table below.

Social class in the UK

Socio-economic group	Type of job	Examples
1	Professional and higher administrative	Lawyers, accountants, doctors, directors of large companies
2	Intermediate professionals and administrative	Teachers, managers, librarians
3NM	Non-manual skilled workers	Nursery nurses, clerks, policemen, sales representatives, office clerks
3M	Skilled manual workers	Electricians, miners, train drivers, printers
4	Semi-skilled manual workers	Postmen, farm workers, telephonists
5	Unskilled manual workers	Cleaners, refuse collectors, porters, long-term unemployed on benefits

The government and market research organisations use these categories and carry out research into different aspects of people's lives. Research reveals that there are close links between a person's social class and their experience of, and chances in, life. Such research shows, for example, that those from higher groups are more likely to survive infancy, i.e. have lower infant mortality, have better health and live longer. Market research shows that what we buy and how we behave is also closely linked to our social class.

Do this!   *10.3*

Using the table above, work out and record the social class of the following occupations: a Director of Education, a teacher in a primary school, a child-care and education worker, a school secretary, a builder, a cook, a cleaner.

Social mobility and equality of opportunity

The test of how far a society gives equality of opportunity to its members is based on how easy it is for a citizen to move up to a social position with higher status, say from Group 5 to Group 2. In a 'closed' society (for example, the caste system in India, and in feudal Britain) people are ascribed, or given, a role and position in society at birth and can never move from this. In an 'open' society, people can achieve a different status because they are able to move from one social position to another. The ways they can do this are usually through the education system, their job or by marriage.

The extent to which children can move from their social position of birth depends on the relative openness of a society. Many people think that the USA is a more open society than the UK, where many people still find it difficult to be successful and upwardly mobile. This can be especially so of those people in the lowest socio-economic groups and also those who commonly experience prejudice and discrimination, including people from ethnic minority groups and those with disabilities. **Equal opportunities policies** are designed to overcome this, and to provide opportunities for all people to achieve according to their efforts and abilities.

> **equal opportunities policies**
> Policies designed to provide opportunities for all people to achieve according to their efforts and abilities

> **Think about it**
> How can an equal opportunities policy be put into practice in a nursery or school environment?

Do this!	*10.4*

1 Carry out some further research of your own to find out which groups of people in the UK are less likely to be successful. Interpret your information and present the data as a graph.
   Present your information to and discuss it with others. Suggest some reasons for inequality.

2 Find out what is stated in the equal opportunities policy of your place of work.

Children, the education system and social mobility

Children initially take the social status of their family of birth. The day-care and education system provides them with a real opportunity to broaden their experience and, if they wish, to change their social position as adults. The attitudes of their family of origin are very important in determining whether children make use of the opportunities provided for them.

The strong influence of family background becomes obvious when reading the published examination results of individual schools. With slight variations, the children from schools that are in areas where more families are from higher socio-economic groups achieve higher results than children from schools in areas where most families are from lower socio-economic groups. It would seem that, despite the introduction of equal opportunities policies and comprehensive schools in recent decades, social mobility through education is still limited.

Case study: Social mobility

The grandparents of Leroy and Sam were born in Jamaica and were encouraged to come to the UK in the 1950s to work on public transport. Their mother and father were originally left in the Caribbean until their parents were established, and they joined them in their early teens.

Leroy and Sam's mother became a nurse and their father worked in service industries. They lived in a flat in an inner-city area. Both boys attended their local schools. Leroy and Sam were bright children and their parents were very keen for them to do well. They encouraged them to work hard, listened to them read, and made sure that they did their homework. Their teachers encouraged them, and Leroy and Sam passed their exams at school well. Leroy went to university and studied law. He now works as a solicitor. His brother, Sam, did teacher training and now teaches in a local primary school.

1 Have Leroy and Sam been upwardly or downwardly socially mobile?
2 What were the most important things that enabled them to be socially mobile?

Think about it

The published examination results illustrate that many children who come from lower socio-economic groups tend on average to do less well academically at school. What reasons can you think of for this?

✓ Progress check

1 What usually determines a person's social status in the UK?
2 In what ways can a person's social class affect their chances in life?
3 What is social mobility?
4 What is the test of how far a society provides equality of opportunity for its members?
5 Which children tend to achieve better results at school?

Social pressures and social disadvantage

Personal and social pressures and problems

All adults are likely to face some kind of difficulty, problem or pressure in their lifetime. If they are parents, their children will probably be affected in some way by their experiences.

Some problems can be referred to more accurately as 'personal' others as 'social'. The source of personal problems lies very close to the circumstances of an individual person's life. Examples of personal problems are difficulties with or loss of relationships, bereavement, mental and physical ill-health. Other problems are referred to as 'social' when their source can be mainly found in the way the social and physical environment is organised. Examples of social problems are urban decay or rural decline, racial and social discrimination, poverty, unemployment, bad housing and homelessness.

Think about it

What other links may exist between the experience of social and personal problems? Explain the links.

There are often close links between personal and social problems; the experience of social problems often causes personal problems. For example, unemployment may cause stress, worry and feelings of uselessness; these can then lead to anxiety, depression and ill-health.

Sources of social disadvantage and pressure

People can be described as disadvantaged if they do not have an equal opportunity to achieve what other people in society regard as normal. This may be because they are experiencing poverty, unemployment, inadequate housing, homelessness, racial discrimination, an impoverished environment, or are sick or disabled.

Poverty

Lack of money is usually a major problem for people. A family is considered to be living in poverty if their income is less than half the national average weekly wage. This is called the *poverty line*. A Department of Social Security (DSS) report published by the government in 1994 revealed that 14 million people in the UK were living below the poverty line; four million of them were children. This is three times the number recorded in 1979.

Poverty is now usually described as being **relative**. This means that people are considered to be poor 'if their resources fall seriously short of the resources commanded by the average individual or family in the community' (Peter Townsend, *Poverty in the United Kingdom*, 1979). In the past in the UK there were many people living in **absolute poverty**, that is they did not have 'enough provision to maintain their health and working efficiency' (Seebohm Rowntree, *Studies of Poverty in the City of York*, 1899).

relative poverty
Occurs when people's resources fall seriously short of the resources commanded by the average individual or family in the community

absolute poverty
Not having enough provision to maintain health and working efficiency

> **Do this!** 10.5
>
> There are many references to poverty in sociology and social policy books. Read some of these so that you understand clearly the ideas of absolute and relative poverty, and write a report of your findings.

The main causes of poverty are low wages or living on state social security benefits. The people who are most likely to be poor are those who are:

- unemployed
- members of one-parent families
- members of black and other minority groups
- sick or incapacitated
- elderly
- low paid.

The effects of poverty on the family

Poverty can affect every area of a family's life. There may not be enough money for a nutritious varied diet, adequate housing, transport, household equipment, toys. It can cause stress, anxiety, unhappiness and lead to poor physical and mental health. People are limited in their ability to go out, to entertain others, and to have outings or holidays. Family relationships can become strained. People are aware through the media, especially television, that others have a much higher standard of living. All this can result in a feeling of hopelessness and of being outside (excluded from) the main stream of society.

Some sociologists refer to people in extreme poverty as the 'underclass' – a group of people who feel they have no hope of improving their situation. The Social Exclusion Unit works at the centre of government to bring socially-excluded people back into society.

Many people experience the **poverty trap** if they are receiving state benefits – they find that, by earning a small additional amount more, they lose most of their benefits and become worse off. They are trapped in their position. This is of great concern to the government who aim to get people out of this trap through introducing welfare reforms.

> **poverty trap**
> Experienced by people if they are receiving state benefits and they find that by earning a small amount more they lose most of their benefits and become worse off

Unemployment

Unemployment has always varied. It was high in the 1980s and since then it has both fallen and risen again. There is little hope of ever achieving full employment. Unemployment has affected every section of the population, but some people are more vulnerable to it than others. These are:

- people without skills or qualifications
- manual workers
- young and old people
- women
- people who generally suffer discrimination in society; these include people from ethnic minority groups and people who have disabilities
- people who have suffered mental illness or have been in prison.

The effects of unemployment on the family

Unemployment can have profound effects on individuals and families. Those experiencing long-term unemployment are more likely to be living in poverty and suffering its effects. They may also have feelings of shame, uselessness, boredom and frustration that can affect their mental and physical health. Family relationships can become strained, and provide an unhappy or even violent environment for children. Whole communities can become demoralised and run down.

Do this!   *10.6*

Find out what the current level of unemployment is and how this has varied in recent years. Find out who can and cannot register as unemployed.

Make an information factsheet for others.

Inadequate housing

Despite the fact that there has been a massive slum clearance and rebuilding programme since the 1950s, many people still live in accommodation that is damp, overcrowded and unsuitable for children. Some of the high-rise flats that were built to rehouse people in the 1950s and 1960s were very badly built. They contributed to a wide range of personal and social problems. Some of them have since been demolished or redesigned, although many still remain in some urban areas.

There are obvious links between people being poor and living in poor housing conditions. Those who have money buy accommodation that suits their needs. Those who are poor usually have to take anything that is available to them.

The effects of inadequate housing on the family

Damp, inadequate and dangerous housing can lead to bad health, illness, accidents, the spread of infection and poor hygiene. It is difficult to improve broken down houses or keep them clean. Adults may blame each other, feel depressed and worried. This, together with lack of play space, creates a unsuitable environment for children to grow up in.

Think about it
What are the disadvantages to a young family of living in a poorly maintained high-rise block of flats?

Homelessness

There is a national shortage of accommodation at affordable prices. This was caused in part in the 1980s by the Conservative government's policy of giving council tenants the right to buy their houses, while not allowing councils to use the money from sales to build more houses. Private owners are reluctant to let accommodation to families because legislation makes it difficult subsequently to evict them. There is a growing number of homeless people; they mainly become homeless when:

- their relatives are unwilling or unable to continue to provide them with accommodation
- they are evicted for mortgage or rent arrears
- their marriage or partnership breaks up.

The majority are:

- young
- either single or with young families
- on low incomes.

The local authority has a legal duty to accommodate homeless families. The shortage of accommodation means that an increasing number are placed in temporary bed and breakfast accommodation. The conditions for families in bed and breakfast hotels are totally unsuitable. The accommodation can often be overcrowded, dangerous and unhygienic. There is usually a lack of cooking, washing and other basic amenities. There is little privacy or play space. People often suffer isolation from family and friends. In addition, their access to education, health and other services is disrupted. Families can spend several years in this type of accommodation.

The effects of homelessness on the family

Living for a long period in cramped and unsatisfactory conditions can have a very bad effect on family relationships between adults and children. Parents who experience this degree of stress in their everyday existence may have little energy to provide more than the basic necessities for children. It is often difficult for people to maintain good standards of hygiene, and the provision of nutritious food can be a problem if there are little or no cooking facilities. The lack of play space can lead to children being under stimulated and having little access to fresh air and exercise. Their development can be affected in every area. The provision of day care can be of great value for children living in bed and breakfast accommodation.

Do this! 10.7

Produce a chart showing what children's developmental needs are, how they may not be met if a child is living in bed and breakfast accommodation, and how these needs could be met in a good day-care setting.

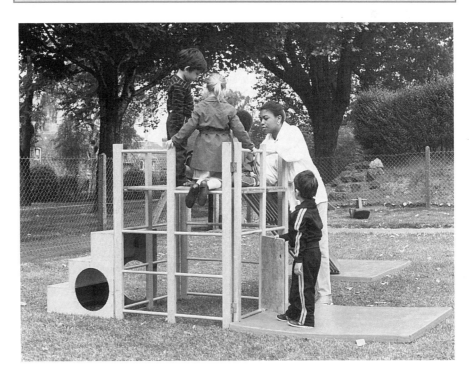

The provision of day care can be of great value for children living in bed and breakfast accommodation

ethnic group
A group of people who share a common culture

ethnic minority group
A group (of people with a common culture) which is smaller than the majority group in their society

Racial discrimination

Race is difficult to define, but the term is used describe a group who share some common biological traits. **Ethnic groups** are people who share a common culture. **Ethnic minority groups** are smaller than the majority group in their society.

There are many ethnic groups in the UK. Some attract little attention, for example the many people of Italian, Polish and Irish origin who live in some parts of the country. The groups that receive the most attention are those who are noticeable because their culture, dress or skin colour make them stand out, particularly those of African-Caribbean, Indian, Pakistani and Bangladeshi origin. They are commonly referred to as black and/or Asian.

The Race Relations Act (1965) made it illegal to discriminate against people, because of their race, in employment, housing and the provision of goods and services. Discrimination occurs when people are treated less favourably than others, either intentionally or unintentionally. In 1976 the Commission for Racial Equality (CRE) was given greater powers to take people to court for both direct discrimination (i.e. that is practised openly) and indirect discrimination (i.e. that is 'hidden', for example rules which exclude particular groups).

> **Think about it**
>
> In what ways might children and their parents experience indirect discrimination in a school?

Patterns of migration

Historically the pattern of **migration** (the movement either to or from a country) in the UK has been that:

> **migration**
> The movement either to or from a country

- there has been a steady flow of people emigrating (leaving)
- there have been noticeable waves of people immigrating (coming in).

Overall the numbers have more or less balanced each other, although some people express racist ideas about being overwhelmed by numbers of immigrants that has no basis in fact.

The problems faced by ethnic minority families

Ethnic minority families, particularly those that are very visible, experience discrimination, prejudice and intolerance, stereotyping and scapegoating as part of their everyday life. Black and Asian people experience discrimination particularly in:

- *employment* – they are more often found in low-status, low-paid jobs with less chance of promotion and more shift work than white people; black people are also more vulnerable to unemployment and poverty
- *housing* – differences between ethnic groups are very noticeable; Asian families have tended to buy their homes, but often the cheaper houses in inner-city areas; people of African-Caribbean origin have been more likely to live in poorer private or council accommodation
- *racial harassment and attacks* – there has been an alarming rise in racial attacks in the UK, some resulting in death; the experience of this can be devastating for an individual and a family. The police are introducing programmes to counteract racism amongst police officers and to encourage a policy of quicker response to racist attacks.

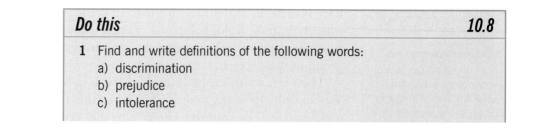

Do this   **10.8**

1 Find and write definitions of the following words:
   a) discrimination
   b) prejudice
   c) intolerance

d) stereotyping

e) scapegoating.

2 Carry out some research into patterns of migration in the UK. You will find references to this in sociology books. Write a conclusion in your own words.

3 Find some more detailed information about the differences in life chances between people from different ethnic groups.

The urban environment

Many inner-city areas in the UK are characterised by environmental pollution and decay, lack of play space and higher crime rates. They have attracted a lot of publicity in recent years. This has resulted in a number of government- and voluntary-funded schemes aimed at improving the environment and the quality of people's lives. The success of these initiatives is varied, partly because of the difficulty of knowing exactly what the problems are.

The UK's inner cities have suffered a loss of population in recent years. Many people have chosen to move from urban centres to the suburbs for gardens and cleaner air. This has been helped by the development of public and private transport. There has also been a loss of industry and employment opportunities in inner cities, and poor planning has contributed to impersonal environments and decay.

In most cases, therefore, with the exception of some sought-after central areas, people who have material resources choose not to settle in the centre of towns, but to live on the outskirts. This leaves a concentration of people in inner cities who have fewer resources, including people experiencing:

■ poverty, unemployment and housing stress

■ physical and mental illness

■ discrimination because of their ethnicity or disability

■ social isolation, being members of one-parent families

■ family problems, including violence and abuse.

There are also more people involved in crime, drug abuse and prostitution in inner-city areas.

In addition, demands on the health and social services tend to be higher, and because of this the quality of these services tends to be poorer.

One way of understanding inner-city problems, therefore, is through the idea of **multiple deprivation**, which emphasises the fact that urban deprivation is not a single problem, but a number of problems concentrated in one area.

> **multiple deprivation**
> The concentration of social problems in one area

The effects of the urban environment on the family

It is important to remember that an urban environment is not necessarily a negative experience for all residents. There are many people who live happy and fulfilled lives and who rear their children successfully in cities and towns. Deprivation is, however, more common than in suburban areas. The lives of some children and their development may be adversely affected in a variety of ways by living in such an environment.

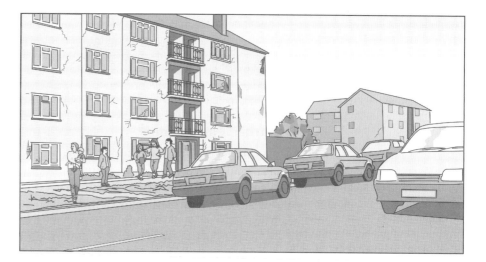

Many of the UK's inner cities are characterised by environmental pollution, decay and lack of play space

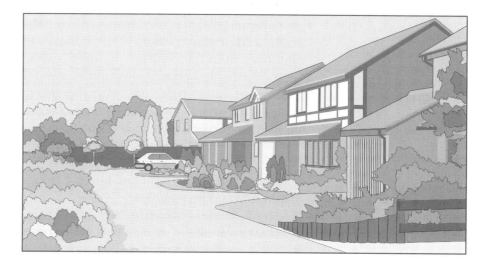

In most cases people who have material resources choose not to settle in the centre of towns, but live on the outskirts

The rural environment

Much less publicity is given to the problems faced by families in rural areas. The UK has a proportionately smaller rural population than many European countries. Some people who live in rural areas are supported by a high income and this buys them desirable housing, land and private transport. Others, for example farm workers, have incomes well below the national average. They may suffer from poverty and unemployment and all the effects that this can bring. They can find housing and transport very difficult to obtain.

The effects of a rural environment on the family
Families living in a rural environment can be subject to similar pressures to those of an urban family if they are on low incomes.

✓ Progress check

1 Which people are most likely to be poor in the UK today?
2 How can unemployment affect people?
3 Why is it very difficult for people to bring up children in bed and breakfast accommodation?
4 In what ways do people from ethnic minority groups experience disadvantage?
5 What are:
   a) discrimination?
   b) prejudice?
   c) intolerance?
   d) stereotyping?
   e) scapegoating?
6 What multiple disadvantages can be experienced by people living in inner cities?
7 How can a family be disadvantaged by living in the country?

Case study: Multiple disadvantage

Sharon is 7 years old and lives with her mother and father and two younger brothers in a fifth floor flat of a six-storey block on an inner-city housing estate. The area around the flats is run down. Piles of rubbish accumulate regularly and graffiti covers many walls and doors. The lifts to the flats, even when working, are inhospitable. Sharon's mother, Sandra, works some shifts in a local factory, but as her father is unemployed most of the money she earns is deducted from their Income Support. Sandra is often tired and depressed, her husband gets angry with her and sometimes hits her. Sharon's younger brothers are 3 and 4 years old, and regularly wet the bed at night. Washing and drying are difficult and, when their mother is at work, the boys sometimes remain unwashed and unfed. Sharon is mature for her age and helps her mother all she can, but she is often tired in the day and her concentration at school is poor.

1 List the problems that this family face.
2 Why is it difficult for the family to get out of the poverty trap?
3 What progress is Sharon likely to make at school, and why?
4 What sources of help might improve things for this family?
5 What are your thoughts about this situation?

People's differing responses to pressures and problems

One of the dangers of describing social problems and people's responses to them is that not *all* people respond to them or are affected by them in the same way. It can be puzzling that some people cope with pressures and others do not. We can only say that people *may* respond to, or *might* be affected in a certain way. Differences in responses can partly be explained by:

- how severe, intense and long-term the pressure is – many people cope reasonably well with short-term pressures in every day life, but are more tested by those which are long-term and severe
- differences in the practical, social and emotional resources that people have to cope with life.

Having resources

Resources are the practical, social and emotional sources of help and strength that people have in varying degrees to help them to cope with life, and bring up their families. Some people have fewer resources to cope with everyday life than others. This means that:

- at times of stress and difficulty they are very vulnerable and can be overwhelmed
- they are less able to protect their children from pressures and problems
- they may at times be unable to provide adequate care for their children. This does not mean, however, that they are irresponsible or lack affection for their children.

Lack of practical resources

Practical resources include reserves of money, material assets, managing skills, mobility. The stress caused by social conditions such as poverty, unemployment or poor housing may affect the capacity of a person to care for their children, either temporarily or permanently. People who have no savings, who worry constantly about money and who endure poor environmental conditions probably experience a higher level of stress in their everyday lives than those who have no such worries.

Lack of social resources

Social resources include a supportive family, friends, a close social network, being a member of a group. People experience social isolation when they have no close family or friends to care about them. It means there is no one to share troubles and anxieties with. There is a saying 'A trouble shared is a trouble halved'. Parents who have warm and caring personal relationships, and have the support of others, may be better able to cope at times of stress and difficulty.

Lack of emotional resources

Emotional resources include having had the experience of stable and caring relationships, having high self-esteem, the ability to cope with stress and frustration, being able to recognise and deal with extreme feelings and having a positive view of life and the ability to trust and give.

Many things may reduce people's emotional resources. A range of personal issues such as low self-esteem, mental ill-health, difficulties with relationships, bereavement, illness, incapacity or other previous life experiences. These issues can profoundly affect a person's view of life and make them vulnerable to stress. This may in turn affect parenting skills. A nursery can help to meet the all-round needs of a child and help to compensate for any disadvantage the child may experience by providing for their all-round needs.

✓ Progress check

1 Why do people respond differently to pressures?
2 What kinds of resources do people have to cope with pressure?
3 Give examples of some of these resources.
4 How can day care help to compensate for any disadvantage a child may experience?

Help available

There are many statutory, voluntary and private organisations that can help people at times of need, and these are described in Chapter 8, *Early years care and education*.

Key terms

You need to know what these words and phrases mean. Go back through the chapter and find out.

absolute poverty
**equal opportunities
    policies**
ethnic group
ethnic minority groups
migration
multicultural society
multiple deprivation
poverty trap
relative poverty
social mobility
**socially deviant
    behaviour**

Now try these questions

1 What kinds of deviant behaviour might affect a family's ability to care for their children and what effect might this have?

2 With slight variations, the children from schools that are in areas where more families are from higher socio-economic groups achieve higher results than children from schools in areas where most families are from lower socio-economic groups. Why do you think this is?

3 How do people get caught in a poverty trap?

4 Describe how social pressures and a lack of resources can affect the healthy development of a child.

Part 4: Child Protection

Children of all ages, male and female, from all cultures and socio-economic groups are the victims of abuse. History reveals that it is not a new phenomena. Although our awareness and understanding of child abuse and child protection within a society that is legally and socially protective of children has developed recently.

All those who work with young children have a unique opportunity and responsibility to recognise the signs and symptoms of abuse and to know and follow the correct procedures if they suspect abuse. Child-care workers may also work to support abused children and their families. All workers have a responsibility to ensure that children develop the skills needed for self-protection.

The responsibility for protecting children from abuse is shared by all. However, it is important to recognise that knowledge alone will not be enough to support workers in their child protection role. In practice, child-care workers will need help and guidance from other colleagues and other professionals to support them in their role.

11 *Understanding child protection*

This chapter includes:

- ■ **Child protection: history and the law**
- ■ **Child protection and the rights of children and parents**
- ■ **Understanding child abuse**
- ■ **Predisposing factors**

The view by any society of what constitutes child abuse within that society varies both between societies and within them at different stages in their history. In nineteenth- and twentieth-century Britain that view evolved considerably, together with ideas about the rights that children have as individuals and the responsibilities of parents towards them. In order to understand child abuse and the way to best protect children into the twenty-first century, we need to understand the current thresholds of what is considered to be abusive, and what leads to abuse.

You may find it helpful to read this chapter in conjunction with:

- ▶ **Book 1, Chapter 15**   Bonding and attachment
- ▶ **Book 2, Chapter 4**   Working with parents
- ▶ **Book 2, Chapter 12**   Types of child abuse
- ▶ **Book 2, Chapter 13**   Responding to child abuse
- ▶ **Book 2, Chapter 14**   Child protection procedures

Child protection: history and the law

The unkind treatment by some adults of children has occurred throughout history. The novels of Charles Dickens paint a vivid picture of the lives of some children in nineteenth-century Britain. In *Oliver Twist*, for example, Dickens shows how cruelty and harsh punishment were both common and acceptable. Many children had to work long hours; they were often beaten and neglected.

The Earl of Shaftesbury was one of the people in the nineteenth century who initiated a series of social reforms that improved the lives of children. However, the amount of abuse that occurs in any society depends firstly on the view that that society has of what child maltreatment is, and this in turn determines the threshold at which society will take action against perpetrators. The nineteenth-century reformers would have had difficulty in recognising some twentieth-century definitions of abuse, and when the state believes intervention to be appropriate. Laws passed since the nineteenth century have

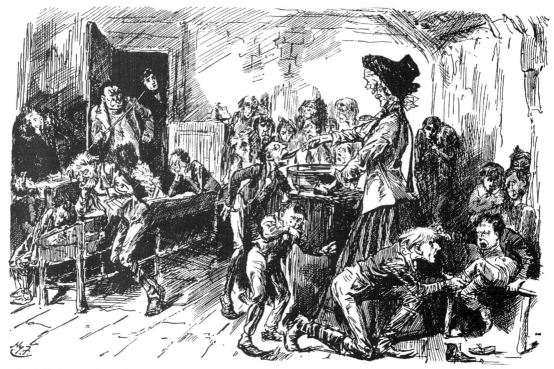

The novels of Dickens paint a vivid picture of the lives of some children in nineteenth-century Britain

increasingly recognised the rights of children to be protected and to have their basic needs met, and the responsibilities of parents to protect children and meet those needs. The most recent child protection law to be passed was the Children Act in 1989.

Recent history

By the 1960s most people thought that the ill-treatment of children was a thing of the past. Whenever cases came to light people thought that they were exceptional and explained as **psychopathic events** carried out by people who lack the ability to put themselves in another person's place and empathise with how that person might be feeling. Such people also lack guilt about, and understanding of, the results of their sometimes violent behaviour.

There was an apparent lack of awareness of the widespread abuse taking place at a higher **threshold of acceptability**. The threshold of acceptability refers to the type of behaviour towards children that is believed to be acceptable by a society at a certain time. For example, at present in the UK parents giving their children a short sharp smack is generally considered acceptable by the majority of people and it is not illegal, whereas the sustained beating of children that used to be acceptable is now both unacceptable and illegal. In other words, the threshold of acceptability has been lowered.

psychopathic events
Actions by people who are unable to put themselves in another person's place and empathise with how that person might feel

threshold of acceptability
The behaviour towards children that is believed to be acceptable by a society at a certain time

There remained also a commonly-held belief that no one should interfere with the rights of parents over their children, especially the right to punish them. Consequently, the law still failed to protect children.

However, during the 1960s, some doctors and social workers began to develop a new awareness of abuse. They took a close interest both in the injuries that they observed in children and the explanations that carers gave for their children's injuries. They asked questions to try to find out whether some injuries were really accidental, and came to realise that certain kinds of abuse were more widespread and could not be explained as psychopathic. They began to develop an understanding of the social and environmental stresses that could prompt people to mistreat children. As a result, they discovered more and more cases of abuse.

In 1962, Dr C.H. Kempe wrote about 'The battered child syndrome'. This drew attention to the problem of 'non-accidental injury' of children by their carers both in the USA and the UK, and the fact that some children were more vulnerable to abuse than others. During the 1970s and 1980s, awareness increased of a range of signs that might indicate deliberate injury to children, and also how certain social and psychological factors interact to predispose people to violent behaviour. Awareness of the occurrence and signs of sexual abuse also increased during the 1980s, followed by awareness of the activities of paedophiles and organised criminal abuse. Today, it is broadly accepted that a combination of social, psychological, economic and environmental factors play a part in the abuse or neglect of children.

> **Think about it**
>
> Why did most people in the UK in the 1960s think that the ill-treatment of children was a thing of the past?

✅ *Progress check*

1 What treatment of children was common and acceptable in the nineteenth century?
2 What is psychopathic behaviour?
3 What awareness did some doctors and social workers begin to develop during the 1960s?
4 What combination of factors is thought to play a part in the abuse or neglect of children?

Child protection and the rights of children and parents

The Children Act 1989

The Children Act 1989 is a major piece of legislation. Previous laws, passed during the nineteenth and twentieth centuries, overlapped and were sometimes inconsistent. This caused confusion and difficulty. The Children Act aims to provide a consistent approach to child protection both by bringing together and changing previous laws.

There was also a concern that recent law, passed before the Children Act, could be used too easily to take rights and responsibilities away from parents. This was thought to be neither in the interests of children nor parents. One of the main aims of the 1989 Act was therefore to balance the needs and rights of children and the responsibilities and rights of parents.

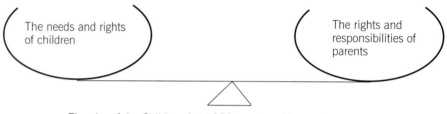

The Children Act 1989

The aim of the Children Act 1989 was to achieve a balance

The needs and rights of children

Cultural differences in child-rearing patterns

The way that children are brought up varies a great deal between different social groups and different cultures. Families have different customs involving children. For example, some groups are traditionally more indulgent towards children, while others are more strict. Some use physical punishment more readily; others are more likely to use emotional forms of control. The Children Act 1989 acknowledges differences and values many of them. It recognises that a positive attitude to working in partnership with parents and understanding their perspective must underpin any action when working with families.

The needs of children

The Children Act 1989 recognises however, that all children have certain needs that are **universal**. These basic developmental needs are the need for:

- physical care and protection
- intellectual stimulation and play
- emotional love and security
- positive social contact and relationships.

The rights of children

All children have certain **rights**. These include the right to:

- have their needs met and safeguarded
- be protected from neglect, abuse and exploitation
- be brought up in their family of birth wherever possible
- be considered as an individual, to be listened to and have their wishes and feelings taken into account when any decisions are made concerning their welfare.

---

universal needs of children
All children have certain needs, whatever their culture, ethnic origin, social class or family background, and are entitled to have them met

rights of children
The expectations that all children should have regarding how they are treated within their families and in society

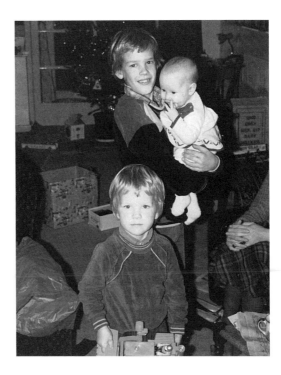

All children have the right to be brought up in their family of birth wherever possible

The rights and responsibilities of parents

Parents' rights

In the past parents had the right of ownership of their children. This right, supported by the law, allowed parents to do more or less as they wished with their children. The law has gradually changed, and it now limits considerably parental rights and powers. It makes the **rights of parents** to bring up their children and make decisions on their behalf dependent on them carrying out their duties and responsibilities towards their children.

rights of parents
To bring up their children and make decisions on their behalf, but they also have duties and responsibilities towards their children

The law gives them the right to be involved throughout any child protection enquiry as long as this is consistent with the welfare and protection of the child. They have the right, for example, to attend a case conference. Research shows that greater parental involvement leads to more purposeful and creative work with families, but that disagreement, real or perceived between social workers and parents greatly hinders the achievement of positive outcomes for children following an enquiry.

Parents' responsibilities

The law includes the idea that parents have rights but that they also have certain duties and responsibilities towards their children.

parental responsibility
The duties, rights and authority that parents have towards their children

The Children Act uses the phrase **parental responsibility** to sum up the collection of duties, rights and authority that parents have concerning their children.

The idea of parental responsibility is a principle that is at the centre of the Children Act 1989. The law does not say precisely how adults should exercise their parental responsibility; it recognises that there is a great variety of ways that they can do this. It emphasises that parents have a duty to care for their children and raise them 'to moral, physical and emotional health'. In this way, the law imposes minimum standards for the care of children and protects their welfare. The 1989 Act recognises that parents have both the right to and responsibilty towards their children for the following:

■ caring for and maintaining them
■ controlling them
■ making sure that they receive proper education.

Parents also have the authority to:

■ discipline them
■ take them out of the country
■ consent to medical examination and treatment.

The people who may have parental responsibility for a child

People have different rights over children at their birth – some people automatically have parental responsibility, others have none but they may acquire (or gain) parental responsibility during the child's life.

These people automatically have parental responsibility for a child at birth:

■ a woman and man who were married at the time the mother gave birth to the child
■ separated or divorced parents – parental responsibility is legally unaffected by the separation or divorce, but there may however be Section 8 Orders in force that say who a child should live with and who can have contact with the child (see Chapter 9, *The family*)
■ an unmarried mother.

These people might acquire parental responsibility during a child's life:

■ an unmarried father – he does not have it automatically; he must either make formal 'parental responsibility agreement' with the mother, or he may apply to court for an order that gives him parental responsibility
■ a non-parent who applies for a Residence Order and can show that they have established a close relationship with the child and are in a position to undertake the role of parenthood, for example a step-father
■ people who are appointed as guardians if a child's parents die
■ carers, following an Adoption Order or a Residence Order
■ a local authority, when a court makes a Care Order or an Emergency Protection Order.

Parents do not now lose parental responsibility for their children (except when they are adopted, or if someone with parental responsibility applies to end the parental responsibility of an unmarried father). They continue to have responsibility even if a court order is made that removes a child from their care.

Case study: Parental responsibility

James was born when his mother Emma was 17 and unmarried. After he was born, Emma made a formal parental responsibility agreement with his father Barry, who was 18, but she and James had no contact with Barry after he moved away when James was 1.

Emma and James continued to live with her parents for four years, after which she married her husband, Steven. James is now 8 and has been living with Emma and Steven since he was 4. Steven, with Emma'a agreement, wishes to acquire parental responsibility for James, and intends to apply for a Residence Order to achieve this. At the same time, Emma intends to apply for Barry's parental responsibility to be brought to an end.

1 Did Emma have parental responsibility for James when he was born, and why?
2 How did Barry acquire parental responsibility for James?
3 Why is it likely that Steven will acquire parental responsibility for James?
4 Why is it possible that Barry will lose parental responsibility for James?

✓ Progress check

1 In what fundamental way have parental rights changed significantly over the last 200 years?
2 What are the universal needs of children?
3 What are some of the duties and responsibilities of parents?
4 What rights does the mother of a child automatically have in law?
5 Does an unmarried father have the same rights?

Understanding child abuse

The importance of understanding

A professional approach

Despite the passing of legislation that makes children's rights and parents responsibilities clear, children are still neglected and abused in different ways. Child-care workers need to understand why this may happen, because understanding is necessary if workers are to develop a **professional approach** to parents and carers. Unless workers understand at least some of the factors that contribute to a case of child abuse, they may be in danger of behaving unprofessionally towards a carer and not treating them with consideration.

This professional approach includes:

■ being considerate, caring and understanding

---

professional approach
How workers deal with and relate to people – they must not allow personal responses to affect their work

- having a non-judgmental attitude towards others
- not stereotyping individuals or groups of people
- respecting confidentiality appropriately.

Partnership with parents

> **partnership with parents**
> A way of working with parents that recognises their needs and their entitlement to be involved in decisions affecting their children

Child-care workers are increasingly involved in working with parents. **Partnership with parents** is one of the principles of the Children Act 1989. The Act recognises that parents are individuals with needs of their own and are entitled to help and consideration. They are also entitled to be involved in decisions affecting their children.

A second reason for the importance of developing an understanding of child abuse is that it helps in planning for work with parents. There are many factors that contribute to parents being abusive to their children. Understanding why abuse occurs increases the ability to understand a carer's needs and to predict the prognosis (the most likely outcome) of working with a carer. The ability of parent to respond to the support given may determine whether the parent is allowed to continue to care for their children.

Why does abuse occur?

> **predisposing factors**
> Factors that make abuse or neglect more likely to occur – usually the result of a number of these factors occurring together

Research shows that abuse does not occur entirely at random, but is more likely to happen in some situations than others. There is a wide variety of **predisposing factors** that make abuse or neglect more likely to occur. Abuse is usually the result of a number of these factors occurring together. In each case, there will be a different combination of factors. The relative importance of each of them will also vary.

The danger in trying to understand abuse is that it might lead to a prediction that if certain characteristics are present abuse *will* happen, or that all people with those characteristics *will* become abusers. This is definitely not so. However, it is possible to look at certain factors, and find that a combination of them is usually present in many cases of abuse. These factors enable us to recognise, understand and work with families where there is a higher risk of abuse.

Do this! 11.1

Prepare an overhead projector presentation for members of your child-care team. Your aim is to develop further the professional approach they have to working with parents and carers. You should aim to review what professionalism means, and outline the reasons why a wider knowledge of the causes of child abuse is significant for their work.

✓ *Progress check*

1 Why do child-care workers need to know why abuse happens?
2 What does the Children Act 1989 recognise about parents?
3 What has research shown about the occurrence of abuse?
4 What is a 'predisposing factor'?

Predisposing factors

Researchers have identified five family types that illustrate the range of background characteristics to be borne in mind when abuse is suspected. They are: multiproblem families, specific problem families, acutely distressed families, those with perpetrators from outside the family, and those with perpetrators from inside the family

Predisposing factors in many cases of abuse may include:

■ factors in the adult's background and personality
■ the presence of some kind of difficulty and stress in the adult's life or environment
■ factors relating to the child.

Factors in an adult's personality and background

A combination of some of the following characteristics has been noticed in abusing parents (remember that non-abusing parents may also have some of these characteristics).

■ *Immaturity* Some people have not developed a mature level of self-control in their reactions to life and its problems. Faced with stressful situations, an adult may lack self-control and react strongly just as a young child might, in a temper or with aggression.

■ *Low self-esteem* Some people have a very poor self-image; they have not experienced being valued and loved for themselves. If they are struggling to care for a child, they may feel inadequate and blame the child for making them feel worse about themselves because they are finding it difficult.

■ *An unhappy childhood where they never learnt to trust others* Parents who have experienced unhappiness in childhood may be less likely to appreciate the happiness that children can bring to their lives. They have not had a good role model to create a happy and caring environment for their children.

■ *Difficulty in experiencing pleasure* An inability to enjoy life and have fun may be a sign of stress and anxiety. This person may also have problems in coping with the stress of parenting and gain little pleasure from it.

■ *Having unsatisfactory relationships* When parents are experiencing difficulties in relationships, whether sexual or other difficulties, this can form an underlying base of stress and unhappiness in their lives. There may also be a general background of neglect or family violence within which there is little respect for any individual.

■ *Being prone to violence when frustrated* The damaging effects of long-term family violence on children has been recognised. Research shows that children who regularly see their mother beaten can suffer as much as if they had been frequently hit themselves.

■ *Being socially isolated* Parents who have no friends or family nearby have little or no support at times of need; they have no one to share their anxieties with, or to call on for practical help.

■ *Adults whose responses are low on warmth and high on criticism* In such families, children can easily feel unloved and negative incidents can build up into violence.

■ *Having a fear of spoiling the child and a belief in the value of punishment* Some people have little understanding of the value of rewards in dealing with children's behaviour; they think children should be punished to understand what is right, they think that responding to a child's needs will inevitably 'spoil' the child. They are more likely to leave a child to cry and not be warm and spontaneous in their reactions to them.

■ *A belief in the value of strict discipline* There are many variations in parenting styles, family structures and relationships; these are not necessarily better or worse than each other. They meet the needs of children in different ways. Some styles of discipline use punishment (both physical and emotional) rather than rewards. This is more likely, however, to lead to abuse when other stressful factors are present.

■ *An inability to control children* Parents under pressure seldom have much time for their children and are more apt to lash out in a rage at the frustrations of everyday interactions.

■ *Not seeing children realistically* This involves having little or no understanding of child development and the normal behaviour of children at different stages; such adults are more likely to react negatively to behaviour that causes them difficulty, rather than accepting it as normal. They may punish a young child inappropriately for crying, wetting, having tantrums or making a mess.

■ *Being unable to empathise with the needs of a child and to respond appropriately* Some people have difficulty in understanding the needs of children; they may react negatively when children make their needs known and demand attention.

■ *Having been abused themselves as children* These parents may have a number of unmet needs themselves and are therefore less likely to be able to meet the needs of a dependent child; they have also had a poor role model for parenting and family life.

■ *Have experienced difficulties during pregnancy and/or birth, or separation from their child following birth* Research shows that difficulties during pregnancy and childbirth, or early separation of a mother from her child, can result in a parent being less positive towards a child. Faced with this child's demands, they may be less able to cope. They may lose their temper more quickly and resort to violence more easily.

Difficulty and stress in the adult's life and environment

Stress of some kind is found in many cases of abuse or neglect. Stress may be short or long-term (sometimes referred to as acute or chronic). It may have many causes.

The experience of stress drains people's energy and leaves them with fewer resources available to cope with meeting the demands of children. The experience of multiple stresses can weaken a person's ability to cope but it does not necessarily mean that they are irresponsible or lack affection for their children. It can however affect the capacity of a person to care for their children.

People who have constant worries and who have to endure long-term difficulties probably experience more stress than those without such worries. This can provide a background of unhappiness that may be significant if it is experienced in combination with other factors outlined in this section.

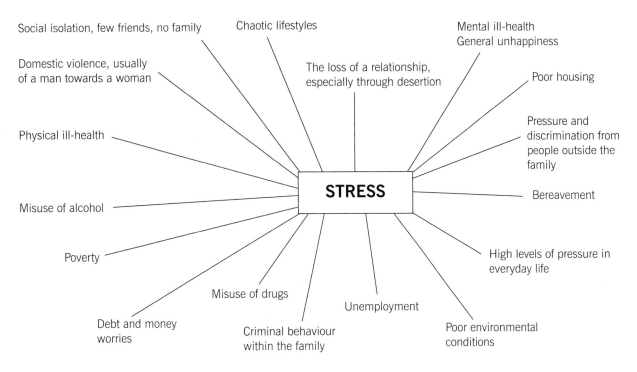

Some factors that create stress in a family

It does not necessarily follow that people who lack coping resources will abuse or neglect their children. In the majority of families they do not. The factors above can, however, help us to understand the different types of stress that may be present in any parent's life and may contribute to abusive situations.

Factors relating to the child

In addition, some things about a child can make them less easy to love by some parents or carers. This does mean that the child deserves ill-treatment but, combined with other factors, it can be significant.

The significant factors about a particular child may include:

■ *a crying child* – most people can sympathise with the stress created by a child who cries a lot; when a carer is tired, and other factors are present, the stress brought about by crying can make a child vulnerable to a violent response

- *interference in early bonding or attachment between carer and child* – there is a wealth of research from Bowlby onwards of the possible ill-effects of early separation of parent and child. Early separation can result in a poor attachment of parent to child. There is evidence that a carer is more likely to abuse a child when the attachment to them is weak rather than strong; it is for this reason that modern antenatal and postnatal care aims to keep parents with their newborn babies and encourage the development of a strong bond between parent and child
- *children who are felt by their carers to be more difficult to care for at a specific stage of development* – some people find babies particularly demanding and difficult, others have more difficulty caring for toddlers or older children
- *children who 'invite' abuse* – these children have learned that the only attention they get is abusive; they learn to bring about certain negative reactions in their carers because this is preferable to having no attention at all.

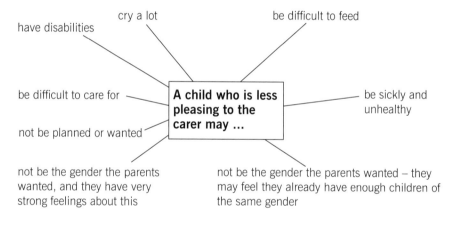

have disabilities · cry a lot · be difficult to feed

be difficult to care for

A child who is less pleasing to the carer may ...

be sickly and unhealthy

not be planned or wanted

not be the gender the parents wanted, and they have very strong feelings about this

not be the gender the parents wanted – they may feel they already have enough children of the same gender

A child who is less pleasing to the carer or who does not meet parents' expectations is statistically more vulnerable to abuse

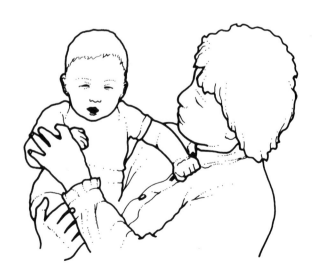

Most people can sympathise with the stress created by a child who cries a lot

Predisposing factors in conclusion

There are many factors that can contribute to the abuse or neglect of children. An awareness of these can help professionals in their work with families and in their efforts to make the best possible decisions for a child in partnership with their parents.

Do this! 11.2

You have been asked to produce a poster for parents on a word processor. It will be placed on the nursery noticeboard. The poster should invite parents to seek help and advice if they are experiencing stress when caring for their children.

a) Select and prepare the information you wish to give them and the graphics to illustrate it. These should show that you understand the various stresses they may be experiencing.

b) Process this information and present it in a suitable format.

c) Evaluate the effectiveness of using information technology for your poster.

Case study: Vulnerable to abuse

Josey is the third daughter of Mr and Mrs Malik. Mrs Malik is 24 years old; Mr Malik is 10 years older than his wife. Mr Malik travels for his work and frequently spends several nights away from home at a time. This makes Mrs Malik anxious and unhappy. They live in an area where nobody has much to do with their neighbours, and she has no close friends. Mrs Malik sees very little of her family who live in the next town. She was unhappy at home as a child; her parents frequently argued and fought. She felt pleased to get away when she married. Although her husband's family lives nearby, she seldom sees them as they disapproved of their son's marriage to her as she is not from his community. Mrs Malik worries because she has never been very good at managing money or the house and her husband blames her for this. Before Josey was born they very much wanted a boy. Her two sisters are 2 and 4 years old. Mrs Malik had high blood pressure during her pregnancy; as a result of this Josey's birth was induced four weeks before term. During the birth she showed signs of fetal distress so a normal delivery was not possible and Josey was born by Caesarian section under general anaesthetic.

Mrs Malik was discharged from hospital two weeks before Josey. She found it very difficult to visit her during this time. When Josey came home, she was very unsettled and cried a lot. She took a long time to take her feed and the doctor diagnosed colic. In recent weeks Josey's mother has seen both her health visitor and doctor several times and reported a series of minor ailments in the infant. Finally Mrs Malik called an ambulance following a long feeding session. They took the baby to the local casualty department, Josey's body was bruised and she was unconscious.

1 What in Mr and Mrs Malik's lives and backgrounds may have contributed to the abuse that occurred?
2 What factors in the child may have contributed to the abuse?
3 What particular stresses may have contributed to the abuse?
4 When this case was discussed at a case conference, what plan of action do you think was agreed, bearing in mind the principles of the Children Act 1989?

Progress check

1 What is a right?
2 What does having a duty mean?
3 What is meant by the term predisposing factors?
4 Name some significant stresses that can be experienced by parents of young children.

Key terms

You need to know what these words and phrases mean. Go back through the chapter and find out.
parental responsibility
partnership with parents
predisposing factors
professional approach
psychopathic events
rights of children
rights of parents
threshold of acceptability
universal needs of children

Now try these questions

1 Describe the development of society's awareness of child abuse.
2 What rights do children have?
3 What duties and responsibilities do parents have?
4 What is a professional approach when working with parents?
5 Why is it possible to predict that some situations are more likely to result in a child being abused or neglected than others?

12 Types of child abuse

This chapter includes:

- Physical abuse and injury
- Neglect
- Emotional abuse
- Sexual abuse
- Disabled children and abuse

Responsibility for diagnosing child abuse rests with GPs and consultants. However, working with young children, you may be in a unique position to notice the signs and symptoms.

Child abuse covers a spectrum of behaviour, from less to more abusive. Early recognition of the indicators may prevent the unacceptable behaviour moving from less to more abusive.

Protecting children from abuse is a responsibility shared by everyone. A first step in protecting children from abuse involves facing up to the fact that it happens at all and understanding the nature and types of abuse. Although identified in this chapter separately, children may be the victim of more than one type of abuse.

You may find it helpful to read this chapter in conjunction with:

- **Book 2, Chapter 11** Understanding child protection
- **Book 2, Chapter 13** Responding to child abuse
- **Book 2, Chapter 14** Child protection procedures

Physical abuse and injury

What is physical abuse and injury?

Physical abuse involves someone deliberately harming or hurting a child. It covers a range of unacceptable behaviour, including what may be described, by some, as physical punishment. It can involve hitting, shaking, squeezing, burning, biting, attempted suffocation, drowning, giving a child poisonous substances, inappropriate drugs or alcohol. It includes the use of excessive force when carrying out tasks like feeding or nappy changing.

Physical abuse also includes Munchausen's Syndrome by Proxy. Munchausen's Syndrome is a condition where a person presents themselves to medical staff for treatment of an illness that they do not have. They seek gratification from the subsequent medical attention, medical tests, care and treatment that they receive. Munchausen's Syndrome *by Proxy* therefore indicates that the sufferer receives gratification from the illness, symptoms, treatment, dependency and resultant need for care of others, including children. A recent case highlighted the damage to children that a sufferer from this condition can inflict.

Think about it

1 Are some forms of physical punishment abusive?
2 Families differ in their attitude to and use of physical punishment. Are these differences based on culture, religious beliefs and/or socio-economic group?

Indicators of physical abuse

Responsibility for diagnosing child abuse rests with GPs and consultants. However, working with young children, you may be in a unique position to notice the signs and symptoms (**indicators**) of child abuse.

indicators
Signs and symptoms

Bruises

Seventy per cent of abused children suffer soft tissue injury, such as bruises, **lacerations** or **weals**. The position of the bruising is important: bruises on cheeks, bruised eyes without other injuries, bruises on front and back shoulders are less likely to occur accidentally, as are **diffuse bruising**, **pinpoint haemorrhages** and finger-tip bruises. Bruises occurring frequently or re-bruising in the same position as old or faded bruising may also be indicators of abuse.

Think about it

Why may you, working with young children, be in a unique position to notice the indictors of child abuse?

The pattern of bruises may also be an indicator: bruises reflecting the cause, for example finger-tip, fist- or hand-shaped bruising. Bruises incurred accidentally do not form a pattern.

It is very important that *mongolian spots* are not confused with bruises. They should not arouse suspicion of abuse. Mongolian spots are smooth, bluish grey to purple skin patches, often quite large, consisting of an excess of pigmented cells (**melanocytes**). They are sometimes seen across the base of the spine (**sacrum**) or buttocks of infants or young children of Asian, Southern European and African descent. They disappear at school age. (See Chapter 16, page 289.)

lacerations
Tears in the skin

weals
Streak left on the flesh

diffuse bruising
Bruising that is spread out

Diagnosis of child abuse is by health care professionals: it is rarely made on the basis of physical indicators alone and may depend on prompt referral to appropriate professionals.

pinpoint haemorrhages
Small areas of bleeding under the surface

melanocytes
Pigmented cells

sacrum
Base of the spine

Think about it

1 Why are some bruises less likely to be caused accidently?
2 Why is prompt referral important?

Burns

Around 10 per cent of abused children suffer burns, but only 2 per cent of these are burnt non-accidentally. Examples are cigarette burns, especially when clear and round and more than one, and burns reflecting the instrument used, for example by placing a heated metal object on the skin.

The pattern and position of scalds can be significant, for example a 3-year-old child with scalds on their feet that are spread like socks. This would imply that the child was placed in hot water and probably held there.

Think about it

Why are some burns less likely to caused accidently?

Fractures

In diagnosing non-accidental injury the following would be significant to a doctor:

- the age of the child – immobile babies seldom sustain accidental fractures
- X-rays revealing previous healed fractures of differing ages
- the presence of other injuries
- the explanation given by child or carer (see *Additional indicators of physical abuse* on page 211).

Think about it

Why is the explanation given by child or carer significant?

Head, brain and eye injuries

Head, brain or eye injuries may indicate that a child has been swung, shaken, received a blow or been hit against a hard surface. The result may be a small fracture or bleeding into the brain (**subdural haematoma**). A small outward sign of head injury accompanied by irritability, drowsiness, headache, vomiting or head enlargement should be treated with urgency, as the outcomes can include brain damage, blindness, coma and death.

subdural haematoma
Bleeding in to the brain

Think about it

What would you do if a child with a head injury was drowsy?

Internal damage

Internal damage, caused by blows, is a common cause of death in abused children.

Poisoning

Any occurrence of poisoning needs to be investigated.

Other marks

Other indicators of abuse may be bites, outlines of weapons, bizarre markings, nail marks, scratches, abrasions, a torn **frenulum**. Damage in a young child usually results from something being forcibly pushed into the mouth, such as a spoon, bottle or dummy. It hardly ever occurs in ordinary accidents. This damage may be associated with facial bruising.

frenulum
The web of skin joining the gum and the lip

Recording the indicators of abuse

If you have noticed the indicators of abuse, your responsibility may also include describing and recording them for referral to, and liaison with,

hearsay
What you are told by others

Think about it

What might you suspect if you saw this pattern of bruising on a small child's face?

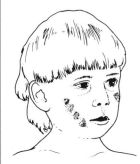

appropriate professionals. Records need to be accurate and dated and should clearly distinguish between direct observation and **hearsay**. The position of the injury, including any pattern, should be recorded as well as the nature of the injury. Physical indicators may be recorded onto a diagram of a child's body to make the position clear and accurate and to avoid misunderstanding.

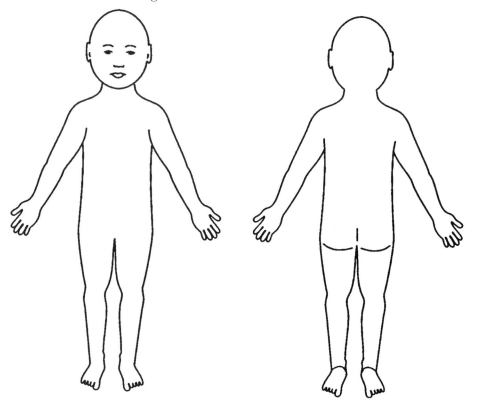

Physical indicators may be recorded onto a diagram of a child's body

All staff in an establishment need to use similar methods of recording and to share the responsibility of this task. Before you are in a position to notice possible indicators of abuse, find out who to report to in the establishment, i.e. the **designated member of staff**. They, or a senior colleague, should always be informed immediately in an appropriate way.

Make sure that you are clear about the rules in your establishment concerning information sharing and confidentiality, and the circumstances under which these may be breached. Remember, if you are unsure about something you have seen or heard, discuss it with the designated person or a senior member of staff. Do not keep it to yourself.

designated member of staff
The person identified in an establishment to whom allegations or suspicions of child abuse should be reported

Think about it

1 Why is it important, in any establishment, to record all accidents and injuries sustained by children?
2 During childhood, most children sustain some injuries accidentally. For each of the indicators outlined above, ask yourself if it is likely that the injury was caused non-accidentally.

Additional indicators of physical abuse

Physical indicators alone may be insufficient to diagnose child abuse. They should, therefore, always be considered alongside other factors. The presence of the following additional indicators increases the likelihood that injuries were sustained non-accidentally; they should be recorded alongside the physical indicators. Some of these additional indicators highlight the need to keep accurate, up-to-date records:

- an explanation by the parent or carer that is inadequate, unsatisfactory or vague, inconsistent with the nature of the injury, considering the age or stage of development of the child
- an unexplained delay in seeking medical attention, or seeking treatment only when prompted by others
- a series of minor injuries to a child which may in themselves have satisfactory explanations
- a history of child abuse or neglect of this or other children in the family
- the existence of certain parental attitudes, such as a lack of concern, remorse or guilt over an accident, blaming others or the child for the injury, denying there is anything wrong or self-righteously justifying the infliction of injury during punishment. For example, if a child aged $3\frac{1}{2}$ was found to have belt marks on their buttocks and lower back, and on being questioned the carer said 'He deserved it. I warned him if he was cheeky once more I'd thrash him. Smacking does no good at all these days.'

Behavioural indicators

In seeking to recognise physical abuse, the following behaviour in an injured child will be significant. This behaviour should be recorded in order to consider it alongside physical and additional indicators, but it cannot be said to prove the existence of abuse:

- fear and apprehension – professionals working with abused children have described a particular attitude or facial expression adopted by abused children and labelled it **frozen awareness** or **frozen watchfulness**. This describes a child who is constantly looking around, alert and aware (vigilant), while remaining physically inactive (passive), demonstrating a lack of trust in adults
- inappropriately clinging to, or cowering from, the carer
- unusually withdrawn or aggressive behaviour (a change in behaviour may be particularly significant)
- the child's behaviour in role-play situations, including their explanation of how the injury occurred.

> ### Think about it
> A 6-week-old baby, with a fractured arm, is said by the carer to have 'just woken up with her arm like that this morning'. Why would you suspect non-accidental injury?

> **frozen awareness/frozen watchfulness**
> Constantly looking around, alert and aware (vigilant), while remaining physically inactive (passive), demonstrating a lack of trust in adults

Case study: Dealing with possible physical abuse

A 2-year-old child often comes to the day nursery with fresh bruises on his arms and upper body. His mother explains these are the result of minor accidents while playing.

1 What might lead you to suspect that the child was being non-accidentally injured?
2 Explain how you would respond to the mother immediately.
3 Describe the procedure you would work through within the establishment, include how and what you would record.

✓ *Progress check*

1 What is physical abuse? What does it include?
2 What is Munchausen's Syndrome By Proxy?
3 Who is reponsible for diagnosing child abuse?
4 a) What percentage of abused children have bruising?
   b) What percentage of burns are caused non-accidentally?
5 What would be significant to a doctor diagnosing physical child abuse?
6 What may head, brain or eye injuries indicate?
7 What do you need to record about the indicators of physical abuse?
8 Describe the possible behavioural indicators of physical neglect.
9 How could a subdural haematoma and a torn frenulum be caused non-accidentally?
10 Where would you expect bruising to occur on a child's back if they had been picked up and shaken?

Do this! 12.1

1 In your workplace, find out who is the designated person for child protection.

2 Design a method of recording all accidents and injuries sustained by children in your workplace.

Neglect

What is neglect?

omission
Not doing those things that should be done, such as protecting children from harm

Neglect involves persistently failing to meet the basic essential needs of children, and/or failing to safeguard their health, safety and well-being.

Neglect involves acts of **omission**, that is not doing those things that should be done, such as protecting children from harm. This contrasts with other types of abuse that involve acts of **commission**, that is doing those things that should not be done, for example beating children.

commission
Doing those things that should not be done, for example beating children

To understand neglect you need to know about children's basic essential needs and their rights. See *The needs and rights of children*, Chapter 11, page 196.

Think about it

1 What are the basic essential needs of children?
2 At what age are children old enough to be left alone in a home for a few hours?
3 What constitutes adequate love and affection?

We will consider neglect under three headings: physical, emotional and intellectual, although in practice these areas will often overlap.

Physical neglect

Physical neglect involves not meeting children's need for adequate food, clothing, warmth, medical care, hygiene, sleep, rest, fresh air and exercise. It also includes failing to protect, for example leaving young children alone and unsupervised.

Emotional neglect

Emotional neglect includes refusing or failing to give children adequate love, affection, security, stability, praise, encouragement, recognition and reasonable guidelines for behaviour.

Intellectual neglect

Intellectual neglect includes refusing or failing to give children adequate stimulation, new experiences, appropriate responsibility, encouragement and opportunity for appropriate independence.

Think about it

Think about how families differ in their standards of care.
a) Are these standards based on culture, socio-economic group or intelligence?
b) Are they related to external forces such as poverty and inadequate housing?

Indicators of neglect

The following signs and symptoms may be observed and should be recorded accurately and dated:

- constant hunger, voracious appetite, large abdomen, emaciation, stunted growth, obesity, failure to thrive (see page 214)
- inadequate, inappropriate clothing for the weather, very dirty, seldom laundered clothing
- constant ill-health, untreated medical conditions, for example extensive persistent nappy rash, repeated stomach upsets, chronic diarrhoea
- unkempt appearance, poor personal hygiene, dull matted hair, wrinkled skin, skin folds
- constant tiredness or lethargy
- repeated accidental injury
- frequent lateness or non-attendance at school
- low self-esteem

- compulsive stealing or scavenging
- learning difficulties
- aggression or withdrawal
- poor social relationships.

It is important to remember, however, that behavioural indicators may be due to causes other than neglect. For this reason, you need to be aware of the background of children in your care. Diagnosis will not be on the basis of behavioural indicators alone. Possible medical conditions that may account for the physical indicators observed will need to be ruled out.

Case study: *Indicators of neglect*

Rachel, aged 2, attends an expensive private day nursery. Her parents, both solicitors, drop her off at 8 a.m. Monday to Friday and are usually the last to pick her up when the nursery closes at 6 p.m. On a number of occasions they have been as late as 7 p.m. Rachel is underweight for her age, unable to manage solid food, preferring a bottle. She takes little interest in the activities of the nursery, preferring to sit alone sucking a toy and rocking rhythmically.

Her mother explains that Rachel was premature, and has never put on much weight, and that her husband's side of the family are all small anyway. Both parents resent being questioned about their child and offer extra payment, to cover the staff's inconvenience, when they are late to collect Rachel.

1   Write a list of the indicators of neglect described in the case study.
2   Describe the kind of on-going records that should be available to confirm each indicator of neglect in this case.
3   Write a description of a child you have known to be physically neglected.
4   Why may the carers of the child you have described be neglecting their child's needs?

Failure to thrive

Failure to thrive describes children who fail to grow normally for no organic reason. Some children are small because their parents are small. Others have a medical condition causing lack of growth. Children may be referred to paediatricians because of concern about growth. Growth charts (**percentile charts**) are used in the assessment of such children. (See Book 1, page 8.)

As a rough guide, any child falling below the bottom line on the graph (the third percentile) should be admitted to hospital for investigation. If in hospital, with no specific treatment, the child gains weight at more than 50 g a day, it is likely that the quality of care has been poor. Most children admitted to hospital for medical reasons tend to lose weight.

percentile charts/centile charts
Specially prepared charts that are used to record measurements of a child's growth. There are centile charts for weight, height and head circumference.

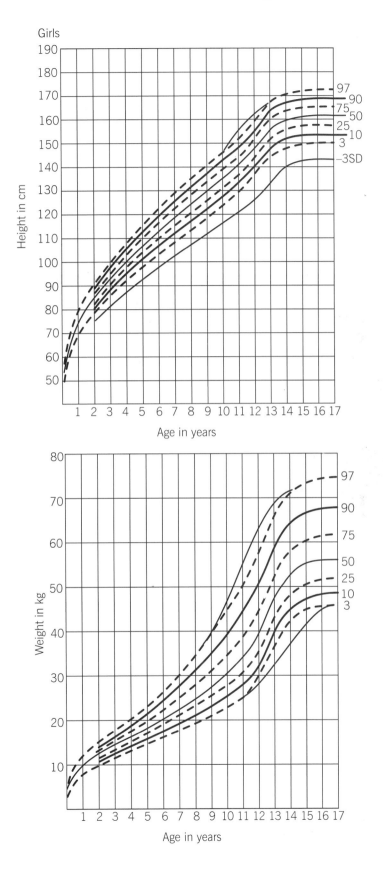

Percentile charts showing (top) height and (below) weight gain in girls up to the age of 17

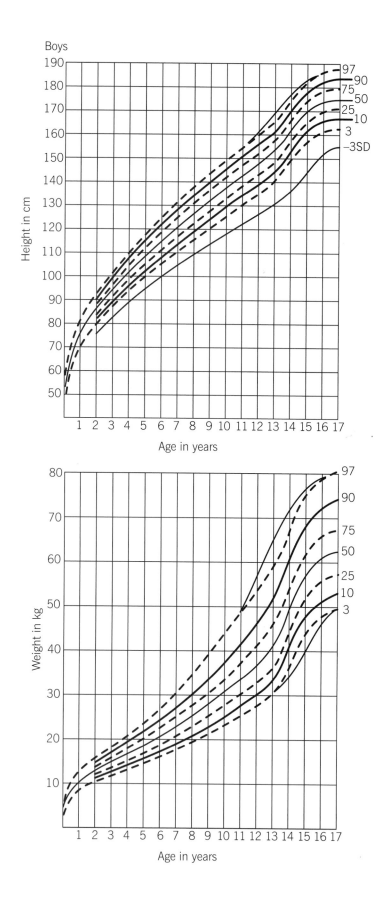

Percentile charts showing (top) height and (below) weight gain in boys up to the age of 17 years

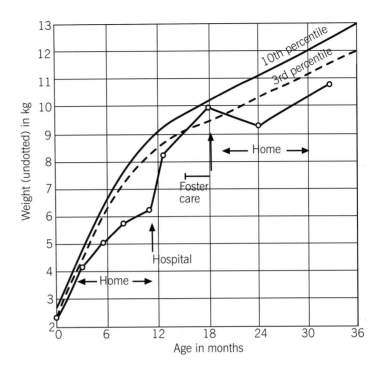

Chart showing a child's weight changes during stays in hospital, foster care and home

The chart above shows the changes in a child's weight when he was in hospital and foster care from the time spent at home.

Think about it

1 What would be your role as a child-care worker in the completion of percentile charts?
2 What factors would you need to consider when completing such charts?
3 How could you ensure that the chart was completed accurately?
4 What might be the results of completing such charts inaccurately?
5 a) Using the chart above, explain what happens to this child's weight in hospital, foster care and at home.
   b) What might lead you to suspect that this child was being neglected?

Progress check

1 What is neglect?
2 Describe three types of child neglect.
3 Describe the indicators of neglect.
4 What is failure to thrive?
5 Why is it important to know about the background of the children in your care?

Emotional abuse

What is emotional abuse?

Failing (omitting) to meet the needs of children in any area of their development, i.e. neglecting children, will cause emotional damage. In addition, it is possible to commit acts of emotional abuse. This occurs when children are harmed by constant threats, verbal attacks, taunting and/or shouting.

Emotional abuse includes the adverse effect on children's behaviour and emotional development as a result of their parent or carer's behaviour, including their neglect and/or rejection of the child. This category is only used in circumstances where it is the only or main form of abuse.

Children may fail to thrive as a result of emotional neglect or abuse, as well as of physical neglect. Children who are neglected are more likely to be victims of other forms of abuse, such as emotional, sexual or physical abuse.

✓ Progress check

What does emotional abuse include?

Case study: Indicators of emotional abuse and neglect

The Wilson family live in a well-maintained detached house in an expensive suburb. They have two children, James aged 6 and Sarah who is 4. Sarah is small for her age, with a thin pale face. She looks sad and wary of adults.

The nursery staff are concerned about Sarah, who seems to be failing to thrive and lacks confidence. Since starting nursery some three months earlier, she has been reluctant to join in structured activities and tells nursery staff that she is no good at anything.

When nursery staff invite the family in for an informal chat, Mrs Wilson constantly compares Sarah unfavourably with her brother, who looks on smugly and agrees with everything his mother says. Mr Wilson doesn't speak directly to Sarah at all, treating her as if she does not exist. In conversation with the staff he refers to her as 'just like her mother'.

The story unfolds, that Sarah was premature, difficult to feed, did not put on weight, was slow to learn and was happy to be left alone to lie in her cot. Mrs Wilson often left her there as James was a rewarding child and demanded a lot of attention. Mr Wilson was away a great deal when Sarah was a baby.

Mrs Wilson made no effort to protect Sarah from the negative comments she was making and said repeatedly to her that she was useless and hopeless, compared to her brother. James referred to Sarah as 'the dummy'. Mr Wilson said he couldn't understand what all the fuss was about, as she was only a girl.

1 Write down the indicators of neglect in this case.
2 Describe how Sarah was being emotionally abused.
3 After reading Chapter 13, *Responding to child abuse*, describe the possible short- and long-term effects on each aspect of Sarah's development.
4 How could staff in the nursery help to alleviate the effects of neglect or abuse?
5 How might the family be encouraged to adopt a different attitude towards Sarah?
6 Describe the roles of other professionals who may become involved with this family.

Sexual abuse

What is sexual abuse?

Sexual abuse is:

'the involvement of dependent, developmentally immature children and adolescents in sexual activities that they do not fully comprehend and are unable to give informed consent to, or that violate the social taboos of family roles.' (Kempe, 1978)

An example of a social taboo of family roles might be incest.

Victims of sexual abuse include children who have been the subject of unlawful sexual activity or whose parents or carers have failed to protect them from unlawful sexual activity, and children abused by other children. Sexual abuse covers a range of abusive behaviour not necessarily involving direct physical contact. It often starts at the lower end of the spectrum, for example exposure and self-masturbation by the abuser, and continues through actual body contact such as fondling, to some form of penetration.

Think about it

1   What does it mean to violate the social taboos of family roles?
2   What does informed consent mean?
3   Why does Kempe include the phrase 'fully comprehend'?
4   What does a range or spectrum of sexual abuse mean?

Who are the victims of sexual abuse?

Child sexual abuse is a universal phenomenon. It is found in all cultures and socio-economic groups. It happens to children in all kinds of families and communities. It is untrue that it is only found in isolated rural communities.

Both boys and girls experience sexual abuse. As far as we know, many more girls are abused than boys. There have been reported incidents of children as young as 4 months old being sexually abused.

Both men and women sexually abuse children. It is becoming clear that the majority of children who are sexually abused know the identity of the abuser. They are either a member of their family, a family friend or a person the child knows in a position of trust, for example a teacher or a carer.

Think about it

1   What does 'Child abuse is a universal phenomenon' mean?
2   What are the implications of the fact that the majority of children who are sexually abused know the identity of the abuser?

How widespread is sexual abuse?

The prevalence of sexual abuse is largely unknown as it is under-reported and we are dependent on estimates. In a study of college students, 19 per cent of women and 9 per cent of men reported having been sexually abused as a child. Out of 3,000 respondents to a recent survey by a teenage magazine, 36 per cent said they had been subjected to a sexually abusive experience as a child.

Think about it

1   Why is sexual abuse under-reported?
2   What are your feelings about child sexual abuse? How could your feelings affect your attitude towards abusers and the victims of abuse?

Indicators of sexual abuse

Early recognition of the indicators of sexual abuse may prevent progression, by the abuser, from less to more abusive acts. If sexual abuse is not recognised in the early stages, it may persist undiscovered for many years.

genital
Sexual organs

Think about it

Why may sexual abuse persist for many years, undiscovered, if it is not recognised in the early stages?

Physical indicators

The following are physical indicators of sexual abuse:

- bruises or scratches to the **genital** and anal areas, chest or abdomen
- bites
- blood stains on underwear
- sexually-transmitted diseases
- semen on skin, clothes or in the vagina or anus
- internal small cuts (lesions) in the vagina or anus
- abnormal swelling out (dilation) of the vagina or anus
- itchiness or discomfort in the genital or anal areas.

In addition, there are signs that are specific to either boys or girls:

in boys:
- pain on urination
- penile swelling

- penile discharge

in girls:
- vaginal discharge
- urethral inflammation, urinary tract infections
- lymph gland inflammation
- pregnancy.

Behavioural indicators

There may be no obvious physical indicators of sexual abuse, so particular attention should be paid to behavioural indicators. The following should be recorded accurately and discussed with the designated person in your establishment or a senior member of staff:

- what the child says or reveals through play with dolls with sexual characteristics, genitals, etc. (anatomically correct dolls, see Chapter 13, page 232)
- over-sexualised behaviour that is inappropriate for the age of the child; being obsessed with sexual matters; playing out sexual acts in too knowledgeable a way, with dolls or other children; producing drawings of sex organs such as erect penises; excessive masturbation
- sudden inexplicable changes in behaviour, becoming aggressive or withdrawn
- showing behaviour appropriate to an earlier stage of development (regression, see Chapter 13, page 228)
- showing eating or sleeping problems
- showing signs of social relationships being affected, for example becoming inappropriately clingy to carers; showing extreme fear of, or refusing to see, certain adults for no apparent reason; ceasing to enjoy activities with other children
- saying repeatedly that they are bad, dirty or wicked (having a poor self-image)
- acting in a way that they think will please and prevent the adult from hurting them (placatory), or in an inappropriately adult way (pseudo-mature behaviour).

✅ *Progress check*

1 According to Kempe's definition, what is sexual abuse?
2 Describe:
   a) the behavioural indicators
   b) the physical indicators
   of sexual abuse.
3 Who are the victims of sexual abuse?
4 Is the abuser likely to be known to the child?
5 Why is early recognition of the indicators of sexual abuse so important?

Case study: *Indicators of sexual abuse*

Claire

During play in the nursery, Claire, aged 3½, is observed to be preoccupied with bedtimes and bathtimes. She places dolls, a teddy and herself into these situations again and again over a period of two weeks. She also acts out being smacked in the bath.

Rangit

When a group is asked to draw themselves for a display, Rangit draws himself with a huge penis and testicles, stating 'Boys have willies, girls have holes instead'.

Helen

Helen indicates that she is sore in the vaginal area. She has spent the previous weekend with her grandfather. Her grandfather was convicted of sexual abuse of the child's mother years ago.

Raymond

Raymond has been displaying over-sexualised play with other children. One 3-year-old boy states he is frightened of Raymond because he keeps asking him to hide and play 'sucking willies'.

Kearan and Liam

Kearan and Liam were playing together in water; both were lying naked on their stomachs. A staff member heard a lot of giggling and saw the boys doing press-ups in the water. When asked what they were doing, one boy said 'We're growing our tails'. Both boys had erections.

1 For each of the cases above, decide whether the behaviour may be an indicator of sexual abuse or not.
2 Explain what influenced your decisions.

Disabled children and abuse

All that has already been written about abuse applies to disabled children, including those with learning difficulties. However, some children are particularly vulnerable to all forms of abuse and have special need for protection.

Why are disabled children more vulnerable?

Some offenders abuse children because they are particularly attracted to their dependency. This, combined with society's negative attitude to disabled people, may increase the risk of disabled children, and those with learning difficulties, being abused. In addition disabled children:

- receive less information on abuse and may be less likely to understand the inappropriateness of it
- are often more dependent on physical care for longer and from different people – this increases their vulnerability
- may receive less affection from family and friends and so be more accepting of sexual attention
- may be less likely to tell what has happened (disclose) because of communication difficulties, fewer social contacts, isolation and the fact that they are generally less likely to be believed
- may have an increased desire to please because of negative responses generally, including rejection and isolation
- may lack assertiveness, vocabulary or skills to complain appropriately
- may find it difficult to distinguish between good and bad touches
- are likely to have low self-esteem and feel less in control
- are likely to have less choice generally, therefore less opportunity to learn whether to choose to accept or reject sexual advances.

> **Think about it**
>
> What extra measures need to be taken to ensure that disabled children are protected from abuse?

Case study: A disabled child and abuse

Wayne Steadman, 7, has learning difficulties. He is looked after regularly by Philip, a long standing friend of Mr and Mrs Steadman. They believe it is good for Wayne to meet older people and are glad of a break when Philip has Wayne to stay at his flat or minds him at home while the Steadmans go out.

Philip has been sexually abusing Wayne for a year. It started with Philip asking Wayne to show him his penis but has now progressed to mutual masturbation and oral sex. Philip gives Wayne sweets and tells him not to tell his parents or else he won't let Wayne stay up to watch TV with him.

Wayne tells a friend at school that he gets sweets from Philip and is allowed to stay up late watching TV if he lets Philip play with his 'willy'. Wayne's friend doesn't understand and asks Wayne to show him what Philip does. The boys are discovered in the library corner at school and asked to explain what they are doing. Wayne explains, but asks the staff not to tell his mother because she will be cross with him for staying up late.

1 Describe how Wayne was being abused.
2 What indicators of sexual abuse may have been evident in this case?
3 After reading *The effects of abuse* in Chapter 13 (page 229), describe the possible short- and long-term effects on Wayne of this abuse.
4 How could staff in school help to alleviate the effects of abuse?
5 Why was Wayne particularly vulnerable to abuse?
6 After reading the section *Prevention and protection* in Chapter 13 (page 235), explain how Wayne could have been helped to protect himself and how the abuse could have been prevented.

Ritual and organised abuse

The media have reported a number of incidents of ritual abuse. The definition used by professionals for this is organised abuse; it often contains bizarre elements which may, or may not, link with satanic practices. Ritual abuse is probably not very common.

✔ Progress check

1 What is ritual abuse?
2 Why are disabled children more likely to be abused?

Do this!   12.3

Develop an information sheet for use by staff in the work setting which gives:
a)   the main forms of abuse
b)   the indicators of each form of abuse.

Key terms

You need to know what these words and phrases mean. Go back through the chapter and find out.

commission
designated member of staff
diffuse bruising
frenulum
frozen awareness/ frozen watchfulness
genital
hearsay
indicators
lacerations
melanocytes
omission
percentile charts
pinpoint haemorrhages
sacrum
subdural haematoma
weals

Now try these questions

1 Describe the main forms of child abuse.

2 Describe the indicators of physical abuse.

3 Describe the possible behavioural signs of sexual abuse.

4 Explain what failure to thrive means and how it may be diagnosed.

5 Explain why it is important to record the indicators of child abuse.

6 Explain the link between emotional abuse and all other forms of abuse.

13 Responding to child abuse

This chapter includes:

- Dealing with disclosure
- The child-care worker's role
- Dealing with the effects of abuse
- Prevention and protection

You will need to develop particular skills for use in situations where abuse is suspected and where it is confirmed.

Children may tell you or show you they are being abused, so you will need to handle disclosure. You may also *observe* and *monitor* abused children. This may involve recording your findings for:

- *referral* to other agencies and professionals
- *liaison* with staff, parents and carers.

Working with abused children will also involve:

- helping to alleviate the effects of abuse and managing difficult behaviour
- having regular contact with families, including those members who commit abuse.

To practise in a professional way it is essential to:

- recognise your own reaction to child abuse issues
- put the needs of children and their families before your own needs
- acknowledge the physical and emotional stress of working in these situations
- make provision to receive support
- form good working relationships with staff team members
- talk about and share your feelings with appropriate people.

Many of the skills required in these situations can be learned and developed during practice, supervised by experienced professionals.

You may find it helpful to read this chapter in conjunction with:

- **Book 1, Chapter 14** The development of self-image and self-concept
- **Book 2, Chapter 11** Understanding child protection
- **Book 2, Chapter 12** Types of child abuse
- **Book 2, Chapter 14** Child protection procedures

Think about it

1 What special skills do you need to work with abused children and their families?
2 What sort of stresses are you likely to experience?
3 Why is emotional support so important?
4 How can you make provision to receive support?

Dealing with disclosure

What is disclosure?

In any day-care setting, it is possible that children will tell you they are being abused; in other words they will disclose, in a full and open way. Alternatively they may, through words or behaviour, hint that abuse may have taken place; in other words they will disclose in a partial, hidden or indirect way. This may happen at inappropriate or pressured times and in awkward situations. You will need to be prepared to respond sensitively and appropriately, both immediately, at initial **disclosure,** and later on.

This section deals with the initial response. For information on follow-up, see Chapter 14, *Child protection procedures*.

disclosure (of abuse)
When a child tells someone (they have been abused)

Responding to disclosure

It is not possible to say exactly what you should do when children tell you they have been, or are being, abused. The points below are only guidelines. You will need to draw on your communication skills and adapt your approach according to the age and stage of development of the child.

- Listen and be prepared to spend time and not hurry the child. Use active listening skills. Do not interrogate them and avoid using questions beginning why? how? when? where? or who?
- Do not ask leading questions, putting words into children's mouths, for example 'This person abused you, then?'
- Reassure them truthfully. Tell them they are not odd or unique; you believe them; you are glad they told you; it is not their fault; they were brave to tell; you are sorry it happened.
- Find out what they are afraid of, so you know how best to help. They may have been threatened about telling.
- Be prepared to record what the child tells you, as soon as possible (within 24 hours), comprehensively, accurately and legibly, with the date of the disclosure.
- Let the child know why you are going to tell someone else.
- Consult your senior (designated person), your agency's guidelines, or if you are working in isolation, for example nannying, an appropriate

professional you think will be able to help. This may be a social worker, a health visitor, a police officer, or an NSPCC child protection officer.

■ Seek support with your personal emotional reactions and needs from an appropriate colleague or professional.

Do not attempt to deal with the issue by yourself. Disclosure is a beginning, but by itself will not prevent further abuse.

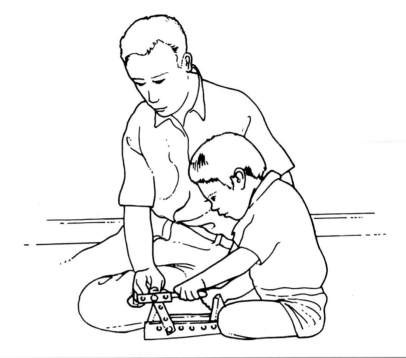

Listen and be prepared to spend time and not hurry the child

Think about it

1 What communication skills do you need to handle disclosure of child abuse?
2 How can you practise these skills in safe conditions?
3 Consider your own need for practical training in the skills required to handle disclosure.
4 What does a child have to lose by disclosing?
5 What might be the impact of disclosure on other family members?

Do this!   *13.1*

1 Check your establishment's procedures for handling disclosure.
2 Talk to staff who have been involved in handling disclosure.

✅ *Progress check*

1 What does disclosure mean?
2 What does partial disclosure mean?

The child-care worker's role

Observation, monitoring and recording

In order to recognise and understand the effects of abuse, skills in observation, monitoring and recording are vital. These skills, useful in the early recognition of abuse, can also be used to monitor progress or **regression** in each aspect of children's development. Careful monitoring can highlight the long-term effects of abuse on individual children, and enable staff to work out plans to alleviate these effects and to monitor their success.

Monitoring is particularly important where progress is slow or erratic, and it is easy to think no progress has been made. It is also important in cases where re-abuse is suspected.

All observations and assessments, including for example percentile charts, need to be recorded regularly and accurately, and dated in order to provide documented evidence for all those involved with the child.

Referral and liaison

Child abuse should never be dealt with exclusively by one person. Recent tragedies highlight the importance of inter-agency co-operation and the need for different professionals to work closely together.

In your establishment you need to know:

- the designated person responsible for child abuse
- who you are directly responsible to
- the roles and responsibilities of the team of people involved with the child, and when to refer to other professionals inside and outside the establishment.

Team work involves liaison, sharing of information and planning. The following guidelines are important when providing information to other professionals about child abuse.

- Information should be relevant, accurate and up-to-date.
- It should also be within your role and responsibility to supply, and provided within agreed boundaries of confidentiality and according to the procedures of the work setting.
- Requests for reports on incidents, disclosures or suspicions of child abuse should be responded to promptly.
- Reports should clearly distinguish between directly observed evidence, information gathered from reliable sources and opinion.
- It should be presented to the appropriate person in the form and at the time requested.
- It is very important that the report remains confidential and is stored securely.

---

regression
Responding in a way that is approriate to an earlier stage of development

---

Think about it

For each of the following professional groups think about what information is most likely to be required, and for what purpose:

- social workers
- NSPCC child protection officers
- police officers
- health visitors
- play therapists.

> ### Do this! 13.2
>
> Find out the procedures of your workplace with regard to:
> a) rules and limits of confidentiality for supply of information to others
> b) arrangements for the security of any documents retained relating to child abuse
> c) the rights of parents to access information held within the setting or passed to other professionals
> d) how and when it is possible to share such information with parents.

✓ Progress check

1 What are the purposes of observation and monitoring of abused children?
2 Under what circumstances is monitoring abused children particularly important?
3 What do you need to know within your establishment in order to refer and liaise?
4 What guidelines should you follow when providing information to other professionals?

Dealing with the effects of abuse

The effects of abuse

self-esteem
Liking and valuing oneself; also referred to as self-respect

As with any trauma, children's reactions to abuse vary. Being subjected to abuse can affect all aspects of children's development: physical, intellectual and linguistic and emotional and social. Perhaps the most significant effect of abuse is the long-term damage to children's **self-esteem,** or self-respect, damage which may persist into adult life. To be abused is to be made to feel worthless, misused, guilty, betrayed. Children's feelings may be translated into observable behaviour patterns.

Martin and Beezley (1977) drew up a list of characteristic behaviour of abused children, based on a study of 50 abused children. The behaviour patterns may also be regarded as indicators of abuse:

- *impaired capacity to enjoy life* – abused children often appear sad, preoccupied and listless
- *stress symptoms*, for example, bed wetting, tantrums, bizarre behaviour, eating problems
- *low self-esteem* – children who have been abused often think they must be worthless to deserve such treatment
- *learning difficulties*, such as lack of concentration
- *withdrawal* – many abused children withdraw from relationships with other children and become isolated and depressed
- *opposition or defiance* – a generally negative, unco-operative attitude
- *hypervigilance*, or frozen awareness or watchful expression (see *Indicators of physical abuse*, Chapter 12)

■ *compulsivity* – abused children sometimes feel or think they must carry out certain activities or **rituals** (sets of activities) repeatedly
■ pseudo-mature behaviour – a false appearance of independence or being excessively 'good' all the time or offering indiscriminate affection to any adult who takes an interest.

Children's reactions can be summarised as either 'fight or flight'. They may respond by becoming aggressive and anti-social (fight), or by becoming withdrawn and **over-compliant** (flight).

Alleviating the effects of abuse

The effects of abuse do not generally make children appealing. Abused children may be very difficult to like. Often they do not attract the love and affection they so desperately need. Alleviating the effects of abuse requires a professional response that puts the needs of children before your own. Caring for abused children may provide you with a deep sense of satisfaction, but abused children are not there to provide this for you. Love and affection should be offered to even the most unattractive, unresponsive personalities. Abused children need consistent, caring adults they can rely on, who will provide unconditional love and affection.

Improving children's self-image

In order to help abused children, you need to have a good understanding of the development of self-image or self-concept. You will need to contribute to the development of a positive self-image, and enhance children's self-esteem. How you do this in practice will vary according to their age or stage of development.

For a thorough understanding of this topic, read Chapter 14 in Book 1, *The development of self-image and self-concept*. The guidelines listed there as *Twenty golden rules* are repeated here for convenience.

Twenty golden rules

1 From the earliest age, demonstrate love and give children affection, as well as meeting their all round developmental needs.
2 Provide babies with opportunities to explore using their five senses.
3 Encourage children to be self-dependent and responsible.
4 Explain why rules exist and why children should do what you are asking. Use 'do' rather than 'don't' and emphasise what you want the child to do, rather than what is not acceptable. When children misbehave, explain to them why it is wrong.
5 Encourage children to value their own cultural background.
6 Encourage children to do as much for themselves as they can, to be responsible and to follow through activities to completion.
7 Do not use put-downs or sarcasm.
8 Give children activities that are a manageable challenge. If a child is doing nothing, ask questions to find out why. Remember that they may need time alone to work things out.

9 Give appropriate praise for effort, more than achievement.

10 Demonstrate that you value children's work.

11 Provide opportunities for children to develop their memory skills.

12 Encourage children to use language to express their own feelings and thoughts and how they think others feel.

13 Provide children with their own things, labelled with their name.

14 Provide opportunities for role-play.

15 Give children the opportunity to experiment with different roles, for example leader, follower.

16 Provide good flexible role models with regard to gender ethnicity and disability.

17 Stay on the child's side! Assume they mean to do right rather than wrong. Do not presume on your authority with instructions such as 'You must do this because I'm the teacher and I tell you to', unless the child is in danger.

18 Be interested in what children say; be an active listener. Give complete attention when you can and do not laugh at a child's response, unless it is really funny.

19 Avoid having favourites and victims.

20 Stimulate children with interesting questions that make them think.

Encouraging expression of feeling

Abused children benefit from involvement in activities that enable and encourage them to express their feelings in an appropriate, acceptable way. Those who work with abused children need to understand the link between feelings and behaviour. They need to be able to see beyond presenting behaviour to children's underlying feelings, and to respond to these rather than to the unacceptable behaviour they may demonstrate.

Observation skills are invaluable in this respect. Information from observations should be carefully recorded and available to all those involved with the care of an abused child. It is not always possible to be

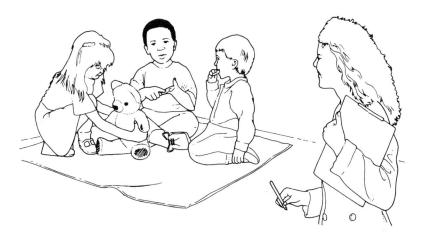

Observation skills are invaluable

certain about children's feelings. The behaviour observed should always be recorded as well as what you think the child was feeling (the evaluation or interpretation).

Play therapy and the use of anatomically correct dolls

Some abused children will need expert professional counselling or play therapy in order to alleviate the effects of abuse. This may be with a child psychologist, a psychiatrist, a counsellor or a play therapist. You may be involved in liaising with these professionals. Under their direction you may be involved in the use of **anatomically correct dolls** with children who have suffered sexual abuse.

Use of the dolls can be helpful because they:
- ease the anxiety involved in discussing sexual matters for the adults as well as the children
- act as an ice breaker to get discussion going, possibly by establishing names for describing the sexual organs and their characteristics
- appeal to a wide age range of children.
- maintain a child-oriented atmosphere
- give the child permission to discuss sexual matters and understand what is natural.

> **anatomically correct dolls**
> Dolls with accurately reproduced body parts including sexual organs

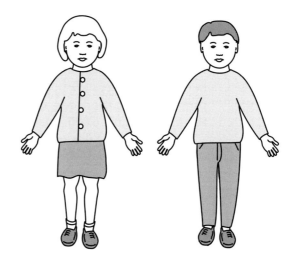

The use of anatomically correct dolls may ease the anxiety involved in discussing sexual matters

The dolls can be used to:
- give children an opportunity to act out, through the dolls, their feelings about what has happened to them
- educate children about sexual matters generally
- describe and demonstrate the events involved in the abuse
- facilitate group or individual play therapy sessions, involving other family members.

They may also be used to encourage and enable disclosure in the investigation of suspected abuse and to obtain evidence of actual abuse. In these contexts their use may be videoed.

Partnership with parents or carers

Part of your responsibility may include working with parents. Your aim will be to enhance, not undermine, the relationship between abused children and their parents or carers. Support and encouragement should be given to parent or carers to motivate them to emulate good methods and practices in relation to their child, rather than to judge and alienate them.

It may be necessary to help particular children to develop positive relationships with their parents or carers. This role will require sensitivity and a real understanding of the importance of the relationship between parent or carer and child. It will require a genuine commitment to partnership with parents.

Think about it

1 Why may abused children be difficult to like?
2 Why do abused children desperately need unconditional love and affection?
3 Take each of the twenty golden rules listed above and explain why they are likely to enhance children's self-esteem and contribute to the development of a positive self-image or self-concept.

Do this!   **13.3**

1 Plan an activity for a group of children aged 3–5, to encourage and enable the expression of feeling.

2 Undertake a number of observations of children of different ages in different settings. Differentiate between their observable behaviour and your understanding of the feelings underlying or causing the behaviour.

Managing difficult behaviour

Emotional damage may well show itself in anti-social behaviour. Even if you understand the reason for abused children's feelings, it may not be easy to cope with their behaviour. The way you respond to difficult behaviour will affect children's self-image and self-esteem. Appropriate responses can help to alleviate the effects of abuse.

It is impossible to give detailed advice about how to respond to all the situations that you may encounter. The table on page 234 summarises the underlying principles for managing difficult behaviour. They may be difficult to live up to in practice, but it is important to set high standards. Abused children may already have suffered considerable emotional damage at the hands of an adult in a position of trust.

Practical points for managing difficult behaviour

Do!	Don't!
Reward positive or acceptable behaviour	Punish aggressive behaviour with violence
Routinely give praise, time and attention	Presume that a child's behaviour is aimed at you personally
Remain calm and in control of your feelings	Pretend that everything is all right if it is not
Respect the child	Presume that you are always right
Reassure the child that you will go on loving them	Promise what you cannot do
Recognise how the child's behaviour makes you feel	
Restrain the child gently if necessary	
Reason with the child	
Respond consistently to similar events	

We all respond more to praise and encouragement than punishment. If punishment cannot be avoided, keep it as low-key as possible. Seek to make punishment a removal of attention from the child, rather than a drama that they will want to repeat because it brings them attention.

Think about it

1 Why does the way you respond to difficult behaviour affect children's self-image or self-esteem?
2 How can appropriate response help to alleviate the effects of abuse?
3 Why is praise and encouragement more effective than punishment?
4 Why is it important to keep punishment as low-key as possible?
5 How can children of different ages be safely restrained to prevent them hurting themselves or others?

Do this!   13.4

1 Before any incidents occur in your workplace, you need to consider how you will control yourself and remain calm under stress.
Discuss with staff in your workplace their experiences of handling difficult behaviour; include the negative as well as the positive experiences.
Draw up a list of ideas, based on their experience of coping, that may help you.

2 Discuss the difficult behaviour of a particular child with an appropriate member of staff in your workplace. After consultation, design a programme to reward or reinforce positive behaviour and deter negative behaviour.

✓ **Progress check**

1 How can children's reactions to abuse be summarised?
2 Describe a professional response to abused children?
3 What are the uses of anatomically correct dolls?
4 What are their potential benefits?
5 What is the child-care worker's role with parent/carers?
6 How may emotional damage in children show itself in practice?

Prevention and protection

A shared responsibility

Parents, professionals and even politicians share responsibility for the prevention of child abuse and the protection of children. Part of this responsibility involves teaching children to protect themselves. This alone will never prevent all abuse, just as teaching children about safety will not prevent all accidents. Nevertheless, it would be negligent to fail in this responsibility. Many adults are reluctant to tackle the subject of protection from abuse because they:

■ feel embarrassed or ashamed
■ do not want to introduce the subject of sex in a negative way
■ are unsure how to tackle the subject.

Principles of child protection

Much insight into the area of protection for children in the UK has come from the work of the Kidscape Campaign for Children's Safety. Kidscape's basic concepts of child protection are:

■ children learning to trust, recognise and accept their own feelings
■ children understanding they have a right to be safe
■ children understanding that their bodies are their own and that no one should touch them inappropriately
■ kisses, hugs and touches should never be kept secret, even if they feel good.

These concepts and the skills that children need to put them into practice can be taught through the existing curriculum in schools. They can also be incorporated into themes and topics in pre-school settings. If taught well, they will encourage children's confidence, assertiveness and communication skills, as well as contributing to their protection. They are relevant to all children, including disabled children and children with learning difficulties, who may be especially vulnerable.

What would you need to ensure before putting the following activities (Do this! 13.5) into practice? Consider parents, colleagues and the children themselves.

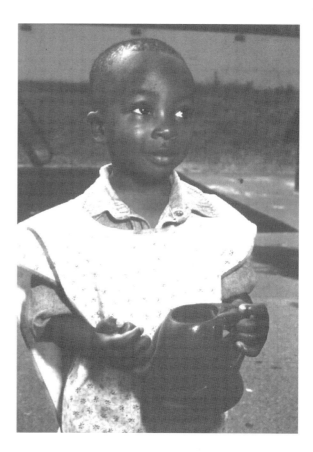

Children need to learn to trust, recognise and accept their own feelings

---

Do this!   **13.5**

1 For the children in your workplace, plan an activity or story that seeks to encourage and enable them to do each of the following:
   - express and trust their feelings – this may include feelings about anything, but particularly things they don't like
   - think and talk about touches that feel good, safe and comfortable and touches that feels bad, unsafe or are secretive
   - say no in an assertive way, even to someone they love, and get help when someone tries to take away their rights, for example through bullying
   - understand that if it is not possible to say no, because of fear or the threat of violence, caring adults will understand and support them
   - get help when they need adult assistance
   - learn that there are times when the rules of being polite do not apply
   - know the difference between safe secrets and unsafe secrets
   - differentiate between telling tales to get someone into trouble and getting help when someone is threatening their safety
   - know how to deal with bullies
   - understand the difference between presents and bribes and to recognise tricks.

> **2** Devise a list of 'What if...?' questions for the children in your workplace to encourage discussion of potentially dangerous or abusive situations. For example, 'What if you were being bullied by someone who made you promise not to tell?' or 'What if a grown-up told you to run across the road and there was a car coming?'

Resources for developing awareness and protection skills

There are a large number of books and resource materials concerning protection (for example, videos) that are available to use with children. In general, they will need to be used in an interactive way if they are to be truly effective. They need to be part of a programme offering children the opportunity to discuss the issues raised. They should not be used by people unprepared for handling children's fears and worries or any disclosure of abuse.

Protecting yourself from allegations of abuse

There may be times when child-care workers are themselves accused of abuse. Sadly, although rare, there are occasions when these allegations are founded. All those who work directly with children need to consider how to avoid allegations. There may already be guidelines in the establishment in which you work. If so you should ensure that you know what they are and follow them. If not, the following common-sense ideas, from *The Kidscape Training Guide* may be used to help you to draw up guidelines for your own workplace.

- In the event of any injury to a child, accidental or otherwise, ensure that it is recorded and witnessed by another adult.
- Keep records of any false allegations a child makes against you. Record dates and times.
- Get another adult to witness the allegation, if possible.
- If a child touches you in an inappropriate place, record what happened and ensure that another adult knows (do not make the child feel like a criminal).
- On school trips, always have at least two members of staff.
- Do not place yourself in a position where you are spending excessive amounts of time alone with one child, away from other people.
- In residential settings, never take a child into your bedroom.
- Do not take children in your car by yourself.
- If you are involved in a care situation, try to have someone with you when changing nappies, clothing or bathing a child.
- Never do something of a personal nature for children that they can do for themselves, for example wiping bottoms.
- Avoid going on your own to the toilet with children.
- Be mindful of how and where you touch a child. Consider using a lap

cushion with young children or disabled children who may need to sit on your knee.
- Be careful of extended hugs and kisses on the mouth from children. This may be particularly relevant to those working with children with learning difficulties.
- Always tell someone if you suspect a colleague of abuse.

Think about it

1 Do you think that all of the above guidelines are necessary or practical in your workplace?
2 Are there some guidelines you would add to this list?

Do this!   13.6

Devise incident report forms suitable for recording:
a) accidental or non-accidental injury to a child
b) allegations made against staff members in your workplace.

✓ Progress check

1 Who is responsible for child protection?
2 Why are many adults reluctant to tackle the subject of protection with children?
3 What are the principles of child protection?
4 How can you protect yourself from allegations of child abuse?

Key terms

You need to know what these words and phrases mean. Go back through the chapter and find out.
anatomically correct dolls
disclosure (of abuse)
over-compliant
regression
rituals
self-esteem

Now try these questions

1 Describe how you would deal with a child's disclosure of abuse.

2 What is the role of the child-care worker with abused children and their families?

3 What are the possible effects of abuse on children?

4 How can the effects of abuse be alleviated?

5 How can the difficult behaviour demonstrated by abused children be managed?

6 How can a child-care worker contribute to the protection of children from abuse?

14 Child protection procedures

This chapter includes:

- **The procedures for the protection of children**
- **Organisations and professionals involved in child protection**
- **Referrals of suspected abuse**
- **Procedures for the investigation of suspected abuse**

In the UK, as in many other countries, there are laws that aim to protect children from abuse and neglect. The Children Act 1989 is the most recent, comprehensive piece of child protection legislation to be passed in the UK. It is based on a number of principles. One of the most important of these principles is that, when considering any action to protect a child, the welfare of the child is the first, or of paramount, importance. The Children Act 1989 also provides guidance to all local authority areas about the steps that should be taken if abuse or neglect is suspected. It requires them to agree and publish these steps, called procedures, and ensure that everyone who works with children in that local authority area is aware of them. Procedures are step-by-step instructions for action for the referral of abuse.

You may find it helpful to read this chapter in conjunction with:

- ▶ **Book 2, Chapter 11**   Understanding child protection
- ▶ **Book 2, Chapter 12**   Types of child abuse
- ▶ **Book 2, Chapter 13**   Responding to child abuse

The procedures for the protection of children

Child abuse is a social and health problem that occurs among people of all social backgrounds, cultures and races. It affects both disabled and non-disabled children. It can take place in a variety of settings including the family, day-care settings and residential homes. The Children Act 1989 recognises the need and right of children from every background and in every setting to be protected from abuse. The Act makes clear recommendations about how this should be done, and requires every local authority to form an **Area Child Protection Committee (ACPC)** to write the procedures for protection for that area.

The child protection procedures for any area include:

- a description of the signs and symptoms of abuse

Area Child Protection Committee
Writes, monitors and reviews the child protection procedures for its area, and promotes co-ordination and communi- cation between all workers

- information needed by each agency about how to refer a concern
- details of the enquiries and protective measures that may follow a referral

The aims of procedures

Child protection procedures aim to:

- protect all children from risk of abuse in any kind of setting
- give clear instructions for action to anyone involved in the care of children if they suspect that a child is at risk
- give details of how agencies, that is social services, the police or NSPCC, should deal with referrals
- promote co-ordination and communication between all workers by providing support and an understanding of their different roles.

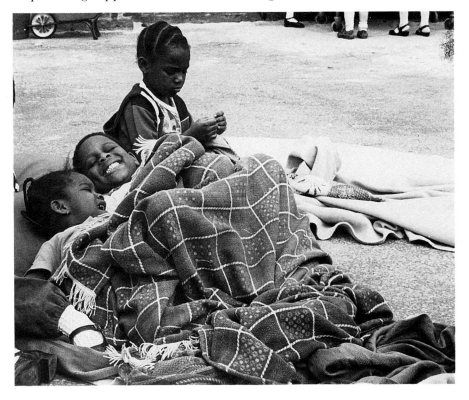

Child protection procedures aim to protect all children from all possible kinds of abuse in any setting

The Area Child Protection Committee

The Area Child Protection Committee (ACPC) consists of representatives of all organisations that may be involved in protecting children. This includes the social services department, police, probation, education, the health service and representatives of voluntary organisations, including the NSPCC. The committee promotes a close working relationship between all professionals. The role of the ACPC is to write, monitor and review the child protection procedures for its area, and to promote co-ordination and communication between all workers. To do this, it uses the guidelines provided by the Children Act 1989.

The principles on which the procedures are based

principle
A basic truth which
underpins an activity

The Children Act 1989 completely revised the law relating to child protection. The Act bases child protection on some key **principles**. (A principle is a belief that something is right and should be used to guide action.) These principles are as follows.

- Children are entitled to protection from neglect, abuse and exploitation.
- The welfare of the child is the first consideration.
- Wherever possible, children should be brought up and cared for by their families.
- The child's wishes should be taken into account when making decisions.
- Unnecessary delay in procedures or court action should be avoided.
- A court order should only be made if it positively contributes to a child's welfare.
- Professionals should work in partnership with parents at every stage.
- Parents whose children are in need should be helped to bring up their children themselves.
- Although the basic needs of children are universal, there can be a variety of ways of meeting them. Patterns of family life differ according to culture, class and community. These differences should be respected and accepted.

✔ *Progress check*

1 In what settings can child abuse occur?
2 What are procedures?
3 What is the principle aim of child protection procedures?
4 What is the ACPC?
5 What is the role of the ACPC?
6 What is one of the most important principles underlying the Children Act 1989?

Organisations and professionals involved in child protection

All people who have contact with children have a duty to protect them. This includes people who work with children in schools, day care and health care. Certain agencies and professionals have a key role in child protection work.

The responsibilities of child protection agencies

Making enquiries

The only agencies with the legal (statutory) power to make enquiries and intervene if abuse is suspected are the social services department, the police, the National Society for the Prevention of Cruelty to Children (NSPCC) and the Royal Scottish Society for the Prevention of Cruelty to Children (RSSPCC). The basis for an effective child protection service must be that all professionals and agencies:

■ work co-operatively on a multi-disciplinary basis
■ understand and share aims and objectives, and agree about how individual cases should be handled
■ are sensitive to issues associated with gender, race, culture and disability.

Promoting equality of opportunity

The Children Act 1989 makes it very clear that although discrimination of all kinds is a reality, every effort must be made to ensure that agencies do not use discriminatory practices or reinforce them. All people have a right to good, non-discriminatory services and equality of opportunity, and in some cases workers may need to take advice about how to achieve this. Child-care workers must take account of gender, race, culture, linguistic background and special needs throughout their working practices. In the opening stages especially, workers involved in child protection must keep an open mind about whether abuse has or has not taken place and avoid making any stereotypical assumptions about people.

There are ways to increase equality of opportunity and some are listed below.

■ Anyone who interviews a child or parent needs to use appropriate language and listening skills.
■ It may help when black families are being investigated to involve a black worker, or at least someone with appropriate cultural knowledge and experience.
■ It may be necessary to make arrangements for children and parents to be interviewed in their home language.
■ If a parent or child has communication difficulties, for example a hearing impairment, assistance must be given during interviews.
■ Remember that children and parents with disabilities have the same rights as any other person.
■ The gender of those being interviewed needs be taken into account: it may be better to involve a worker of the same gender. This is especially true in cases where the victim of suspected sexual abuse is female and the alleged perpetrator is male.

Think about it

Think of times when people might be stereotyped and discriminated against because of their social or cultural background.

Do this! 14.1

Discuss with other child-care workers any difficulties you may have in working in partnership with parents whose child-care practices differ from your own. Record the main points of your discussion and compile an action plan for working with parents and avoiding discriminatory practices.

The role of the child protection agencies with the power to investigate

The social services department

Prevention

Social services departments have a wide range of statutory duties and responsibilities to provide services for individuals and families. The child protection work of social services departments is only a part of its child-care services. Social workers are also involved in prevention, by providing services such as referral for day care, and giving advice, guidance and support to families with children and other client groups. They have a broad awareness of the facilities that are available to help and support all families and prevent neglect and abuse.

Making enquiries following a referral

Local authorities, through their social services departments, have a statutory duty under the Children Act 1989 to investigate any referral of a situation where there is reasonable cause to suspect that a child is suffering or is likely to suffer significant harm. They take the leading role both in enquiries, in child protection conferences, and keeping the child protection register (all described later in this chapter). To fulfil this role, some social services departments have appointed social work specialists to advise and support other social workers in child protection work.

Social services departments also have a system for people to refer their concerns about individual children to them. They provide a telephone number for the public and children to contact them.

Working in partnership with parents

Local authorities must now involve parents throughout the child protection process, as long as this is consistent with the welfare and protection of the child. They must:

- give parents full information about what is happening
- enable parents to share concerns openly about their children's welfare
- show respect and consideration for parents' views
- involve parents in planning, decision-making and review.

The NSPCC (RSSPCC in Scotland)

The National Society for the Prevention of Cruelty to Children is the only voluntary organisation that has statutory powers to investigate and to apply for court orders to protect children. To do this, it has teams of qualified social workers, called *child protection officers*. The society works in close liaison with the social services departments in the areas in which it is active.

The NSPCC is involved in the prevention of abuse, working with vulnerable children and their families, and in research and publication.

The police

Police officers have a duty to investigate cases of suspected child abuse that are referred to them. Their focus is to determine and decide whether:

- a criminal offence has taken place
- to follow criminal proceedings if there is sufficient evidence
- to prosecute if that is in the best interests of the child and the public
- to consider the best way to protect a child victim.

The police share their information with other agencies at child protection conferences. Co-operation and understanding at this level are essential.

The police also have a unique emergency power to enter and search premises and to detain a child in a place of protection for 72 hours, without application to a court.

The role of other workers in child protection

Guardian *ad litem*

The Children Act 1989 recognises that children can find it difficult both to speak for themselves in court and to understand the decision-making process. A **guardian *ad litem*** will help with both of these. They also provide a valuable second opinion in court about what outcome is likely to be in the best interests of a child.

Guardians are people appointed by the courts to safeguard and promote the interests and welfare of children during court proceedings. The guardian is an independent person, usually with training in social work. They have a number of powers, including being able to instruct a solicitor to legally represent a child in court if necessary.

> **guardian *ad litem***
> Person appointed by the courts to safeguard and promote the interests and welfare of children during court proceedings

The probation service

Probation officers have responsibility for the supervision of offenders. Through this, they may become involved in cases of child abuse, for example if an offender is released from prison. They will inform social services if they are concerned about the safety of a child who is in the same household as an offender.

The health service

Prevention

All health service workers are committed to the protection of children. They play an important role in supporting the social services department and provide ongoing support for children and their families. General practitioners and community health workers play an effective part in the protection of children. They identify stresses in a family and signs that a child is being harmed; they may make an initial referral and attend a child protection conference. Health visitors and school nurses record and monitor children's growth and development. They are in a good position to identify children who are being neglected and harmed or who may be at risk.

Treatment and examination

Where a child's health is the immediate issue, in an emergency the first duty of a doctor is to give treatment to the child as a patient. However, in situations where abuse is alleged or suspected, but there is no immediate medical emergency, a doctor's role is to examine a child who has been referred and record evidence that may be used in any legal proceedings. This is a skilled task and best undertaken by a designated doctor with a specialist knowledge of child abuse. Parents may try to prevent such an examination, but if they do, steps can be taken to protect the child, for example by calling the police to used their powers.

The education service

Prevention

Schools may also be involved in prevention through a personal and social education programme. They can help children to increase their personal safety by developing assertiveness skills, raising their self-esteem and giving them an understanding of unacceptable adult behaviour.

Observation and referral

Teachers and other staff in schools have daily contact with children. They are therefore in a good position to observe both physical and behavioural signs of abuse. The education service is not an investigative agency; it must refer any suspicions to the social services department. All school staff need to know the referral procedures within their setting. Each school should have a trained senior member of staff who is given specific responsibility for referral and liaison with social services. This person is called the designated teacher.

Schools should be notified of any child whose name is on the child protection register (see page 253). This alerts them to observe the child's attendance, development and behaviour.

Educational welfare officers and educational psychologists also have important roles to play. They help and support the child in the school and home environment. They may contribute at child protection conferences.

Other voluntary organisations

There is a wide range of national and local voluntary organisations that provide services to support children and their families. National voluntary organisations, such as Barnados, the Children's Society and NCH Action for Children, all provide and run family support centres. Parentline and ChildLine provide telephone counselling and support services for parents and children.

There are many voluntary organisations that are locally based. Some of these specifically support families and children from ethnic minority groups.

✓ Progress check

1 Which three agencies have the power to make child protection enquiries?
2 Name three things that a guardian *ad litem* may do.
3 Why may a doctor with specialist skills be needed in a child protection investigation?
4 What important role do child-care workers in schools have?
5 What is a designated teacher responsible for?

> ### *Do this!* 14.2
>
> Find out about any national and local voluntary organisations in your area that help to protect children and support their families. Using a word processor, produce a small poster that could be used in a child-care setting to inform parents.

Referrals of suspected abuse

Referrals

> **referral**
> The process by which suspected abuse is reported by one person to someone who can take action if necessary

Referral is the process by which suspected abuse is reported by one person to someone who can take action if necessary. Referrals of suspected abuse come from two main sources:

- members of the public, including family members – just over 51 per cent of all enquiries begin by someone, usually the child or member of the family, disclosing their concerns to a professional
- the identification by professionals who work with children in a range of settings – about 39 per cent of enquiries begin in this way.

The remaining 10 per cent of enquiries are suggested during unrelated events, such as home visits or arrests.

Referrals by members of the public

Members of the public are entitled to have their referrals investigated. If any person either knows or suspects that a child is being abused or is at risk of harm, that person should inform one of the agencies with a statutory duty to intervene (that is the police, social services department or the NSPCC/RSSPCC).

Referrals by professionals

Professionals have a duty to refer any case of suspected abuse. In order to be able to respond to signs of abuse and make referrals, professionals need:

- appropriate training to recognise the signs of abuse and neglect
- to know the procedures for the setting in which they work, including their own role, how to respond and their responsibility for referral, including whether it is appropriate either to report this to a designated person or to refer it themselves
- to be aware of the local procedures that will follow a referral of suspected abuse
- to be able to recognise and evaluate the difference between different sources of evidence, and the relative value of these including:
  - directly observed evidence (i.e. evidence they see or hear themselves)
  - evidence from reliable sources (i.e. the evidence of other professional colleagues)

- opinion (i.e. what people think, which must be used very cautiously)
- hearsay (i.e. evidence that is second-hand or more and may have been changed when passed between people).

Do this!   14.3

a) Obtain and read a copy of the child protection procedures for your child-care setting. They should be available through your place of work or local authority outlets.
b) Make notes about what you should do if you suspect abuse.
c) Check your understanding by asking your supervisor.
d) Summarise the information you have obtained by giving an oral feedback to your colleagues/peers.

Record-keeping

When making a referral, the person involved must make a clear record. Well-kept records are essential for good child protection practice. They provide accurate facts that can be used as evidence. Good practice in keeping records can be achieved by:

- the person in charge of a setting (for example, a head teacher or an officer-in-charge) ensuring that staff make accurate records of any observations made or action taken
- making the records immediately, or at least within 24 hours – this is especially important, because only then can they be used as evidence in court
- each agency having a policy stating the purpose and format for keeping records
- being clear about how to maintain confidentiality and safeguard the information, as well as knowing with whom they can share it.

Case study: Working in a family and nursery centre

Jaswinder is a child-care worker in a busy family and nursery centre. Leanne, a 3-year-old child in her group, is giving cause for concern partly because of her irregular attendance.

Leanne's young mother, Carly, has been attending the centre and until recently staff had been pleased with the gradual maturing of her parenting skills. However, recently she started bringing Leanne late or not at all. She has also begun to make excuses about why she cannot stay on the mornings there are parenting classes. Jaswinder observes and records that Leanne now seems very hungry at meal times, she eats quickly and wants more, she falls asleep sometimes while playing, and is wearing small summer dresses into the late autumn. The manager of the centre has already contacted the child's health visitor who is concerned about Leanne's recent weight loss.

One morning her mother arrives late and obviously has a bruised eye herself. Leanne clings to her and cries, but Carly leaves her quickly saying she bumped into a cupboard. Another mother, Marie, is in the room at the time. She tells Jaswinder that Carly has a new boyfriend, and that the whole street knows about him because he plays loud music late into the night and is abusive to anyone who complains. She says that apparently he was in prison until earlier this year and neighbours say it was for assault. She says she thinks he is knocking Carly around and taking her money.

Jaswinder makes a full record of all she has seen and heard and signs and dates it. She reports all her evidence and concerns to the manager.

1 What are the main causes for concern in this case?
2 Why is it important that the child-care worker signs and dates her report?
3 Give an illustrated example from this case study of observed evidence, evidence from a reliable source, opinion and hearsay evidence.

Medical emergencies

Any member of staff who discovers that a child has an injury, whatever its cause, should first decide whether the injury requires immediate medical treatment or not. If it does, the child must be taken to the accident and emergency department of the local hospital. It is better to have parental permission and involvement, although it may be appropriate in child protection cases to consult social services about gaining this.

Do this! 14.4

Imagine you are the child-care worker in the previous case study. Write a factual report of what you have seen and heard.

If possible obtain a sample of the actual recording documentation that is used in a child-care setting and use this. Make sure that you write clearly at the top that this is an imaginary case study.

✓ *Progress check*

1 What do professionals have a duty to know and do in any case of suspected abuse?
2 Why are well-kept records are essential?
3 What should a member of staff who discovers that a child has an injury first decide?
4 Why is it important to make records at least within 24 hours?

Procedures for the investigation of suspected abuse

The procedures for the investigation of suspected abuse involve a series of steps, as outlined below.

The first enquiry – Consultation

Following a referral the social services department, the NSPCC and the police will consult one another, according to whom the referral was made. Records are checked, other agencies and professionals involved with the family are contacted, and the register will be checked. Those involved at this stage will decide whether there are grounds for further investigation and agree their respective roles in any subsequent enquiry. This first enquiry may be undertaken without the knowledge of the parents. Of the 160,000 referrals received in an average year 40,000 result in no further investigation or enquiry.

Enquiry

Following a referral and consultation, if there are reasonable grounds to suspect that a child is suffering or is likely to suffer significant harm, a local authority has a duty to carry out an **enquiry**.

> **enquiry (into suspected abuse)**
> A local authority has a duty to carry out an enquiry if there are reasonable grounds to suspect that a child is suffering or is likely to suffer significant harm

The aims of the enquiry are to:

- establish the facts
- decide if there are grounds for concern
- find out the source of the risk and assess how great it is
- decide what action, if any, to take to protect the child.

The enquiry must establish in particular whether there is an emergency and whether the police or the authority needs to exercise any of its powers under the Children Act to protect the child from any person or situation.

In order to establish the facts, social workers will make a home visit – approximately 120,000 home visits are made a year. They will interview the child, the parent(s), carers, anyone who has a personal interest in the child and any appropriate agencies and professionals. This may include a medical examination by a designated doctor. This is when the enquiry becomes public and the effect of this on a family can be devastating. Parents can be shocked, scared, and confused. Real care needs to be taken to work in partnership with them. Accurate recordings of any interviews are made. As with any records, the difference between fact, hearsay and opinion must be very clear. New provisions under the Criminal Justice Act 1991 allow a video recording of an interview with a child to be used as a child's main evidence in criminal proceedings.

If cause for concern is established during an enquiry, an initial child protection conference will be held. This should take place within eight days of the initial referral, but in practice may not happen for a month.

Case study: The home visit

Aneka attends her local infants school. Her teacher is concerned about a recent decline in her general appearance. Her clothes and her body are frequently unwashed. At milk time she seems very hungry and asks for biscuits. Her mother's neighbour has recently been bringing her to school and implies that all is not well in the family.

The class teacher discusses Aneka with the designated teacher who decides to refer their concerns to social services. Social workers make an initial enquiry and establish that staff at the older children's school is also concerned. They decide to proceed with the enquiry and to visit the family. A social worker makes a home visit and tells Aneka's mother of the referral. She learns that Aneka is one of three young sisters who live with their mother. Her father has recently left the family home. Her mother is a shy woman, slow to tell anyone about her difficulties, but since the loss of her husband she has found it hard to cope, and this has led to some neglect of the children's physical needs. A decision is made not to refer the family to a case conference, but the social worker is able to suggest some services that will offer them help and support.

1 Why were the school concerned about Aneka?
2 What were the causes of the problems?
3 Why do you think that social services decided not to refer the case to a conference?

Police protection

If it is considered that there is an emergency, the police can take a child into police protection. They can remove a child to suitable accommodation (for example, foster care or a community home), or ensure that the child remains in a safe place (for example, a hospital).

Police protection cannot last for longer than 72 hours. During this time, an officer who has special training (a designated officer) will inquire into the case. The officer must inform the child, those with parental responsibility, and the local authority of the steps taken. An appropriate court order (for example, an Emergency Protection Order, see below) must be obtained if the child continues to need protection.

Emergency Protection Order

> **Emergency Protection Order**
> A court order which enables a child to be removed to safe accommodation or kept in a safe place

If it is decided that a child needs further protection during an enquiry, the police or the local authority can apply for an **Emergency Protection Order**. To make this order, a court must be satisfied that:

- the order is in the child's best interests
- the child is likely to suffer significant harm if not removed from their present accommodation.

This Order enables a child to be removed to safe accommodation or kept in a safe place. The court can also say who is allowed to have contact with the child while the order is in force.

An Emergency Protection Order lasts for a maximum of eight days. An authority can ask a court to extend the order for a further seven days if it needs more time to investigate. If the parents of a child were not in court when the order was made, they can, after 72 hours, put their own point of view to the court and apply for the Emergency Protection Order to be removed. The court may appoint a guardian *ad litem* to protect a child's interests during this period. In one year, approximately 1,500 emergency separations are made.

Child Assessment Orders

If during the investigation a child is not considered to be in immediate danger, but the authority wish to make an assessment of the child's health, development, or the way the child has been treated, the authority can apply to the court for a Child Assessment Order, providing that:

- the parents or carers of a child are unco-operative during the investigation
- there is sufficient concern about the child
- the authority believes that the child may suffer significant harm if an assessment is not made.

The authority has to convince the court that they have made reasonable efforts to persuade parents or carers to co-operate with an assessment.

An Child Assessment Order has to say on which date the assessment will begin. It will then last for a maximum of seven days. The court may appoint a guardian *ad litem* to protect the child's interests during the period of the order. Children can refuse to undergo any assessment or examination (providing they have sufficient understanding to make an informed decision about this).

The initial child protection conference

initial child protection conference
Brings together the family, professionals concerned with the child and other specialists to exchange information and make decisions

Following an enquiry, if there is enough cause for concern, an **initial child protection conference** is called. The Guidance to the Children Act 1989 says that this should be held within eight working days, and *must* be held within 15 days. However, research shows that the average interval between referral and conference is 34 days.

The initial child protection conference brings together the family, professionals concerned with child protection (social services, health, the police, schools, probation), and other specialists who can give advice (psychiatrists, psychologists, lawyers). It enables them to:

- exchange information in a context within which sensitive information can be shared
- make decisions about the level of risk
- decide whether the child needs to be registered and how best to protect the child
- agree a child protection plan for the future and ensure that vulnerable children are subject to regular monitoring and review.

One of the ways that you may contribute to the protection of children is by providing information to other professionals at a child protection conference. This may take the form of a general report about a child's development, or a more specific report of something you have observed or witnessed.

Working with parents

The principle of working in partnership with parents must form the basis of the child protection conference. Parents and carers will, as a matter of principle, be included in conferences. There may, however, be occasions when parental involvement may not promote the welfare of the child and they will be excluded them from all or part of the proceedings. Research shows that in practice nearly a third of parents do not attend or are not invited to attend a conference. Children are encouraged to attend conferences if they have sufficient understanding. They can take a friend to support them.

The conference must assess risk and decide whether a child is suffering or likely to suffer significant harm. The conference may decide to register the child. It will appoint and name a key worker and also recommend a core group of professionals to be involved in a child protection plan. The key worker will be from the social services department or the NSPCC. However, it may agree that other workers from the core group will have more day-to-day contact with the child and family. Of the 40,000 cases that go to a conference in a year, 25,000 are placed on the child protection register. In 96 out of 100 cases the children remain at home with relatives.

Case study: Reporting to a case conference

Jackie is 3 years old and attends a local authority family and nursery centre. Her grandmother has made a referral to social services claiming that Jackie's mother's partner shouts at her a lot and that he makes her spend long periods locked in her room. An enquiry has resulted in a decision to call an initial child protection case conference. Marcia, her key worker at the centre, has been asked to present a written factual report about Jackie to the conference. The manager of the centre will be giving an overview report of the child including facts about the family. Marcia is told that her factual report should be based primarily on her recorded observations of the child's development, and that it should also include:

- how long the child has been with her
- how often the child is with her during the week
- a description of the child when she arrives and leaves the nursery, including her physical and emotional state
- how the child responds when leaving and greeting her mother
- the stage of the child's physical, intellectual, language, emotional and social development
- the nature of her contact with the child's parents or carers

■ whether she works alongside the parents in the nursery
■ any special cultural, gender, physical or educational needs of the child.

1 Why has Marcia been asked to write this report?
2 What will she base her report on the child's development on?
3 Why should she be able to describe accurately how the child responds to her mother, and what will she base this on?
4 What should she avoid including in her report?

Do this! 14.5

a) Produce a report based on the imaginary situation in the previous case study. The report should cover all the things requested of Marcia.
b) Imagine you are the manager of the centre. Write the overview report of the child including facts about the family that has also been requested for the conference.

The child protection register

> **child protection register**
> Lists all the children in an area who are considered to be at risk of abuse or neglect

The **child protection register** lists all the children in an area who are considered to be at risk. A child's name is only registered following agreement at a child protection conference. The register must be kept in each social services area office.

The four main categories of registration are:
■ neglect
■ physical injury
■ sexual abuse
■ emotional abuse.

But other labels are also used, including:
■ failure to thrive
■ a child living in the household of a previous abuser.

Following a decision to register, a child's name will be put on a central child protection register. The register is seen by professionals as an essential tool that gives a case conference a focus, and encourages co-operation between agencies. The registration of a child means:
■ the protection plan for the child will be formally reviewed at least every six months.
■ that if a concerned professional believes a child is not being adequately protected, or that the plan needs to be changed, they can ask the social services department (or the NSPCC) to call a child protection review
■ any professional who is worried about a child can quickly refer to the register to see if the child is registered and therefore considered to be at risk, and if there is a protection plan in force.

Case study: The child protection register

As a nursery officer in a day nursery, you have observed a child being reluctant to go home with her mother. She clings to you at home time, and you hear her mother speaking aggressively to her when leaving the nursery. A few weeks later you notice the child sitting astride a broom handle and rubbing herself and also touching herself inside her pants. You record these incidents and discuss them with colleagues. The next day you notice some finger-tip bruising on the child's upper arms. You know that they were not there the day before. You report the matter to your officer-in-charge. She tells you that she will follow the child protection procedures and refer the matter to the social services department. She instructs you to write a factual report about everything you have heard and seen, and to draw on a diagram where the bruises are. Following an enquiry, the child is referred to a case conference. Investigations and discussions reveal that the mother has had a succession of male partners, and has poor parenting skills. The child is placed on the child protection register and an initial child protection plan is agreed.

1 What were the signs that made the staff of the nursery concerned?
2 Why do you think the officer-in-charge decided to refer the matter to the social services department?
3 Why was the child placed on the child protection register?

Initial child protection plan

The initial child protection plan that is made by the core group of professionals after the conference will:
- include a comprehensive assessment of the child and the family situation
- form the basis for future plans of work with the child and family.

A Care Order

If a conference concludes that a child is at risk, the social services department may apply to a court for a Care Order. If made, this places the child in the care of the local authority. It also gives the authority parental responsibility, in addition to the parents. A Care Order gives the local authority the power both to care for the child and to determine the extent that parents can be involved with their child. A child may either be placed in the care of foster parents or in a children's home.

An Interim Care Order

If assessments are not complete enough to decide on making a full Care Order, the court may make an Interim Care Order. This cannot last initially for more than eight weeks; a subsequent order can only last for four weeks to avoid extending delays in the decision-making process.

A Supervision Order

If it is considered that a Care Order is not necessary, the court may make a Supervision Order. This gives the local authority the right to supervise, advise, befriend and direct the care of a child who remains at home. It is effective for a year.

A child protection review

To ensure that registered children continue to be protected from abuse, and that their needs are met, a review of the child protection plan by those involved must be held regularly, at least every six months.

De-registration

De-registration (the removal of a child's name from the child protection register) should be considered at every child protection review. Alternatively, a conference can be called by any agency to consider de-registration. The grounds for de-registration are:

- the original factors which led to registration no longer apply, the home situation may have improved or the abuser has no further contact with the child
- the child and family have moved to another area (when this happens the other area will have to accept the responsibility for the case)
- the child is no longer a child in the eyes of the law: this follows an 18th birthday or marriage before this age
- the child dies.

Discovery of injury, disclosure, or suspicion of abuse or neglect
↓
Immediate medical treatment if necessary
↓
Referral
↓
Consultation and initial enquiry
↓
Subsequent enquiry
↓
Police protection, Emergency Protection Order or Child Assessment Order
↓
Initial child protection conference
↓
Child protection register
↓
Initial child protection plan
↓
Care Order or Supervision Order
↓
Child protection review
↓
De-registration

The possible path of child protection procedures

Do this!   14.6

The following statistics for child protection referrals are taken from *Child Protection – Messages from Research* (HMSO, 1995).

- There are approximately 160,000 child protection referrals made annually to social services departments.
- Out of these, there are around 1,500 emergency separations.
- Research estimates there is no further investigation into around 40,000, and a family visit is made to the remaining 120,000.
- Of those visited, there is no further investigation into 80,000 cases, but around 40,000 then proceed to a child protection conference.
- Of the 40,000 that are conferenced, fewer than 25,000 are placed on the child protection register.
- Of the 25,000 registered children, around 3,000 are taken into care, and a further 3,000 accommodated voluntarily.

a) Read the information above and record it yourself on a data collection sheet.
b) Calculate the following:
    i)   the percentage of referred cases that need emergency separations
    ii) the ratio of referrals that need no further investigation
    iii) the percentage of referrals that have a home visit
    iv) the fraction of referred cases that proceed to a child protection conference
    v) the percentage of children altogether that are taken into care and accommodated.
c) Explain the main features of the data by presenting it in a bar chart

---

✓ Progress check

1 What takes place at the initial enquiry stage?
2 What is a case conference?
3 What is the child protection register?
4 Briefly describe the reasons that a child might be de-registered.

Key terms

You need to know what these words and phrases mean. Go back through the chapter and find out.

Area Child Protection Committee	**guardian *ad litem***
child protection register	**initial child protection conference**
designated teacher	**principle**
Emergency Protection Order	**referral**
enquiry	

Now try these questions

1 Describe the *particular* powers of the social services department, the NSPCC and the police in protecting children that are not shared by other organisations.

2 Describe the role of designated person for child protection in a work setting.

3 What are the difference between observed evidence, evidence from reliable sources, opinion and hearsay evidence?

4 Describe a situation that might lead to a child being referred to a case conference.

5 What are the possible outcomes of referrals of suspected abuse or neglect to social services departments?

Part 5: Babies 0–1

Information about preconceptual and antenatal care increases awareness of the factors which influence health, growth and development before and after birth. Child-care workers need to understand the significance of internal and external factors which influence a baby's health.

High standards of care in the early days lay the foundations of good health and are vitally important. Child-care workers need to establish sensible and effective caring routines to meet the individual needs of all babies in their care.

A thorough knowledge of early development will enable carers to recognise the stages of development and to promote and stimulate babies' development successfully. Carers need to be able to predict a baby's needs and know how to meet them.

Babies are very vulnerable to infection because of their immature immune systems. Their good health depends upon high standards of hygiene and care to prevent infection, and on observational skills to note any deviation from the norm.

Some conditions are far more common in babies, or only occur during the first year of life. Child-care workers who care for young babies must be aware of these so that appropriate care and reassurance can be offered.

Part 5 should be used in conjunction with a great deal of 'hands on' care of babies, which will increase both knowledge and practical skills.

15 Care before birth

This chapter includes:
- **Preconceptual care**
- **Pregnancy**
- **Antenatal care**

Pregnancy is a period of rapid change. The growth and development of the fetus is dependent upon the good health and well-being of the mother, so attention to health is important before pregnancy begins and throughout its duration. This chapter contains information about the importance of preconceptual care and includes details of the necessary steps which should be taken to maintain, and even improve, maternal health before conception occurs. Care in pregnancy is offered to promote good health and to detect the earliest signs of abnormality, so that appropriate care can be provided to resolve any problems, if possible, and to prevent further difficulties. The services provided by health care professionals include emotional and practical advice which recognises the value of support from family and friends.

You may find it helpful to read this chapter in conjunction with:

▶ **Book 1, Chapter 2** Development from conception to birth
▶ **Book 1, Chapter 6** Factors affecting physical development

Preconceptual care

preconceptual care
Attention to health before pregnancy begins

Preconceptual care is the phrase used to describe attention to health and lifestyle before pregnancy. It begins with a decision to have a baby and ends when conception occurs.

When a couple decide to have a baby, they should try to make sure that they are both in a good state of health. Although it is impossible to guarantee a healthy outcome, this will help to ensure that their baby is given the best chance to be born in a healthy condition.

During the first three months of pregnancy, the baby is developing very quickly and all the systems of the body are formed. All the major congenital abnormalities (disorders that the baby is born with, but which are not necessarily inherited conditions), such as spina bifida, heart disorders, blindness and deafness, will occur during this time of rapid growth and development. The fetus is very vulnerable to substances which can cross the placental barrier (such as drugs and viruses) and harm it.

For the first few weeks of pregnancy, a woman may not realise that conception and implantation have occurred, because by the time menstruation stops the embryo is already growing rapidly inside the uterus (see Book 1, page 18). So it is of great importance that the woman and her partner are in the optimum (best) state of health before conception takes place.

Some health clinics run courses for prospective (future) parents offering advice and guidance about important areas of health care (Book 1, page 112). They also refer couples to the appropriate agencies for advice about financial matters or social factors which may affect pregnancy or future child-rearing. It is important that both partners attend the preconceptual care clinic. Women are usually the centre of attention and concern during pregnancy and men can feel isolated and left out of the process. They have an important role to play in supporting their partners and taking an active part in planning a family. There may be specific areas of health care that the future father needs to consider before pregnancy begins. The preconceptual care clinic is able to prepare both partners for a healthy pregnancy.

General health factors

Basic screening checks are made at the preconceptual care clinic. The following areas of health should also be checked.

Weight

It is advisable for a woman to begin pregnancy as near to her ideal weight as possible. The average weight gain in pregnancy is 12–15 kg , and often it is substantially more. The higher the weight at the beginning of pregnancy, the more difficult it is to achieve a healthy weight afterwards.

Blood pressure (BP)

hypertension High blood pressure

High BP (**hypertension**) is a health risk to everyone and can cause problems to mother and baby in pregnancy. If it is detected before pregnancy begins, it may be possible to find the cause and treat it.

Dental care

dental caries Tooth decay

Regular dental checks are important for everyone. Tooth decay (**dental caries**) is a source of infection which can affect the whole body and should be treated before pregnancy begins. Poor dental health before pregnancy will get worse during it, as the fetus takes its calcium requirement from the mother. For this reason, dental care is free to all pregnant mothers and for a year after the birth.

Cervical smear

This is an ideal time for a woman to have a cervical smear test to detect any changes in the cervix, which could later become cancerous. Pregnancy can increase the growth rate of abnormal cells present before conception.

Long-term illness

It is essential for women who receive ongoing treatment for any illnesses to see their GP to discuss the advisability of pregnancy, any changes in their medicines and the best care for them during pregnancy.

Blood tests

Rubella

rubella
German measles, a mild viral infection which damages the fetus in the first 12 weeks of pregnancy

Rubella (German measles), although not itself a serious disease, has a catastrophic effect on the developing fetus in the first 12 weeks of pregnancy, and perhaps until 24 weeks. The virus crosses the placental barrier and damages the eyes, the brain, the heart and the ears. It may result in fetal death and is certainly responsible for more than half of the cases of congenital deafness which occur in children.

If a woman is not immune to rubella (if her blood does not contain antibodies), she will be offered immunisation against this condition and advised not to become pregnant for at least three months, to allow time for her body to make antibodies to the virus.

Anaemia

haemoglobin
A red oxygen-carrying protein containing iron present in the red blood cells

Haemoglobin is a protein in red blood cells which contains iron and carries oxygen. Iron-deficiency **anaemia** is revealed by a low haemoglobin level in the blood. This is usually treated with a diet rich in foods containing iron (green vegetables, egg yolk, raisins, wholemeal bread, baked beans, liver), combined with a course of iron tablets.

The fetus will take its iron and oxygen requirements from the mother, so if she is anaemic, not only will the fetus suffer but the mother may become seriously ill.

anaemia
A condition in which the blood lacks adequate amounts of haemoglobin

Types of haemoglobinopathies (inherited disorders of the haemoglobin) may be screened for preconceptually: sickle cell anaemia may be found in black or mixed race people whose ancestors originated in Central or West Africa or parts of Asia (see Book 1, Chapter 18, page 335); thalassaemia is most common in people of Mediterranean origin.

Being aware that a mother is affected by one of these conditions will ensure that doctors and midwives give the appropriate care in pregnancy.

The prospective father should also be checked for these conditions because the baby may inherit the affected genes from both parents and be affected itself.

Genetic counselling

genetic counselling
Specialist service to provide advice and support for parents who may carry genetically inherited conditions

A couple may be aware that one or both of them have a family history of an inherited condition, such as Duchenne muscular dystrophy, sickle cell disease, cystic fibrosis or Down's syndrome. They may already have a child who is affected by an inherited condition, such as phenylketonuria or haemophilia. A preconceptual care clinic would refer the couple for **genetic counselling**, which is available to all prospective parents who need it. It is usually a hospital-based service with a team of experts who will be able to give the couple some idea of the risks to a future pregnancy, so that they can make an informed decision (knowing all the risks and weighing them against the benefits). (See *Heredity*, in Book 1, Chapter 6, page 112.)

Contraception

Before pregnancy begins, a decision must be made to discontinue all forms of contraception. Barrier methods (the condom and the diaphragm) are easy to stop: a couple will simply no longer use them. The intra-uterine contraceptive device (the coil) needs to be removed by a doctor. These methods do not affect the hormonal cycle, unlike the oral contraceptive pill. It is best for women to stop taking the pill three months before pregnancy begins:

- to allow the body's natural hormone cycle to return to normal
- so that accurate dates can be used to assess the length of the pregnancy, which is always measured from the date of the first day of the last menstrual period (LMP).

Drugs

Any substance taken for its effect on the workings of the body is a drug. Alcohol is a drug; so is nicotine which is present in tobacco; medicines prescribed by a doctor or purchased over the counter without a prescription, or drugs acquired illegally may all cross the placenta and affect the developing fetus.

Smoking

It is much better for both parents to stop smoking before conception takes place. Research has shown that smoking in pregnancy can lead to a higher risk of:

- miscarriage
- premature birth
- low birth weight (on average 200 g less)
- stillbirth or death in the first week of life (**perinatal** death)
- sudden infant death syndrome (SIDS, see Chapter 17, page 334).

After birth, babies who are regularly exposed to cigarette smoke are more likely to suffer from respiratory (breathing) problems. Smoking can also affect the male sperm, so the future father should also be encouraged to give up smoking.

Positive help to stop smoking can be given in the form of guidance, counselling, support groups and referral to other agencies. Smoking is an addiction which is not easy to curb, but it may be easier when it is for the sake of a future baby.

Alcohol

Evidence suggests that moderate and high levels of alcohol consumption during pregnancy affect fetal growth and development. **Fetal alcohol syndrome** is a condition caused by excessive alcohol intake resulting in:

- poor growth, before and after birth
- developmental delay

perinatal
The period of time during birth

fetal alcohol syndrome
A condition affecting babies whose mothers are alcoholic or 'binge' drinkers in pregnancy

■ congenital abnormalities
■ intellectual impairment.
The baby is born addicted to alcohol and has to be weaned off it.

Women are advised to cut out alcohol altogether before conception occurs. A session of heavy drinking after conception, but before pregnancy is diagnosed, could seriously damage the fetus.

Excessive alcohol consumption in men can cause infertility and abnormalities in the sperm, so it is better if they too moderate their drinking habits before a pregnancy is commenced.

Medicines

Women are advised not to take any medicines at all during pregnancy. Even such widely used drugs as paracetamol and aspirin are best avoided. Only those medicines prescribed by a doctor should be taken, and only when the doctor has confirmed that they do not damage the fetus.

Those who are on regular medication would be advised to consult their GP regarding the safety of the drug(s) in pregnancy, and whether an alternative would be advisable.

Illegal drugs

All addictions to potentially dangerous substances should be treated before pregnancy begins. Heroin, cocaine, opium, morphine and other illegal drugs in their various forms, and solvents such as glue or lighter fuel, are not only dangerous for a woman to take but could risk the life of a baby. The prospective mother would be given help and guidance about the services available to treat her addiction before she becomes pregnant.

Diet

A well-balanced diet is important at all times and especially in pregnancy. Women who are significantly over- or underweight may have difficulty in conceiving, and should be given dietary advice about how to achieve a suitable weight before pregnancy begins. Eating disorders such as anorexia nervosa and bulimia must be treated by experienced doctors.

A diet rich in vitamins, minerals and protein is preferable before conception takes place. Folic acid supplements should be taken for three months before a pregnancy begins and for at least three months after it has started. This mineral may help to prevent a neural tube defect, such as spina bifida (see Book 1, Chapter 18, page 336).

The growing fetus lives off its mother, as a parasite, taking all the essential nutrients in preference to her needs. So it is essential that the mother has good dietary advice and acts upon it before becoming pregnant. This advice should also include a warning to avoid soft cheeses and pate which may contain listeria, and to cook food thoroughly to prevent toxoplasmosis (see Book 1, Chapter 6, page 121).

Communicable diseases

Sexually-transmitted diseases (STDs), such as gonorrhoea and syphilis, can be detected and treated before pregnancy begins to avoid the possibility of the baby being affected. If they are not treated, babies can be born with congenital syphilis, which is eventually fatal. Gonorrhoea can cause blindness as the baby's eyes can be infected during delivery.

Human immunodeficiency virus (**HIV**) is not yet curable, nor is it routinely tested for before or during pregnancy. Women who think that they may be infected with this virus need professional counselling to help them to decide whether to have a test or not. Women who are HIV positive can pass on the virus to their babies during pregnancy, and should be discouraged from breastfeeding as the virus is present in breast milk.

> **HIV**
> Human immunodeficiency virus

Lifestyle

The way women live their lives affects their general health; this includes the amount of exercise taken and the type of work done. Regular exercise and a stress-free environment will help to improve the general health and well-being of both partners.

Although it may be difficult to achieve in a busy life, this is the time for them to consider their lifestyle and perhaps try to change the parts which can lead to difficulty or stress. This is not always possible, but sometimes an awareness of the causes of difficulties can help.

Case study: Preconceptual care

Jessie and Richard lost their first baby in the eighteenth week of pregnancy when the ultrasound scan revealed that the baby had died in the uterus. Jessie was induced and when the baby was delivered it was obvious that the little boy had a severe spina bifida.

The doctors said that this was probably nature's way of dealing with a baby who may find life very difficult. Jessie and Richard grieved for their son, but they knew that they still wanted to have children eventually. When the doctor told them that there was no physical reason why they should not have a healthy child, they decided to try again. They both attended a preconceptual care clinic at the local health centre and within three months Jessie was pregnant again.

1 What particular advice from the preconceptual clinic may help to prevent spina bifida occurring in this pregnancy?
2 How may genetic counselling help this couple?
3 What sort of emotional pressures may Jessie and Richard experience during this pregnancy?

Think about it

Make a list of all the social factors you can think of which may affect a decision to have a baby. Include positive and negative points and remember to include the influence of family and friends, and local, national and global issues.

✓ *Progress check*

1 a) What is preconceptual care?
   b) Why is it important to prospective parents?
   c) Why should men be encouraged to attend for preconceptual care?
2 What health checks may be made at the preconceptual care clinic?
3 How long after rubella immunisation should a woman wait before becoming pregnant?
4 a) What is anaemia?
   b) Why is the haemoglobin content of the blood important?
5 Which foods are rich in iron?
6 What is genetic counselling?
7 a) How long before trying to conceive should the contraceptive pill be stopped?
   b) Why is this length of time recommended?
8 a) What is a drug?
   b) Why is smoking in pregnancy discouraged?
   c) Why is heavy alcohol consumption a health risk for both prospective parents?
   d) What condition can alcohol cause to the fetus?
9 Why are soft cheeses and pate best avoided in pregnancy?
10 What problem could maternal gonorrhoea cause to the fetus?

Do this! 15.1

1 Make a chart of your findings from the *Think about it* exercise opposite.

2 Design a booklet or a poster about the benefits of preconceptual care.

3 A friend and her partner have been talking about having a baby. Your friend has heard about preconceptual care and is keen to go to the clinic. Her partner refuses to go with her and she asks you to have a word with him. How would you try to convince him of the benefits of the clinic? Why might some men be reluctant to attend?

4 Research the facilities in your area:
   ■ How many clinics are there near to your home?
   ■ Who are they organised by (for example, GP, health visitor, practice nurse or midwife?)
   ■ How often are clients invited to attend?
   ■ Are men welcome at every session?
   ■ Are the clinics publicised and if so, where?

   Write a report of your findings. Evaluate it in terms of the acceptability of the service offered and, if necessary, how it may be improved.

Pregnancy

Pregnancy begins when fertilisation of the ovum and sperm takes place, usually in the fallopian tubes. It is impossible for a woman to be aware of this happening inside her body. It is only after the embryo (fertilised ovum) has implanted in the wall of the uterus that the signs and symptoms of pregnancy appear.

These early changes noticed by the mother are caused by the action of the two female hormones, oestrogen and progesterone, produced by the ovary for the first 12 weeks of pregnancy and then by the mature placenta (see Book 1, Chapter 2).

Pregnancy is usually confirmed by using a simple urine test to detect **Human chorionic gonadotrophin** (**HCG**). This a hormone produced by the implanted embryo which is excreted in the mother's urine.

| **Human chorionic gonadaotrophin (HCG)** |
| A hormone produced by the implanted embryo, which is excreted in the mother's urine; its presence confirms pregnancy |

Signs and symptoms of pregnancy

Amenorrhoea

Amenorrhoea (stopping of menstruation) is a very reliable symptom of pregnancy in an otherwise healthy woman, who has had a regular menstrual cycle and is sexually active.

Breast changes

Breast changes which take place during pregnancy are summarised in the table below.

Breast changes during pregnancy

Weeks	Changes
3–4	Prickling, enlarging sensation
6	Breasts feel enlarged and tense
8	Surface veins are visible; Montgomery's tubercles appear
12	Darkening of the primary areola; fluid can be expressed
16	**Colostrum** can be expressed; secondary areola appears

| **colostrum** |
| The first breast milk containing a high proportion of protein and antibodies |

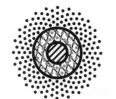

/// Nipple

XXX Primary areola

Montgomery's tubercules

Secondary areola

Frequent passing of urine

Due to hormonal action and the enlarging uterus, women need to empty their bladders more often in early pregnancy.

Nausea and sickness

Often referred to as 'morning sickness', nausea (feeling sick) can occur at any time of the day or night, or be present all the time. Sometimes nausea can be due to particular smells, or foods. This usually passes by the end of the third month.

Tiredness

Lethargy (lack of energy) is common in early pregnancy but usually improves as the pregnancy progresses.

Vaginal discharge

A white, mucousy vaginal discharge, which is not offensive, is normal and is caused by increased hormonal activity.

Later signs of pregnancy

Although the early signs of pregnancy are fairly conclusive in a healthy woman, they can all be due to other causes than pregnancy. Later signs are known as the positive signs of pregnancy – they are objective signs which can be detected by an observer – fetal parts, fetal movements and the fetal heart.

At 12 weeks, the uterus is above the pelvic bone and can be felt by a midwife or doctor. At 16–20 weeks, the mother may begin to feel the baby move (quickening), and it is possible to feel parts of the baby when she is examined at antenatal clinic. The fetal heart can be heard using a stethoscope.

The growth of the uterus during the weeks of pregnancy

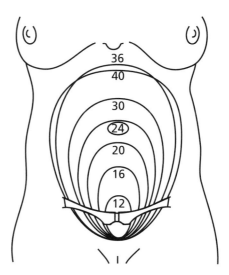

Fundal heights at various weeks during pregnancy

✓ Progress check

1 What are the signs and symptoms of pregnancy?
2 Which hormones are responsible for the early signs of pregnancy?
3 When can colostrum be expressed?
4 What are the positive signs of pregnancy?

Antenatal care

antenatal care
Care of the pregnant mother and developing fetus during pregnancy

The concept of **antenatal care** was introduced as recently as 1915, but was not available to all women free of charge until the National Health Service was created in 1948. Antenatal care has been greatly responsible for:

■ the reduction in the **maternal mortality rate** – the number of women whose death is caused by pregnancy or childbirth. Until about 1935, 40–50 women died per 10,000 total births. The current rate is 1 death per 10,000 births

maternal mortality rate
The number of women who die as a result of pregnancy within a year of the birth

infant mortality rate
The number of deaths in the first year of life calculated per 1,000 live births

■ the reduction in the **infant mortality rate** – the number of children who die in the first year of life. In 1900, out of 100 children born alive, 14 would die before their first birthday. Today the statistics show that 1 out of 100 will die in the first year.

Antenatal care alone cannot take all the credit for these large reductions. Improvements in living conditions since the turn of the century are also responsible for the improved health of the population; but people who live in poverty and deprivation today still suffer from higher than average maternal and infant mortality rates.

The aims of antenatal care

Antenatal care is care offered free of charge by professionals to a woman and her partner during pregnancy. The professionals might be a midwife, general practitioner, health visitor or obstetrician, who specialises in care of the mother and unborn child. The care includes all aspects of health and social conditions to promote well-being. Its aims are:

■ to maintain and improve health in pregnancy
■ to find any abnormality as early as possible and treat it
■ to prepare both parents for labour and a safe, normal delivery which is a pleasurable experience
■ to encourage breast-feeding
■ a live, healthy mature baby who is happily accepted into the family
■ health education of the parents.

Early pregnancy

Women are encouraged to see their own doctor (GP) as soon as they think that they may be pregnant. The doctor may confirm their condition by doing a simple urine test for HCG (see page 268). It is important to see a doctor as early as possible in pregnancy so that:

- a baseline of recordings and observations can be made. It is much easier then to see if any abnormalities occur later
- advice can be given about health and lifestyle to promote a healthy pregnancy.

The doctor should explain to the mother about the choices available to her regarding antenatal care and where she wants her baby to be born. A general health check may be performed (weight, blood pressure and urine test) and advice given about diet, smoking and lifestyle. Blood tests may be performed for rubella antibodies, haemoglobin estimation and grouping.

If the woman chooses to have a hospital delivery, the doctor will refer her to the local maternity unit, and she will be sent an appointment to attend the booking clinic.

Booking clinic

> **booking clinic**
> The first visit to the hospital antenatal clinic

The **booking clinic** is the first visit to the hospital antenatal clinic (ANC). A bed is booked for the time the baby is due. Several observations, tests and recordings are made at this clinic and the information is put into the woman's hospital notes.

History taking

General particulars

Accurate records of the woman's name, age, address, GP and midwife are taken.

Present pregnancy

- Calculation of the expected date of delivery (EDD) – The woman is asked the date of the first day of her last menstrual period (LMP). Nine calendar months are counted forwards and seven days added, for example:

    LMP: 1.1.99, add 9 months and 7 days → EDD: 8.10.99

- Health during this pregnancy is assessed, for example the mother may report excessive sickness, vaginal bleeding or any other abnormality.

Previous pregnancies

Details of previous pregnancies are recorded, because this may affect the care given during this pregnancy, for example:
- date of birth of previous children
- type of delivery
- weight and sex
- method of feeding
- miscarriages, terminations, stillbirths, abnormal babies.

Medical history

Any illnesses affecting the mother are recorded, especially if they may affect the baby, for example diabetes or heart disease.

Family history

Twins, multiple births, genetic conditions or medical problems are recorded.

The midwife's examination

Weight

Weight is recorded as a base measure for future weight gain. The average gain in pregnancy is 12–15 kg.

Height

Height may indicate the size of the pelvis.

Urine test

The urine is tested for protein, ketones and sugar. These substances are not usually found in the urine; if they are present further investigation will be required:

- protein – possibly an early sign of toxaemia of pregnancy (see Book 1, Chapter 6, page 122), or it may be caused by an infection or contamination of the specimen
- **ketones** – produced by the breakdown of body cells to provide energy. Dieting or constant vomiting may be the cause
- sugar – not uncommon in pregnancy because the kidneys are less efficient than usual; it could, however, be an early sign of diabetes.

> **ketones**
> Excreted in the urine as a result of the breakdown of body cells to provide energy

Blood pressure (BP)

This again provides a baseline for future recordings. High BP in pregnancy may be the first sign of toxaemia of pregnancy (Book 1, page 122).

Medical examination

A full medical examination will be performed by an obstetrician. This will include examination of:

- teeth
- breasts
- heart and lungs
- abdominal examination (see illustration on page 269)
- lower limbs, for varicose veins or swelling (**oedema**)
- internal vaginal examination to check the size of the uterus; an ultrasound scan (see page 275) will give an even more accurate assessment. A cervical smear will be done if necessary.

> **oedema**
> Swelling of the tissues with fluid

Blood tests

At this first visit to the ANC, a sample of blood is taken for a variety of tests:

- *ABO group and Rhesus factor* – with information from this test, blood can be cross-matched without delay in the case of anaemia or bleeding during pregnancy, when a transfusion may be needed (see Book 1, page 125 for the importance of the Rhesus factor)
- *serology* – to detect syphilis (a venereal disease), which can be treated to prevent damage to the baby
- *haemoglobin* – the iron content of the blood is recorded and is taken at monthly intervals thereafter. All mothers of African, Asian or Mediterranean descent have their blood tested for sickle cell disease and thalassaemia
- *rubella* – blood is tested for rubella antibodies
- ***serum alpha-fetoprotein (SAFP)*** – this test is taken at 16 weeks of pregnancy when a raised level of SAFP indicates that the baby may have spina bifida; this high level could mean, however, that it is a multiple pregnancy or that the date of the LMP is incorrect. An amniocentesis (see page 275) is offered to mothers with a raised SAFP, and a detailed ultrasound scan will usually be performed to check for twins, or more, and to examine the spine
- ***triple test*** – this test may be offered to women over 35 years of age, or it may be requested. It measures levels of serum alpha-fetoprotein (SAFP), human chorionic gonadotrophin (HCG) and oestriol (placental hormones). In conjunction with maternal age, the test calculates the risk of the baby having Down's syndrome and spina bifida. An amniocentesis may be offered to mothers if necessary.

serum alpha-fetoprotein (SAFP)
A protein found in the maternal blood during pregnancy; a high level requires further investigation

triple test
An antenatal blood test to measure levels of serum alpha-fetoprotein (SAFP), human chorionic gonadotrophin (HCG) and oestriol

The co-operation (co-op) card

co-operation card
A record of pregnancy carried by the mother and used at each antenatal appointment

Every pregnant woman is given a **co-operation card** to record every antenatal assessment made by the hospital, GP or midwife. As its name implies, the card is to enable co-operation between all the providers of ANC as well as the mother. She should carry it with her at all times because pregnancy is not predictable – a problem could occur at any time, even when out for the day or on holiday. Whoever cares for her will need to know the progress of the pregnancy so far, so that the best treatment can be offered.

As the pregnancy progresses, it will be possible to record the fetal heart and feel the fetal parts when the mother is examined. The mother will begin to feel the baby move, at about 20 weeks for a first baby, and earlier for subsequent pregnancies because an experienced mother will recognise the sensation of fetal movement. These observations will be recorded at each antenatal visit together with records showing:

- weight
- urinalysis
- blood pressure
- height of the fundus
- fetal heart
- oedema.

An example of a co-operation card is shown overleaf.

ANTE - NATAL RECORD

INVESTIGATIONS

	DATE	RESULTS
A.B.O. Blood Group		A Rh +
Rhesus Blood Group	24/8/98	
Antibodies		
WRKJAHN	3/12 10668	
X-Ray Chest		
Other		

IMPORTANT NOTE - in the event of a transfusion this record of the blood grouping should always be checked and cross-matching should always be carried out

FIRST EXAMINATION — Date

Height 5. 6".
Teeth
Breasts
Heart } NAD
Lungs
Varicose veins
Pelvis
Cervical smear — Avg. 96

Special observations
URINE CULTURE
CERVICAL CYTOLOGY
K.P. INDEX
SERUM ALPHA
FOETO - PROTEINS

RUBELLA A/B

Sig. — Wishes to breast feed

EXAMINATION 33/37 week — Date
Head/Brim relationship
Pelvic capacity
Sig.

Signature of Doctor

This patient is fit for inhalation analgesia
Date

DATE	WEEKS	WEIGHT	URINE ALB SUGAR	B.P.	HEIGHT FUNDUS	HISTORY (Oedema, Headache, Bowels, Micturition, Discharge, Date of quickening) PRESENTATION AND POSITION	RELATION OF P.P. TO BRIM	F.H.	OEDEMA	Hb	NEXT VISIT	SIG	NOTES e.g. antibodies, other tests, infections, drugs
26. 7. 98	7	57 kg	n o.d.	95/60					nil			SB	Well
24.8.98	11	59.8	Nad	100/65	Just palp				Nil	12.6	2 wk	Jo Harris	SAFP here
20.9.98	15	59 kg	NAD.	94/60	16				nil		4 wk	SB	BKD MRS BAKER CHN
18.10.98	19	59 kg	N A.D.	100/60	19			FHH	nil		4 wk	SB	Well
5.11.98		Home visit Community midwife.			Home conditions suitable for 24 hr discharge							Coxsey	Breasts examined : satisf Br care advise
15.11.98	22+	60½ kg	NAD	95/60	23			FHH	nil		4 wk.	SB	
13-12-98	27	65 kg	N.A.D.	100/60	27	Ceph.	Free	≥	nil		4 wk.	SB	Well
10. 1. 99	31	69 kg	NAD	90/50	31	Ceph.	Free	H	nil		31st Jan	SB	well - Asthma tabs
19/1/99	32	67 kg	NAD	100/60	32	Vx mobile	LOT	FHH	nil	11.4	4 wk.	B	
31.1.99	34	67 kg	NAD	90/50	34	Vx mobile		H	nil		2 wk.	SB	Well
6/2/99	36	69.35	NAD	100/60	36	Vx at brim LOT		FHH	nil		2 wk	B	
21.2.99	37	69 kg	N.A.D	90/54	37	''	LOT.	FHH	nil		1 wk.	SB	Well
28.2. 99	38	69.5 kg	N.A.D	88/54	38	Vx.	LOT.	FHH	nil	11.7	1 wk.	SB	Well
5 - 3 - 99	39	70.0 kg	NAD	96/55	39	Vx.			nil.		1 wk.		Well
13 - 3 - 99	39+	70.0	NAD	95/55	40	Vx.		✓	nil.		1 wk.	SB	Well

A co-operation card

The position of the baby

The following abbreviations are used to describe the way the baby is positioned in the uterus:

O = occiput – the crown of the baby's head
A = anterior – in front
P = posterior – at the back.

So:

ROA = right occiput anterior
ROP = right occiput posterior
LOP = left occiput posterior
LOA = left occiput anterior.

Frequency of antenatal visits

Visits should be made as shown in the following table.

Frequency of antenatal visits

Until the 28th week of pregnancy	Every four weeks
From week 29 to week 36	Every two weeks
From week 37 until delivery	Weekly

Common tests and investigations during pregnancy

Ultrasound scan

The ultrasound machine is an echo-sounding device which uses high-frequency sound waves. An **ultrasound scan** can be used to:

- check the position of the fetus in the uterus
- measure the size of the fetus
- find the position of the placenta
- detect and confirm multiple pregnancies
- diagnose some fetal abnormalities.

At 18 weeks of pregnancy women are offered a detailed scan for doctors to look at the structure of fetal organs.

> **ultrasound scan**
> A check made during pregnancy using an echo-sounding device to monitor the growth and development of the fetus

Placental function tests

A healthy placenta is essential for a fetus to grow and develop normally. It is possible to test the health and strength of the placenta by checking the amount of pregnancy hormones it produces, for example oestrioles.

Hormones are carried in the blood and then excreted in the urine. Blood or urine tests, to test the presence and amount of hormone, will indicate how well the placenta is working.

Amniocentesis

Amniocentesis involves the removal of a small sample of amniotic fluid from the uterus, via the abdominal wall. It may be performed after the

> **amniocentesis**
> A sample of amniotic fluid is taken via a needle inserted into the uterus through the abdominal wall; used to detect chromosomal abnormalities

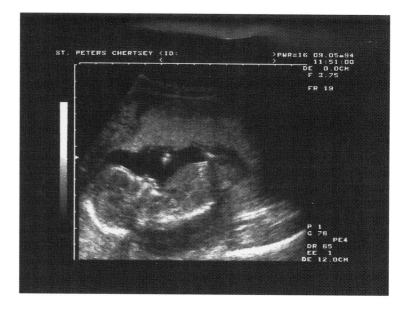

An ultrasound scan taken in the eighteenth week of pregnancy

sixteenth week of pregnancy, when it is possible to check that the chromosomes, including the sex chromosomes, are normal.

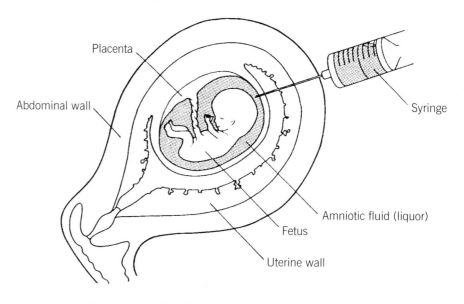

Amniocentesis

Amniocentesis may be offered to women who have:
- a history of chromosomal abnormalities, such as Down's syndrome
- raised SAFP
- a history of sex-linked disorders, such as Duchenne muscular dystrophy
- passed the age of 35 years (the risk of chromosomal abnormalities, especially Down's syndrome, increases with age).

Chorionic villus sampling

Chorionic villus sampling (CVS) is carried out between eight and 11 weeks of pregnancy. With the help of an ultrasound scan to find the

chorionic villus sampling (CVS)
A small sample of placental tissue is removed via the vagina; used to detect chromosomal and other abnormalities

position of the placenta and the fetus, a small sample of placental tissue is removed via the cervix. CVS is used to detect inherited disorders such as:

- Down's syndrome
- haemophilia
- thalassaemia
- sickle cell disease
- cystic fibrosis.

It can also be used to detect the sex of the fetus if there is a family history of sex-linked conditions.

A couple may decide to terminate a pregnancy because of the results of amniocentesis or CVS. Whatever their decision, they will need a great deal of support and empathy from all the professionals involved in their care.

Needs of expectant parents

Physical needs

Physical needs include:

- housing
- equipment
- finance
- information.

Emotional needs

Emotional needs include:

- security – feeling secure reduces stress and promotes well-being
- communication, with professionals, to understand the process of care
- family support, to minimise worries and concerns
- reassurance, from family and professionals
- self-confidence, to ask questions and be assertive
- a stable relationship
- maturity, to cope with the inevitable changes that pregnancy produces
- a compassionate midwife.

Professional guidance

The midwife, doctor and health visitor will provide a great deal of emotional support, as well as physical care. As the pregnancy progresses, they will be available to discuss, advise and give reassurance on any issues which may be causing the parents concern.

Parents will be invited to preparation for parentcraft classes towards the end of the pregnancy, when a mother who has been in employment will by that time be on maternity leave. These classes are organised by the local health authority and are run by the local midwife and/or health visitor in the health centre or hospital. They usually last for two hours and take place once a week for six to eight weeks, and include evening sessions which the mother's partner can attend.

Parentcraft classes aim to:

- educate the parents about pregnancy and childbirth

- reduce any anxieties
- educate parents about child development and child-rearing practices.

Areas covered include:

- relaxation, to help towards an easier labour
- signs of labour
- what happens in labour and what to do
- methods of feeding
- details of layette
- home safety
- child development
- the immunisation programme
- the role of the health visitor
- future family planning.

The classes usually include a visit to the local maternity unit, to look at the labour suite and postnatal wards and the neonatal ICU (intensive care unit). This visit helps to reduce anxiety about going into hospital.

Case study: A concealed pregnancy

Bianca is 15 and, although she started her periods when she was 12, they are very irregular, sometimes eight or nine weeks apart. She and her boyfriend, Steve, have been having a sexual relationship for almost a year, but they keep it a secret because their parents would not approve. They go to the same school and their families are registered with the same GP. Although Bianca realises she may get pregnant because they are not using any contraception, she feels that she cannot risk going to her doctor or to the school nurse in case her family find out.

When she had not had a period for 16 weeks and her breasts started to feel sore, Bianca thought she may be pregnant but was too scared to tell anybody. She thought that if she ignored the signs they may go away. She started to gain weight and wore loose jumpers to cover her growing abdomen. One evening at home she had terrible abdominal pains that came and went, her parents were out for the evening and her younger sister was in bed. Bianca took some paracetamol and went to bed. At 2 a.m. she went to the toilet and delivered a baby girl. Her mother heard the baby cry and fainted when she saw her daughter in the bathroom.

1 If the pregnancy had been planned, what particular care should Bianca and Steve have taken before conception took place?
2 Which important antenatal tests has Bianca missed?
3 Why do you think that concealed pregnancies are not uncommon in teenage girls?

✔ *Progress check*

1 What are the aims of antenatal care?
2 a) How often are visits made to the antenatal clinic?
  b) What is the midwife looking for when she records the BP at each visit?
  c) What observations are made at each antenatal visit and why?
3 a) Study the co-operation card on page 274. Find out what the following abbreviations mean: NAD, PP, BP, FHH, Vx, Hb.
  b) Which two dates on the co-operation card should roughly correspond?
4 Assuming that the following dates are the first day of the last menstrual period (LMP), work out the expected date of delivery (EDD):
  a) 28.4.99
  b) 25.9.99
  c) 15.11.2000
  d) 25.12.2001
  e) 6.5.2001
  f) 29.1.2002.
5 What is the fundus?
6 What tests are made on the urine sample and how often is the urine tested?
7 Why is the position of the head in the uterus so important?
8 Describe oedema.
9 Explain the value of:
  a) ultrasound scan
  b) blood test for serum alpha-fetoprotein (SAFP)
  c) amniocentesis
  d) chorionic villus sampling (CVS).
10 a) What are the needs of the expectant parents?
   b) How can these needs best be met?

Do this!   *15.2*

1 Write a detailed report describing the importance of antenatal care for mother and baby. Describe the reasons why some women may need investigations during pregnancy.

2 Try to find out what antenatal services are like in another country.

3 Research the antenatal care offered to women from different generations; for example ask a friend or relative aged:
  a) 70 or over
  b) about 50
  c) about 30.
Make a list of questions to ask them about their experiences of antenatal care:

- Who gave the care?
- Where was it given?
- Was it the same midwife or doctor all the time?
- How often was she examined?
- Where was the delivery?
- Was the father present?
- Types of investigations, and so on.

Report on your findings of the differences in antenatal care. Has it improved? If so, how and why?

Key terms

You need to know what these words and phrases mean. Go back through the chapter to find out.

amniocentesis
anaemia
antenatal care
booking clinic
chorionic villus
 sampling
co-operation card
colostrum
dental caries
fetal alcohol syndrome
genetic counselling
haemoglobin
HCG
HIV
hypertension
infant mortality rate
ketones
maternal mortality rate
oedema
perinatal
preconceptual care
rubella
serum alpha-
 fetoprotein
triple test
ultrasound scan

Now try these questions

1 Explain the value of preconceptual care.
2 What are the dietary needs of an expectant mother?
3 Describe the blood tests taken in pregnancy and when they are taken.
4 What is the value of the co-operation card?

16 Care and stimulation of early development

This chapter includes:

- **The birth process**
- **Immediate care at birth**
- **Postnatal care**
- **Low birth-weight babies**
- **Early development**

During pregnancy most women find it difficult to think very far beyond the moment of birth, especially if this is the first baby and each experience is new. Labour and delivery are the focus of their attention. Although the birth of the baby is very important, it is usually over very quickly. It is after the birth that parents begin their continuing commitment to care for a totally dependent infant and child.

You may find it useful to read this chapter in conjunction with:

- **Book 1, Chapter 3**   Physical development
- **Book 1, Chapter 6**   Factors affecting physical development
- **Book 1, Chapter 18**   Conditions and impairments
- **Book 2, Chapter 15**   Care before birth
- **Book 2, Chapter 17**   Physical needs in the first year

The birth process

labour
The process by which the fetus, placenta and membranes are expelled from the birth canal

Labour is the process by which the fetus, placenta and membranes are expelled through the birth canal.

Signs that labour has started

- The onset of strong and regular contractions
- A 'show' – the discharge of blood-stained mucous from the vagina
- 'Waters breaking' – rupture of the membranes resulting in some amniotic fluid escaping via the vagina

One, or any combination of these, may indicate that labour has begun. A woman should contact her midwife for advice as soon as she thinks that she may be in labour. The rupture of the membranes may allow infection to enter the uterus, so she should contact the hospital immediately if the baby is to be born there.

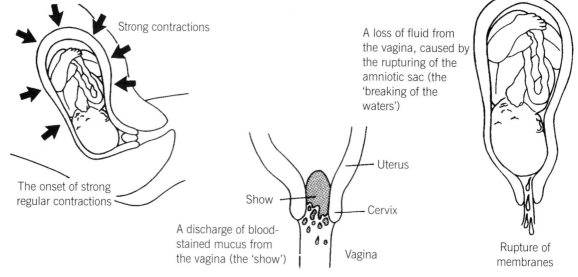

There are three signs that labour has started

Strong contractions

The onset of strong regular contractions

A discharge of blood-stained mucus from the vagina (the 'show')

Show

Uterus

Cervix

Vagina

A loss of fluid from the vagina, caused by the rupturing of the amniotic sac (the 'breaking of the waters')

Rupture of membranes

The onset of labour

Normal labour

A normal labour will have the following characteristics.

- It starts spontaneously (naturally) without any help from the doctor or the use of drugs.
- It starts at **term**, that is between 38 and 42 weeks of pregnancy.
- There is a cephalic (head-first) presentation.
- It is completed in 24 hours.
- The baby is born alive and healthy.
- There are no complications.

term
Between the 38th and 42nd week of pregnancy

Stages of labour

Labour is divided into three stages.

Stage 1

The first stage of labour begins with the onset of regular uterine **contractions**, during which the cervix dilates (widens or gets larger) to allow the baby to be delivered. It ends with full dilatation of the cervix, when it is about 10 cm dilated and cannot get any bigger.

contraction
Involuntary, intermittent muscular tightenings of the uterus

Stage 2

The second stage of labour begins with full dilatation and ends with the birth of the baby.

Stage 3

The third stage begins with the birth of the baby and ends with the complete delivery of the placenta and membranes.

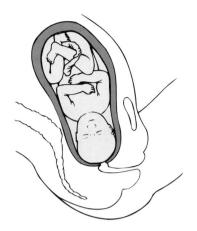

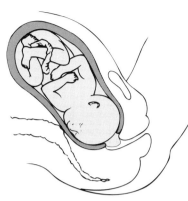

The cervix dilates

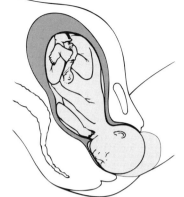

When the cervix is fully dilated,
the head is about to be delivered

The first stage of labour

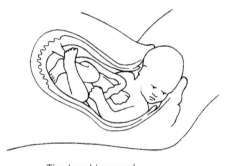

The head 'crowns'

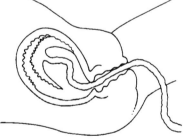

Delivery of the baby

The second stage of labour

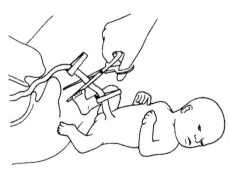

The cord is clamped and cut

The placenta is delivered

The uterus contracts

The third stage of labour

Types of delivery

Some babies and mothers need help with the birth process, and some type of medical intervention may be necessary to make sure that both mother and baby are healthy at the end of labour.

Induction

Induction means starting labour by artificial means. Labour may need to be induced if:

- the baby is very overdue
- the mother is ill, for example with toxaemia
- the placenta is failing.

Labour may be induced by rupturing the membranes and/or giving artificial hormones to stimulate contractions.

Episiotomy

An **episiotomy** is a cut made in the perineum (the area between the vagina and the rectum) during the second stage of labour. It is a fairly common procedure performed for two main reasons:

- to allow the baby to be delivered more quickly
- to prevent a large tear which may involve the rectum.

Forceps delivery

Delivery may be with **forceps** if the baby is becoming distressed. Forceps are spoon-shaped and fit around the baby's head so that the doctor can help with the delivery of the head.

Ventouse extraction

A **ventouse** extraction involves the use of a cup-shaped instrument which fits onto the baby's head and which is attached to suction equipment. The baby is gently helped down the birth canal with the help of suction.

Caesarian section

A **Caesarian** section is a surgical operation to remove the baby, placenta and membranes via the abdominal wall. It may be performed when the mother is awake, but under an epidural anaesthetic or spinal block, which prevents any feelings of pain. Some women may prefer to have a general anaesthetic. Caesarians are performed for many reasons. Some are 'elective' which means that they are done before labour starts, and some are done as an emergency procedure because of an abnormality occurring during labour.

Pain relief in labour

The best form of pain relief in labour is having a positive attitude and knowing what is happening. Women who have been to parentcraft/relaxation classes usually cope well, and their partners are aware of how best to help. Having a familiar hand to hold, a sympathetic midwife and remembering breathing techniques may help to prevent the use of analgesics (painkillers) and anaesthetics. The following are, however, used by many women:

- *pethidine* – a strong drug which can be injected every four hours, to take the edge off contractions

epidural
Anaesthetic injected into the epidural space in the spine to numb the area from the waist down

transcutaneous nerve stimulation (TENS)
An electronic device to control pain in labour

- *nitrous oxide and oxygen (NO$_2$ and O$_2$)* – a gas which the mother can breathe in to help with contractions; she controls the amount she takes, so that she cannot be given too much
- *epidural* – the injection of a painkilling drug into the space around the spinal cord; it numbs the pain of contractions by anaesthetising the nerves that carry sensations to the brain. This type of anaesthetic does not harm the baby and leaves the mother fully conscious
- *transcutaneous nerve stimulation (TENS)* – consists of equipment that produces electrical impulses which block any sensations of pain before they reach the brain; the equipment is loaned to the mother before labour begins so that she can begin to use it as soon as she thinks that labour has begun. It is most effective if it is started very early in labour.

> ### ✓ Progress check
>
> 1 What are the three signs that labour has begun?
> 2 What do you understand by 'normal labour'?
> 3 What are the three stages of labour?
> 4 Why may labour be induced?
> 5 What is an episiotomy?
> 6 What types of pain relief may be offered in labour?

> **Think about it**
>
> 1 Think about how women may be encouraged to feel relaxed during labour.
> 2 Why do women remember the events of childbirth so clearly, years after the event?

Immediate care at birth

The newborn baby

The arrival of a new baby is a time for celebration. Parents are usually overjoyed with the new addition to their family. The first question they ask, however, is usually 'Is she alright?', closely followed by 'How much does she weigh?'

To make sure that the baby is in the best of health and that her progress continues, the midwife and doctor will be making sure that the baby is alright and will eventually get the baby weighed!

Establishing respiration

As soon as the head is delivered, the midwife will wipe the baby's nose and mouth so that when the first breath is taken it is not contaminated with mucus or blood. She may use a mucus extractor to gently suck away

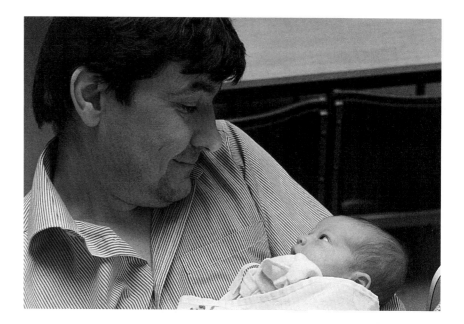

The arrival of a new baby is a time for celebration

the debris of delivery. Most babies breathe spontaneously, but specialised equipment is available in the delivery room for resuscitation if necessary.

Maintaining body temperature

Babies are wet at birth and lose heat very quickly. That is why hospital delivery suites are so hot! It is important to dry the baby as quickly as possible, usually by wrapping her in warm towels to be cuddled by her mother. Radiant heaters over the cot will warm it in preparation for the baby.

The temperature of the baby is taken within an hour of birth using a rectal or digital thermometer.

Bonding

It is extremely important that the parents have close contact with their new baby, so that their relationship can begin positively. Bonding can be encouraged by:

- the mother helping with the delivery, by holding the baby's shoulders and lifting him out
- the baby being delivered into the mother's arms, or onto her tummy if possible
- the mother or her partner cutting the umbilical cord if they wish; this is a symbolic gesture of the start of a new life
- the mother being encouraged to breast feed as soon as possible after delivery, if that is her chosen method of feeding.

Identification

The baby will be labelled immediately after she is born by attaching small bracelets to one wrist and one ankle. These labels contain the name and hospital number of the mother and the date and time of birth. The baby's cot will also be labelled.

Observations

The Apgar score

While all this is happening, the midwife will be closely observing the baby. She will be looking at the vital signs:

- heart rate
- respiration
- muscle tone
- response to stimulus
- colour.

From observing these specific areas she will be able to assess the **Apgar score**. This is an internationally used system for assessing the condition of babies at birth. Each of the five areas above is observed and the baby is given a score of 0, 1 or 2 points according to their condition. These points are added to give a maximum score of ten. (See the table below.)

> **Apgar score**
> A method of assessing the newborn baby's condition by observing the vital signs

The Apgar score

Sign	0	1	2
Heart rate	Absent	Slow (below 100)	Fast (above 100)
Respiration	Absent	Slow, irregular	Good, crying
Muscle tone	Limp	Some flexion of extremities	Active
Response to stimulus (stimulation of foot or nose/mouth)	No response	Grimace	Cry, cough
Colour	Blue, pale	Body pink/dusky, well oxygenated; extremities blue	Completely pink/healthy colour, well oxygenated

The heart and respiratory rate are the most important.
Babies of black, Asian or mixed parentage are a dusky pink colour at birth because the melanin under the skin, which is responsible for their eventual colour, has not yet reached its full concentration. All babies are assessed by monitoring the oxygenation of the blood to the skin.

The test is first performed when the baby is 1 minute old, then 5 minutes later, and every 5 minutes afterwards until the maximum of 10 is achieved. A score of 8–10 indicates that the baby is in good condition at birth. Most babies score 9 at 1 minute, losing a point for colour, as the fingers and toes often remain blue until the circulation becomes fully established.

The Apgar score may be referred to later in childhood if the child shows any signs of developmental delay which may have been caused by their poor condition at birth. A record of the score is kept in the child's health records held by the parents, the health visitor and later by the school nurse.

Measurements

The baby will be weighed soon after birth and the weight recorded in kilograms.

The circumference of the head is also recorded to give a baseline reading against which to measure future growth.

Some centres may continue to measure the length of the baby, but this is now generally thought to be of little value.

Temperature

The temperature is taken to ensure that the baby is warm enough.

Stools and urinary output

It is very important that the midwife observes and records whether the baby has passed urine, and passed meconium (a greenish-black soft stool – see page 291). Failure to do one or either indicates an abnormality which will need investigation.

Examination

The midwife will perform a detailed examination of the baby in the presence of the parents, starting at the head and working downwards, checking for any abnormalities in the baby, and making sure that everything is normal.

General observations

The midwife will check for regular, effortless breathing and skin colour – a healthy bloom will indicate that blood is circulating oxygen around the body.

All babies are varying shades of pink at birth, regardless of their racial origin. There may be **lanugo** (soft, downy hair mainly found in pre-term babies, but some may still be present in babies born at term). **Vernix caseosa** is a white, greasy substance that protects the skin in its watery environment in the uterus. In mature babies, it may be found in the skin creases, but may also be present on the trunk if the baby is premature.

The midwife will note the baby's activity, whether the limbs are moving.

Detailed observations

The head

Fontanelles and suture lines are felt; the eyes are examined to confirm their presence and that formation is normal. The ears are checked for

lanugo
The fine hair found on the body of the fetus before birth and on the newborn infant; mainly associated with pre-term babies

vernix caseosa
White creamy substance found on the skin of the fetus, in the skin creases of mature babies and on the trunk of pre-term infants

skin tags and the mouth for cleft lip and palate, tongue tie (if the frenulum – see Chapter 12 – is attached near the tip of the tongue) and for the presence of teeth.

The arms and hands

The arms and hands are checked for full movement; fingers are counted (an extra digit is not unusual) and webbing (rare, but it may be missed in a check) noted.

The body

An umbilical cord clamp is applied; external genitalia is noted and checked.

The anus is checked by taking the temperature. With the baby in prone (face down), the back is examined to look for any evidence of spina bifida. There may be an open lesion (wound) or a small dimple to signify the presence of a hidden lesion.

The baby may have **mongolian blue spots**, areas of blue tingeing to the skin which look like bruising. They are commonly found at the base of the spine (the sacrum), although they can be anywhere on the body. They are usually found in babies of Asian, African-Caribbean or Mediterranean descent or in babies of mixed race. They disappear before the age of 5 years, but should be recorded to prevent any later allegations of child abuse (see Chapter 12).

The legs

The baby's hips are tested for congenital dislocation (see Book 1, Chapter 18, page 324). Leg movements are noted, to exclude paralysis, and **talipes** (club foot, an abnormality of the foot) is noted. The toes are counted.

Within 24 hours of birth the baby should be examined by a paediatrician (a doctor who specialises in the care of children). This check will include listening to the heart and lungs and palpating (feeling) the abdominal organs.

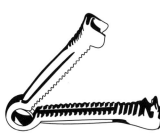

An umbilical cord clamp

mongolian blue spot
Smooth, bluish grey to purple skin patches consisting of an excess of pigmented skin cells

talipes
An abnormal position of the foot caused by the contraction of certain muscles or tendons

> ### ✓ Progress check
>
> 1 What immediate care is given to the baby at birth?
> 2 Why are delivery rooms kept very warm?
> 3 Why is the Apgar score such an important observation?
> 4 What measurements of the baby are recorded after birth?
> 5 What is the first stool called?
> 6 What is lanugo?
> 7 What is vernix caseosa?
> 8 What is a mongolian blue spot?

Do this!   16.1

1 Describe the Apgar score.
2 Briefly describe the midwife's first examination of the new baby.

> ### *Case study: A normal delivery*
>
> Jocelyn has just delivered her second baby. It was a much easier birth this time – her partner, Barry, was with her and she appreciated his presence and concern throughout. The first stage only lasted four hours and after 20 minutes of pushing their son, Jake, was born. When the head was delivered, the midwife encouraged Jocelyn to feel his head and to help to lift his shoulders out with the next contraction. The baby was placed on Jocelyn's abdomen and Barry cut the cord, supervised by the midwife. Jocelyn was cuddling the baby when the midwife told her that his Apgar score was 9 at 10 minutes, but she was too busy counting his fingers and stroking his hands to ask for an explanation.
>
> 1 What did the midwife and parents do to encourage bonding during the delivery?
> 2 How else can bonding be encouraged?
> 3 How could you explain the Apgar score to Jocelyn?

Postnatal care

Security in obstetric units

Most hospitals now employ strict security measures to keep babies safe during their hospital stay. These measures include the use of locks on ward doors, video cameras to record what happens in hospital corridors and wards, extra security personnel, and electronic tagging of babies to monitor their whereabouts and to prevent abductions.

Daily observation and care

Registered midwives have a legal right and responsibility to examine all mothers and babies for a minimum of 10 days after birth. They may continue to visit for 28 days, if necessary.

During the first 24 hours, most abnormalities and illnesses will be identified. It may be considerably longer before some disabilities, such as deafness or developmental delay, are confirmed. Daily observations, as well as noting temperature, respiration and feeding patterns, should include the following areas.

The skin

Many babies have **milia** (tiny, white, milk spots) over the nose. These disappear in time, but occasionally they become infected and need treatment.

Birthmarks may appear in the first few days after birth; not all are present at birth.

> **milia**
> 'Milk spots' – small white spots on the nose of newborn babies caused by blocked sebacious glands

Stools

Meconium is the first stool passed by the baby. It is dark green and sticky, composed of the contents of the digestive tract accumulated during fetal life. After milk feeds, it becomes greenish-brown, then yellowish-brown. These are called *changing stools*, as the last of the meconium is excreted together with the waste products of the milk feeds. This normally takes place around the fourth day.

The stools of a breast-fed baby are typically watery, bright yellow and passed three or four times a day (although the frequency will vary). There is little or no odour. Those of a bottle-fed baby are firm, paler, putty-like, with odour. Green stools occur naturally in some babies, depending on the mother's diet if she is breast-feeding, or the type of artificial milk. Yellow or green, watery frequent stools may indicate gastroenteritis. Small dark green stools are usually due to underfeeding.

meconium
The first stool passed by the newborn infant – a soft black/green motion which is present in the fetal bowel from about the sixteenth week of pregnancy

The eyes

Sticky eyes (ophthalmia neonatorum) are common, because a new baby cannot yet produce tears. They are easily treated with antibiotic drops if discovered early. The eyes are examined daily and cleaned, using separate swabs for each eye.

sticky eyes
A discharge from the eyes in the first three weeks of life

The mouth

The mouth is checked for oral **thrush**, a common fungal infection. It looks like milk residue on the tongue and cheeks.

thrush
A fungal infection of the mouth and/or nappy area

The umbilical cord

The cord should be checked daily and kept clean and dry to avoid infection. The cord stump usually drops off by the sixth day.

Feeding

Whether breast- or bottle-fed, babies will establish their own routine. Demand feeding when the baby is hungry rather than on a strict four-hourly schedule (see Chapter 17) is recommended.

Bathing

Babies can be bathed daily and the midwife will teach the new mother the correct procedure. However, topping and tailing (washing the face, hands and bottom) is quite adequate with a full bath every two or three days, if this fits in more easily with the home routine.

Crying

All babies cry during the early weeks. The cause can usually be detected by process of elimination: the carer checks whether the baby is hungry, thirsty, in pain (wind) or uncomfortable (too hot, too cold, soiled nappy, uncomfortable position).

Screening tests

Various **screening** tests are performed in the early neonatal period to check for specific abnormalities that can be successfully treated if detected early enough.

The Guthrie test

The **Guthrie test** is performed on the sixth day of milk feeding, to detect phenylketonuria (PKU) and cystic fibrosis (see Book 1, Chapter 18, pages 334 and 326 respectively). A sample of blood is obtained by pricking the baby's heel. This sample is also checked for levels of thyroxine so that hypothyroidism (cretinism) can be treated.

Barlow's test

This hip test is performed by the midwife and later by the doctor, to check for congenital dislocation of the hip (see Book 1, Chapter 18, page 324). The health visitor will repeat the test, and so will the GP when the baby has a 6-week medical and development check.

> **screening**
> Checking the whole population of children at specific ages for particular abnormalities

> **Guthrie test**
> On the sixth day after birth, a sample of the baby's blood is taken, usually by pricking the heel, to test for phenylke-tonuria, cystic fibrosis and cretinism

Low birth-weight babies

Not all babies are born at term; some are born early and an increasing number of these are surviving because of improved neonatal care. **Low birth-weight** babies can be divided into two main categories:

- **pre-term** (premature) – these babies are born before 37 completed weeks of pregnancy, i.e. at 36 weeks gestation or less
- **light-for-dates** (small-for-dates) – these babies are below the expected weight for their gestational age – the length of the pregnancy, according to percentile charts.

Some babies are both premature *and* light-for-dates.

Seven to 8 per cent of all babies are low birth-weight, but almost half of all deaths in the first month occur in this group. This shows how important the birth-weight of a baby is. There is a greater chance of a baby surviving if he weighs more than 2.5 kg.

> **low birth-weight**
> Babies born prematurely or below the 10th centile for their gestation, usually weighing less than 2.5 kg at birth

> **pre-term**
> A baby born before 36 completed weeks of pregnancy; also referred to as premature

> **light-for-dates**
> Babies born weighing less than the 10th centile for their gestation period

Pre-term babies

Pre-term (or premature) babies are immature and are not yet ready to survive alone outside the womb. They have a better chance of survival if their weight falls between the 90th and 10th percentile.

Characteristics of pre-term babies

There are several characteristics common to pre-term babies.

- The head is even larger in proportion to the body than usual.
- The face is small and triangular with a pointed chin.
- The baby looks 'worried'.
- They may be reluctant to open their eyes.

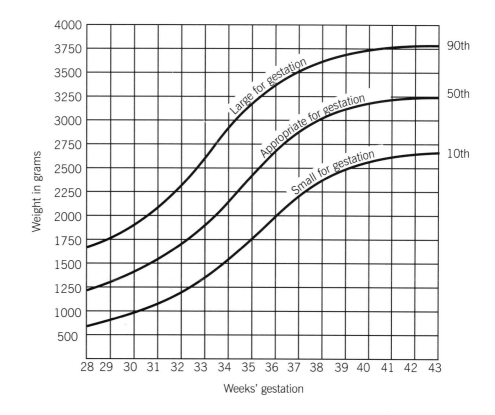

A percentile chart, showing weight and gestation

- The sutures and fontanelles are large.
- The skin may be red.
- The veins are prominent.
- The baby may be covered in lanugo.
- The limbs are thin.
- Nails are soft.
- The chest is narrow.
- The abdomen is large.
- The umbilicus is low-set.
- There are small genitalia, poorly developed.
- Muscle tone is floppy.
- Arms and legs are extended.
- They are feeble and drowsy.
- Reflexes are poor, the baby may be unable to suck.

Causes of prematurity

Causes of premature delivery are often unknown, but are commoner in mothers who smoke and in those with pre-eclampsia (toxaemia of pregnancy, see Book 1, Chapter 6, page 122) or with a multiple pregnancy. Prematurity is also associated with poverty and deprivation which may indicate the importance of a good diet and healthy lifestyle in pregnancy.

Complications of prematurity

Complications which might arise for a pre-term baby are:

- **birth asphyxia** – pre-term babies may be slow to breathe at birth due to an immature respiratory centre in the brain
- respiratory problems – immaturity of the lungs may make breathing difficult
- intracranial haemorrhage (bleeding in the brain) – fragile blood vessels in the brain may bleed easily. This may cause long-term damage.

The care of premature babies is a highly specialised field; they are prone to many difficulties. For example, like all babies they cannot control their temperature, but the smaller the baby the greater the risk of hypothermia. They are more likely to become jaundiced or anaemic and are vulnerable to infections. Some pre-term babies do survive and develop well, but some suffer long-term damage as a direct result of their prematurity.

Possible effects on development are:

- *generalised developmental delay* – this 'global' delay may affect all areas of development, with milestones being achieved at a much later age, if at all
- *specific developmental difficulties* – there may be a particular problem with one area of development, such as motor or communication skills
- *sensory loss* – blindness and deafness are much more common in children who have been born very early.

Special Care Baby Unit (SCBU)

Some pre-term infants will require the specialised care of the SCBU to provide the highly skilled and technological support that they need. These units are usually divided into high-dependency and low-dependency areas.

High dependency

In the high-dependency area, babies are cared for in **incubators**. These are enclosed, transparent cots which automatically adjust the temperature to maintain the baby's body temperature at 36.5–37.2° C. Babies may be covered with a heat shield and dressed in hat, mittens and bootees to retain their warmth as long as they can be observed for any changes in their condition. An apnoea mattress will monitor their breathing and an alarm will sound if respiration stops or become irregular.

Small, pre-term babies are handled as little as possible but very gently. They are fed and cared for through perspex doors in the side of the incubator. Strict attention to hygiene in the SCBU helps to prevent infection – handwashing before and after handling each baby is vital.

Low dependency

As the baby's condition improves, they are transferred into the low-dependency area where they are nursed in a cot. Their progress is monitored before discharge to the postnatal ward or home.

Support for parents

At the time of birth the mother may be able to hold the baby for a short time before transfer to the SCBU. She and her partner can visit the baby at any time and should be encouraged to touch and stroke the baby and hold its hand. Parents are always supported and encouraged to provide as much care as possible – early contact and touching is essential if bonding is to occur and a healthy emotional relationship to continue.

Case study: Premature delivery

The ambulance rushed to 24 Hazel Grove. The ambulance station had received a distressed call from Jim Ludlow telling them to hurry, his wife was pregnant and had started to haemorrhage (bleed).

The midwife was at the house, trying to reassure a very anxious and almost hysterical Anthea Ludlow. She couldn't lose this baby – she had miscarried four times already and had never before got to the 28th week. She had been in the shower when she noticed that she was bleeding. Her husband had responded immediately to her screams of anguish, and taken her gently to the bed before calling the midwife and ambulance.

At the hospital, the doctors knew that the baby must be delivered – the bleeding had not stopped and the fetal heart rate was dropping. Anthea signed a consent form and was hurriedly prepared for an emergency Caesarian section. Jim waited anxiously outside the operating theatre. It seemed like an eternity until a nurse and paediatrician came out and showed him his daughter inside a portable incubator. He went with them to the special care unit where he held her briefly and was given a Polaroid picture to give to Anthea when she came round from the general anaesthetic.

1 Describe what you think the physical appearance of the baby is like.
2 What care will the baby require?
3 How can bonding be encouraged for this family?
4 What possible complications might affect Anthea and Jim's daughter?

✓ *Progress check*

1 For how long after a birth does a midwife have the responsibility to visit a mother and baby?
2 What are milia?
3 Describe the typical stool of:
   a) a breast-fed baby
   b) a bottle-fed baby.
4 Why are a baby's eyes vulnerable to infection?
5 What is demand feeding?
6 Why do babies cry?
7 When is the Guthrie test performed? Why is it done?

8 What are the two categories of low birth-weight babies?
9 Why is the birth-weight of a baby important?
10 a) What may be the cause(s) of prematurity?
   b) What are the characteristics of pre-term babies?
   c) What effects may prematurity have on future development?
11 What specialised care is provided in a SCBU ?
12 Why is parental involvement so important if a baby is in SCBU ?

Early development

There are wide variations in the ages at which babies will develop particular skills. Parents and carers will inevitably compare their child to others of the same age to assess progress. It is common to hear conversations concerning the ages at which particular goals are reached, for example 'John smiled at 3 weeks', 'Shazia sat up at 4 months'. If another child has not made similar progress, it can arouse parental anxiety. It is important to remember that all children develop in a very individual way (see Book 1, Chapter 3), and that their progress should be measured against:

- what is typical for their age range
- cultural/biological origin
- parental/genetic background
- social group
- gestational age
- level of stimulation
- medical background
- their own achievements, that is whether or not any new skills have been learnt by them within a period of time.

It is important to remember that all areas of development are linked and dependent on each other, and should not be viewed in isolation.

Stimulating development

All babies need to be stimulated in order to progress through the developmental stages. Stimulation can be as simple as talking to a young baby and achieving or maintaining eye-contact. Babies need a lot of physical contact with adults who will spend time with them, caring for them and meeting their needs. This will enable babies to communicate and feel secure.

Stimulation does not mean a hot-house of toys and activities which are often beyond the capabilities of the child, although some toys do make learning through play exciting and challenging. It is possible to over-stimulate a baby which can cause stress, anxiety and unhappiness in the child, and so defeat the purpose.

Above all, babies need close and secure contact with adults. It is through this trusted relationship that development will proceed and skills will be learnt. A feeling of security and of being well cared for is essential for a child to reach its full potential.

The table on pages 298–301 summarises activities and toys that are appropriate to the different ages and stages of development.

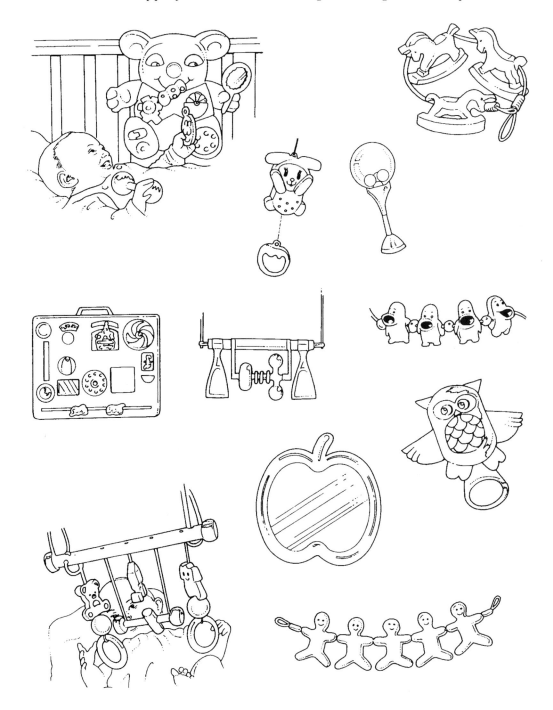

Some stimulating toys for a baby's pram or cot

Methods of stimulating development

Age	Area of development	Stage of development	Stimulating activities/toys
0–3 months	Gross motor	Head control developing; kicking legs with movements becoming smoother and more symmetrical in supine; enjoys being held sitting; begins to support head and chest on forearms in prone	Time for lying on the floor to kick and experiment with movement; opportunity to be without nappy or clothing to encourage co-ordination; change positions from prone to supine so that the baby feels comfortable in either; sitting supported on carer's knee and in bouncing cradle
	Fine motor	Fascinated by human faces; grasp reflex diminishing; outwards direction of development progressing; trying to co-ordinate hands and eyes to control environment; finger play: beginning to discover the hands; may begin to hold objects for a few moments when placed in the hand	Bright colourful objects to encourage focusing within the visual field of 20–25 cm, e.g. mobiles, watching the washing line, pictures of faces around the cot, toys with facial characteristics; opportunity to watch what is happening around her; use of noise to attract attention, e.g. rattle placed in her hand or objects strung over the cot, which make a noise when touched; baby-gym, or other objects within reach of waving arms
	Hearing and speech	Recognises main carer's voice; vocalising in conversational pattern; beginning to look for the origin of the sound; cries to indicate need	Opportunity to bond with main carer and recognise their voice; lots of physical contact and cuddles with loving conversations which maintain eye contact and give the baby the opportunity to respond; carers need to show lots of pleasure when they do; enjoys being sung to
	Social and play	Smiles from about 5 to 6 weeks; enjoys all caring routines and responds to loving handling; imitates some facial expressions, e.g. beginning to recognise situations, e.g. smiles, vocalises and uses total body movement to express pleasure at bathtime or feeding time	Lots of contact with adults and children to widen the social network, but mainly with primary carer, to strengthen the bond; routines for meeting needs to ensure security and comfort; stimulating areas of development, as above; opportunity for eye contact and to watch faces and mimic them, e.g. sticking tongue out
3–6 months	Gross motor	Head control established; beginning to sit with support; rolling over; playing with feet in supine, and raising head to look around; supporting head and chest on extended forearms in prone; weight bearing and bouncing when held standing	Opportunity to practise sitting, on carer's knee, then protected by cushions for a soft landing when she topples! Physical play: bouncing on the knee with suitable songs, rough and tumble on the bed, rolling and bouncing (NB Never leave a baby alone on the bed or other high surface); carer's knee is ideal gymnasium at this age: some babies love to stand and bounce up and down for long periods of time; baby bouncer may be useful purchase; time to practise and experiment skills on the floor

(Continued on facing page)

	Fine motor	Beginning to use palmar grasp and transfer objects from hand to hand; watches all activity with interest; moves head around to follow people and objects	As baby is finding her hands, toys which rattle are essential; as she holds an object, the noise it makes will attract her attention and she will see the clever thing she is doing; colourful, small, safe toys which can be grasped by tiny fingers are invaluable, e.g. soft animals, box of bricks, chiming ball, home-made toys, e.g. transparent plastic bottles with coloured water inside or half-filled with sugar or dried beans which rattle (lid must be tightly on and baby supervised); old plastic cotton reels strung together provide useful tactile experience; baby needs things to reach out for and things to hit
	Hearing and speech	Turns immediately to familiar sounds; screening hearing test may be performed from 6 months onwards; tuneful vocalisations, sing-song sounds, laughs and squeals with pleasure; responds to different emotional voices in carer	Lots of physical contact and play using songs and voice; conversations with carers and others, who give baby time to respond, reinforce responses by showing pleasure and repeating sounds; enjoys listening to nursery rhymes and finger games with tune and rhythm; This little piggy and This is the way the farmer rides encourage listening and fun
	Social and play	Beginning to put all toys in mouth to explore them and investigate the world by object; recognising objects which make a noise, trying to utilise them; finding the feet as a source of investigation and pleasure; enjoys strangers if they are friendly and gentle	Safe, non-toxic toys to put in the mouth; some babies may enjoy finger feeding too; make bean bags with various fillings, e.g. dried peas, crunchy cereals, to give oral experience; make books suitable for chewing, using photographs and/or pictures in plastic covers; waterproof bath books useful purchase; opportunity to play and investigate both alone and in the company of other children
6–9 months	Gross motor	Can sit unsupported for lengthening periods of time; may begin to crawl; may stand and cruise holding on to furniture or other stable objects; some may begin to walk with hands held or even alone	Needs to be given time to play on the floor, placed in sitting position, with support until stability is established; fun toys big enough to see and attract attention, just out of reach to stimulate mobility, but not enough to increase frustration; surround baby with toys in sitting position to encourage balance skills as he reaches to grasp to sides and the front; time spent bouncing on feet and encouraging strength in legs; stable furniture for baby to pull to stand
	Fine motor	Visually very alert to people and objects; developing pincer grasp with thumb and index finger; uses index finger to poke and point; looks for fallen objects	Needs lots of exciting visual activity, e.g. going to the park, shopping; toddler group good opportunity for observing other children play; smaller objects can be introduced with supervision, (remember that everything will go into the mouth), e.g. small pieces of biscuit or bread, hundreds and thousands to encourage a pincer grasp and yet be safe to eat; build towers of bricks to be knocked down with glee; look at picture books, encouraging baby to point at familiar objects with you; encourage baby to look for and find items 'lost' over side of highchair, to help make sense of the world and cause and effect, e.g. something dropped does not disappear forever

(Continued overleaf)

Methods of stimulating development (continued)

Age	Area of development	Stage of development	Stimulating activities/toys
	Hearing and speech	Babbles loudly and tunefully, repeating sounds again and again, e.g. da da da; beginning to understand commonly used words and phrases, e.g. No, Bye bye; varies volume and pitch depending on mood, whether happy or cross; still cries for needs	Talk to baby about what is happening all the time; repeat their interpretations of words; sing repetitive songs, encouraging them to vocalise with you; finger rhymes encourage language; read books together, naming objects; encourage imitations of verbal and non-verbal language; name objects and people baby points at
	Social and play	Now wary of strangers; plays games like Pat-a-cake, Peep-bo; claps and waves; offers toys to others; finger-feeds; attempts to use cup and/or bottle; looks for partly hidden toys	Games and activities to encourage language development also stimulate play and social skills; as baby now discovers values of objects, she will need things that respond differently when same thing is done to them, e.g. ball will roll when pushed, brick will not; biscuit will crumble when squeezed, bread will not, toys that squeak, bricks that do not; safety mirror in plastic frame to allow the baby to recognise herself; post table-tennis balls down kitchen-roll tube; toys or safe household items that can be banged to make a noise, wooden spoon, saucepan or xylophone; babies are beginning to make music and be delighted by achievements
9–12 months	Gross motor	Will now be mobile, crawling, bottom-shuffling, bear-walking or walking; may be able to crawl upstairs; mobility has frustrations as well as pleasures: baby can reach areas previously out-of-bounds, so needs attention in providing suitable playthings within reach	Large-wheeled toys fun to push around, brick-trolley or similar push-along toy to help develop skills of getting around corners, reversing, etc.; small climbing frames used with supervision to increase balance and co-ordination; swimming; walking outside with reins
	Fine motor	Mature pincer grasp; throws toys deliberately; points to desired objects; bangs toys together	Pull-string musical box or similar to encourage dexterity and also teach cause and effect; nesting toys, building bricks, etc. will encourage balance and concepts of shape, size and colour; roll balls for baby to fetch, she will soon roll them for you; tin or basket filled with interesting objects to take out and put back in; plastic jars and bottles with removable lids to encourage investigation of what is inside, or simple delight at removing lid
	Hearing and speech	Understands several words and phrases; obeys simple commands; lots of vocalisations with sounds for certain objects, e.g. dud may mean cup	Talk to baby constantly, repeat names of people and objects, sing songs, games and rhymes, read stories with familiar situations and few characters; baby must be surrounded by language to develop communication skills effectively

(Continued on facing page)

| Social and play | Usually loving and affectionate, likes to be near someone familiar; can drink from cup with a little help; tries to use spoon; likes to put objects in and out of containers; participates in routines | Make sure that care is consistent and familiar; give opportunity to learn to feed, e.g. allow practice with cup and spoon, regardless of inevitable mess; valuable for sensory experience; offer lots of opportunity for play with interaction from adults, e.g. taking turns, stop and go; baby sometimes acquires a new skill by making something happen by mistake – if it is fun he will want to do it again; adult must observe this and reinforce positive actions; opportunity to watch and imitate others, perhaps in routine domestic chores; small dustpan and brush or similar to encourage this and make help valued; needs own equipment, e.g. flannel, toothbrush, cup, spoon to foster feeling of personal identity, and encouragement to take part in caring routines |

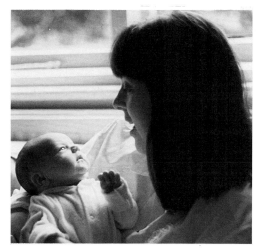

Babies are fascinated by human faces

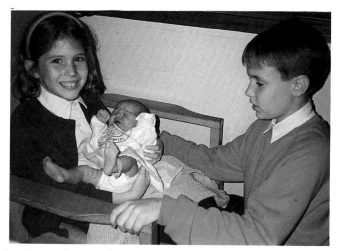

The baby cries to indicate a need

All methods of stimulating development can be achieved without great financial cost. Not all families can afford frequent shopping trips to purchase the latest toy or aid to development. Manufacturers can make parents or carers believe that development cannot be maintained unless a certain article or gadget is purchased, often at great cost. But this is a fairly recent phenomenon. For thousands of years, babies have developed with little more than parental care and home-made equipment, so however attractive and necessary the latest toys appear, parents should be reassured that their children are not deprived if they cannot afford to purchase them all. A little ingenuity and imagination, combined with an awareness of safety, can provide a multitude of learning experiences with everyday household articles.

There are facilities for loaning, renting or giving children the opportunity to play with different toys at a specific venue. It may be possible to purchase toys second-hand. The following should be investigated as possible sources for varied play experiences:

- toy libraries
- toy loan facilities
- playgroups
- mother and toddler groups
- jumble sales and car boot sales
- newspaper and shop advertisements.

It costs a great deal to buy new clothes and equipment for a new baby, but looking through the small advertisements section of any local newspaper will show that all the necessary items can be purchased at a fraction of the retail price. Nor do all toys and equipment need to be purchased: some organisations will loan the necessary items or make a small weekly charge for rental. The health visitor, social services department or Citizens' Advice Bureau should be able to give details of such charitable organisations in any area.

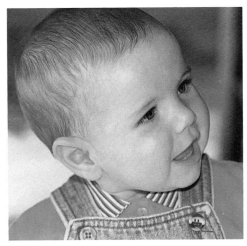

The hearing test may be performed from 6 months when the baby turns to sounds

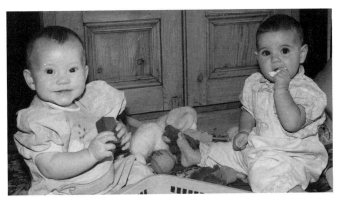

At 6–9 months, babies will sit unsupported for longer periods

Case study: Advice for a new mother

Sonya Middleton has recently come home from hospital with her first child, Logan. Her head is in a whirl with thinking about feeding and changing and why this baby does not seem to sleep! She used to be so organised, working for a merchant bank and making important financial decisions that would affect the lives of hundreds of people on a daily basis. She is completely baffled about how such a tiny creature can turn her world upside down and make her feel like a gibbering wreck. She is due to return to work when Logan is 3 months old and she cannot imagine how she will be able to function as a working, single mother who can provide suitable stimulation for her child. Questions keep going through her head – What should she do to make sure that he develops in all areas? What should he be doing and when? How will she know if something is wrong?

1 Devise a plan of activities for this baby to stimulate all areas of development in the first six months of life.
2 How could a nanny support this mother and baby?

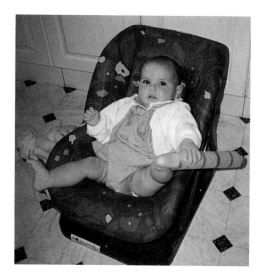

Everyday household articles can easily provide learning experiences

✅ *Progress check*

1 What factors should be taken into account when assessing development?
2 Why is personal contact especially important to a young baby?
3 How could you stimulate:
   a) gross motor development from birth to 3 months?
   b) fine motor development from 3 to 6 months?
   c) social and play from 6 to 9 months?
   d) hearing and speech from 9 to 12 months?
4 Where are toys and equipment available for families who do not wish to purchase them?

Think about it

1 Think of three activities to encourage all-round development in a baby from 6 to 12 months.
2 Think of all the household items you could use to provide stimulation during the first year.

Do this!   16.2

1 Make an item for a baby to provide sensory experience. Observe the baby using your toy and encourage them to use all aspects of it.

2 Collect together several safe items for a baby from 6 to 12 months to explore to stimulate all areas of development. Observe babies playing with these items and evaluate how effective they are.

3 Make a playbox full of interesting and safe items for a baby to examine.

4 a) Select toys from a shop or catalogue that are suitable for a baby during the first year. Make a chart to display their prices.

   b) Give reasons for your choices and include methods of adapting these toys for the baby as she goes into the second and third year.

Key terms

You need to know what these words and phrases mean. Go back through the chapter to find out.

Apgar score
birth asphyxia
Caesarian
contraction
epidural
episiotomy
forceps
Guthrie test
incubator
induction
labour
lanugo
light-for-dates
low birth-weight
meconium
milia
mongolian blue spot
pre-term
screening
sticky eyes
talipes
transcutaneous nerve stimulation (TENS)
term
thrush
ventouse
vernix caseosa

Now try these questions

1 Describe the forms of pain relief available to women in labour.

2 List the screening tests in the first year and explain why they are important.

3 Explain the possible effects of a prolonged stay in a Special Care Baby Unit on a child's emotional development.

4 Make an outline plan to stimulate gross motor development between 6 and 12 months.

17 *Physical needs in the first year*

This chapter includes:

- **Equipment**
- **Layette**
- **Clothing for the first year**
- **Feeding**
- **Weaning**
- **Routines for care**
- **Nappy care**
- **Care of black skin**
- **Signs and symptoms of illness**
- **Sudden infant death syndrome**
- **Positive health for babies**

In the first year of life, babies require care which will meet both their individual needs and the particular needs of all infants. All babies are unique and special and, because of their age and stage of development, they require highly skilled care from their parents or qualified child-care workers. This chapter explains the value of specialised types of care and equipment used in the first year of life.

You may find it helpful to read this chapter in conjunction with:

- ▶ **Book 2, Chapter 19**   Physical care
- ▶ **Book 2, Chapter 23**   Caring for sick children

Equipment

Having a baby will necessarily incur some financial cost, unless the family has a baby already and has kept all the required items. Even so, they will need to ensure that the equipment is still suitable and safe to use. There are many factors to consider, the well-being of the infant being of prime importance. Some of these factors are outlined below.

Safety

All equipment bought, loaned or rented, new or second-hand, must comply with safety legislation and carry the BSI safety kitemark.

Lifestyle

If, for example, the family uses a car for most journeys, a pram may not be an essential item, but a car seat will be.

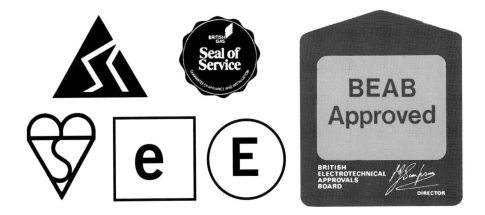

Marks of safety

Accommodation

The family may have plenty of space for large equipment, or may be living in a small flat, bedsit, or perhaps with extended family. Carers may need to consider, for example, how to cope with transporting the baby up several flights of narrow stairs.

Adaptability and durability

Equipment that is to be purchased must be justified in terms of long-term usefulness and be strong enough to withstand normal wear and tear. A cot, for example, will be in use for two years and perhaps more. It should be strong enough to continue to be safe for this and subsequent babies.

Prams and pushchairs must be suitable for continued use as the baby becomes a toddler, to avoid having to replace it unnecessarily early.

Practicality

It is easy to fall for the pretty items that look so appealing but are of little practical value. The frilly pram may prove difficult to clean when the baby has vomited on it! Highchairs with fabric seats may look lovely in the shop, but are not practical when the baby begins to feed himself.

Essential items

All babies need:
- a place to sleep
- provision for feeding and hygiene routines, such as bathing and changing nappies
- to be safely transported.

The tables on pages 308–311 summarise the advantages and disadvantages of different types of essential items.

Essential items for sleeping and transport

Item	Features	Advantages	Disadvantages
To try to prevent avoidable cot deaths, current research recommends that all babies should sleep: ■ on their backs ■ without a pillow ■ without a duvet for the first year; sheets and blankets prevent overheating by removing a layer when necessary.			
Moses basket	Wicker basket with decorative lining and covers, with or without a canopy; usually with two handles for transport; may have a stand or be placed on the floor	Baby feels secure in small, enclosed space; easy to carry from room to room; looks pretty and appealing	Cannot be used to transport baby outside; unsafe for use in the car; unsuitable for older/heavier babies due to lack of internal space; may topple as baby moves around
Cradle	Wooden crib with rocking mechanism, either on rockers or suspended between two upright supports	As for Moses basket, except for ease of use between rooms; baby may respond well to being rocked to sleep	As for Moses basket
Carrycot	Rigid structure with mattress, waterproof cover and hood and carrying handles; covered in washable fabric or plastic	Enclosed space so baby feels comfortable and secure, used for night and daytime sleeping; easy to transport from room to room using handles; suitable for use outdoors, may be available with transporter (wheels) to convert to pram; restraining straps for transport by car	Babies will grow out of a carrycot sooner than a full-size pram; may be heavy and cumbersome to lift when the baby is older
Pram	Rigid, frame-built structure with hood and waterproof cover on wheels, with brakes, washable fabric, plastic or metal exterior and fabric interior with mattress; harness fixing points	Baby feels comfortable, safe and secure; can be used for sleeping downstairs at home; ideal for use outside, for journeys on foot or for letting the baby sleep in the fresh air; suitable for use in all weathers; large enough to carry the baby for the first year and longer; shopping tray makes transporting groceries easier; possible to transport a toddler as well on a specially designed pram seat	Unsuitable for getting up and down stairs, so alternative night-time sleeping arrangements required; may be a problem in a block of flats if lifts not working; unsuitable for transportation by car; may create storage problem in a small house/flat or bedsit

	Features	Advantages	Disadvantages
Cot	A purpose-built sleeping area for a baby and toddler; should be strong and stable; bars should be no more than 7 cm apart to prevent hands, feet and head getting stuck; waterproof, safety mattress that fits tightly within the frame; dropside cots should have childproof safety catches; option of high or low mattress position, depending on age/stage of the baby	Safe secure sleeping environment individual to each baby, whether room is shared or not	No disadvantages provided that all specifications under Features are met
Rearward-facing baby car seat	Designed for safe car travel using standard inertia seat belts; contains harness to restrain the baby within it; carrying handle to move the seat to and from the car	Safe transportation in a car; easy to carry with a sleeping baby in it; back support for a very young baby; can be used from birth until about 9 months; useful for babies who need motion to get to sleep; can be used in the house as a first seat	Can be expensive; will need replacing with a fixed car seat at about 9 months; some models can be difficult to carry and attach car seat belts to
Bouncing cradle	Soft fabric seat for a baby from birth to about 6 months; may include a row of toys	Used from birth; baby can be transported from room to room and can see what is happening everywhere; babies can rock themselves to sleep; easy to wash fabric cover	Dangerous if left on a bed or worktop when the baby can bounce themselves off; not suitable when babies can sit unsupported
Carrying slings	Fabric baby slings, attached to the carer's body to enable the baby to be carried in an upright position on the chest	Baby feels comfortable and secure, can hear carer's heartbeat and feel body warmth; comfortable sleeping position; babies can be carried indoors and out, invaluable for fractious ones who find sleep difficult or crave constant contact; leaves two hands free to cope with a toddler or other children needing supervision and attention; allows carer to continue with routine tasks	May be difficult to put on and take off depending on the mechanism; may strain the back as baby gets heavier; flat shoes and careful posture essential to prevent injury to the baby by falling

Essential items for bathing

Item	Features	Advantages	Disadvantages
Warmth is essential when bathing a new baby. A wall thermometer will ensure that the room is at least 70° C before you start.			
Baby bath	Plastic, purpose-built baby bath, usually bought with a stand	Large enough to use until the baby is about 6 months; can be used in any room where there is sufficient heat; comfortable for baby and carer, who can sit in a chair to bath when the bathstand is in use	Limited life, and of little use when the baby is bathed in the big bath.; difficult and heavy to carry when full of water; storage may be difficult in small accommodation
New washing-up bowl or storage box	Large plastic container	Can be used for its original purpose when no longer needed for bathing; easy to transport to a warm environment when full of water; large enough to bath a baby in the early weeks; avoids expense of purpose-built models	Baby will need to transfer to the big bath by 2 to 3 months

A large plastic bowl or box for bathing is efficient and cost effective

Essential items for feeding

It is largely personal preference which will decide whether a mother will begin to breast- or bottle-feed her baby.

Advantages and disadvantages	Breast-feeding	Bottle-feeding	Other essential equipment
The advantages and disadvantages of breast-and bottle-feeding are discussed later in the chapter.	It is advisable to have some bottle-feeding equipment to provide extra water or fruit juices, even if the baby is being breast-fed; two or three bottles and teats should be sufficient.	If the baby is being bottle-fed, then eight to ten bottles and teats will be required to make up enough feeds for a 24-hour period.	Sterilising equipment will be essential, and a good supply of formula milk; there are many brands available

✅ **Progress check**

1 Which factors need consideration when buying equipment for a new baby?
2 How should babies be put to sleep to try to prevent cot death?
3 What are the features of a Moses basket?
4 List the advantages of a carry cot.
5 Why should a bouncing cradle always be placed on the floor?

Do this!   **17.1**

1 Prepare a booklet for parents to show the range of equipment available for a new baby. Include diagrams or photographs to illustrate each item. Draw attention to the advantages and disadvantages of each item.

2 Visit shops in your area to price all the essential items. Look through the small advertisements section of the local paper and cost similar second-hand equipment. Work out the savings to be made by buying in this way. What factors must be taken into account when buying second-hand articles for a baby? Why do some parents reject the idea of buying previously used equipment?

Layette

layette
First clothes for a baby

The **layette** is the first set of clothes provided for a baby. Some guidelines for purchasing baby clothes are given below.

■ Avoid ribbons, ties and bows which can trap tiny fingers and toes and be very difficult to take on and off. They may cause a strangulation hazard. Garments of a loose weave (for example, hand-knitted) can be similarly hazardous.

■ Buttons are a dangerous choking hazard as well as being fiddly for large fingers.

■ Choose clothes that are easy to launder; babies need changing often.

■ Natural fibres are the most comfortable; cotton, for example is more absorbent than synthetic fabrics.

■ Clothing should be comfortable, to allow for ease of movement, and not too tight, especially around the vulnerable feet. Clothes made of stretch fabric and with raglan sleeves make dressing and undressing much easier. Avoid suits with feet as it is tempting to continue using them after they have been outgrown. A footless suit with a pair of correctly sized socks is a better alternative.

■ Garments should have a flame-retardant finish.

Clothing for a newborn

■ Six vests – bodysuits prevent cold spots and help to keep the nappy in place

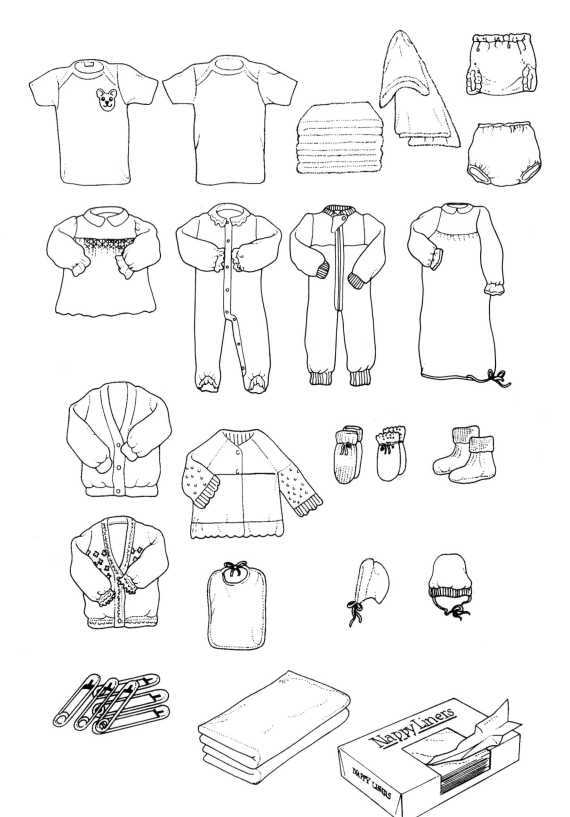

A baby's layette

- Six all-in-ones – babygros, preferably footless
- Three pairs of socks or bootees
- Three cardigans (matinee jackets)
- Hat – sunhat in the summer and bonnet for colder weather
- Outdoor clothing – type will depend on method of transporting the baby. A knitted pramsuit may suffice or a quilted all-in-one may be required
- Warm mittens and scratch mittens
- Nappies – whether disposable nappies or terry nappies are to be used a good supply is required. Do not buy more than one pack of first size nappies until the baby is born and its size is known. Dial-a-nappy services are available in some areas.
  Twenty-four terry nappies are sufficient, and will perhaps last for a subsequent baby. Nappy pins, nappy liners and plastic pants will also be required.

Clothing for the first year

- Babies grow very quickly, so it is sensible not to buy too many clothes of the same size. There will be little chance to wear them all before they are outgrown.
- Shoes are unnecessary until a child needs to walk outside. Bare feet are preferable, even to socks, if it is warm enough and the flooring is safe.

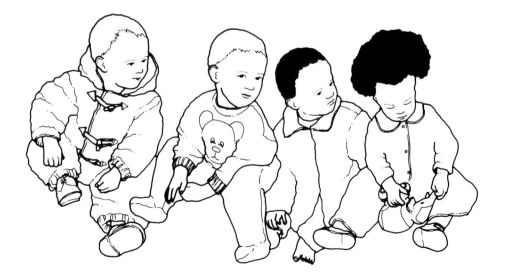

Clothing for the first year: garments should allow for ease of movement and be easily washable

- Choose clothes that will help development and not hinder it; baby girls trying to crawl in a dress, for example, will become increasingly frustrated as they crawl into their skirts.
- Clothing needs will vary according to the season.
- Sort out clothes regularly and remove all that has been outgrown from the baby's drawers. This will prevent anyone who does not dress the baby often trying to squeeze them into garments that are too small.

✓ Progress check

1 What is a layette?
2 What guidelines should be followed when preparing a layette?
3 What special considerations are necessary when buying clothing for a baby in the first year?
4 When are shoes necessary?
5 Give three examples of clothing hindering development.

Think about it

Think of all the available methods of clothing a baby on a small budget. Are there any national organisations or services in your area, which may be able to help a family to meet all the unavoidable costs of caring for a young baby?

Do this!   17.2

1 Prepare a list of all the essential clothing items for a baby during the first year. Include the various items for a winter as well as a summer birth.

2 Find out how much the average baby costs to clothe during the first year. Visit local shops selling infant clothing and use catalogues to prepare your costings.

Feeding

All babies should be fed on milk only for at least the first three months of life, so parents must decide how the baby will be fed. The decision to breast- or bottle-feed is a very personal one. Most women have an idea of how they will feed their babies before they become pregnant. This may be influenced by how their mother fed them, how their friends feed their babies, health education at school, the influence of the media and how they feel about their body.

There are advantages and disadvantages to both methods, but it is agreed that breast milk:

- is the natural milk for babies as it is the ideal source of nutrients for the first months of life
- should be encouraged as the first choice for infant feeding.

However, breast feeding may not be possible for a number of reasons and women should not feel inadequate if they bottle-feed their babies.

Breast-feeding

The primary function of the breasts is to supply food and nourishment to an infant. During pregnancy, the breasts enlarge by about 5 cm and prepare for feeding. Successful breast-feeding does not depend on the size of the breasts; women with very small breasts can breast-feed just as successfully as those with large breasts.

Each breast is divided into 15–20 lobes containing alveoli which produce milk. Each lobe drains milk into a lactiferous duct which widens into an ampulla (small reservoir) just behind the nipple. It narrows before opening on the surface of the nipple.

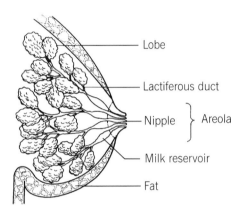

The lactating breast

From the sixteenth week of pregnancy, the breasts produce colostrum. This will feed the baby for the first 2–3 days after birth. It is a thick, yellowish fluid which has a high protein content but is lower in sugar and fat than mature human milk. Only a few millilitres are produced at each feed but it satisfies the baby, it helps to clear the meconium from the intestine and is very easy for the new baby to digest.

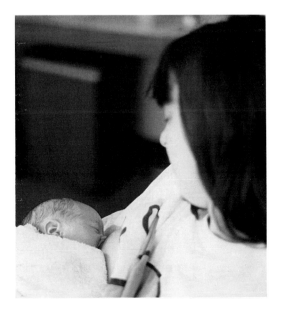

Breast-feeding

On the third or fourth day the milk comes in and a mother may notice that her breasts become fuller. Breast milk is not fully mature until about three weeks after birth.

Advantages of breast-feeding

■ Breast milk from a well-nourished mother is the ideal food: it is made especially for babies. It contains all the right nutrients in exactly the right proportions to meet the changing needs of the baby. It is easily digested.

■ Colostrum has a high concentration of maternal antibodies so it protects the baby from some infections.

■ It is sterile (contains no germs) and reduces risk of infection.

■ There are fewer incidences of allergies, for example asthma (see Book 1, Chapter 18) or eczema (see page 330), in babies who are breast-fed.

■ It is always available at the correct temperature.

■ It is more convenient: there are no bottles to prepare or heat.

■ It is less expensive than purchasing modified milks.

Management of breast feeding

demand feeding
Feeding babies when they are hungry in preference to feeding by the clock

■ **Demand feeding** (the baby is fed when hungry) is preferable to a strict regime of feeding by the clock, every 4 hours. Babies have differing requirements and although they may feed often in the first few days, they will often have established their own 3–5 hourly feeding routine by 3–4 weeks. Some days they will require feeding more often – the only way they can stimulate the breast to produce more milk is by sucking for longer.

■ Avoid giving **complementary feeds** in a bottle.

complementary feeds
Additional bottle feeds as well as breast feeds

■ The mother must be taking a well-balanced diet, especially high in fluids. Her diet will affect the composition of the breast milk and some foods may cause colic. The baby will not need extra vitamins if the mother is taking a healthy diet.

■ Breast-feeding is tiring in the early weeks, so mothers should be encouraged to relax. Extra help at home until breast-feeding is established will benefit mother and baby.

■ Allow the baby to finish sucking at one breast before offering the other. Avoid timing the feeds on each side because the more filling milk – the hind milk, with higher fat content – is the last to be expelled from each breast. This will help the baby to settle for longer between feeds.

■ Breast milk can be expressed using the hands or a breast pump for use when the mother is unavailable. The expressed breast milk (EBM) can be stored for up to three months in a domestic freezer and offered in a bottle.

Breast feeding can continue for as long as the mother desires (feeding for even a few days is better than none at all). Weaning onto solid foods (see page 322) should begin between 4–6 months and milk consumption will gradually reduce, but some mothers may feed for two or three years, mainly as a comfort rather than a source of nutrients.

Bottle-feeding

Most modern infant formulas (modified baby milks) are based on cow's milk, although some are derived from soya beans, for babies who cannot tolerate cow's milk. Manufacturers try to make the constituents as close to human breast milk as possible. All modified milks must meet the standards issued by the Department of Health. There are, however, basic differences between breast and modified milks. Cow's milk:

- is difficult to digest; it has more protein than breast milk, especially casein, which the baby may be unable to digest. The fat content is also more difficult to digest and this may cause wind or colic
- has a higher salt content; salt is dangerous for babies as their kidneys are not mature enough to excrete it. Making feeds that are too strong, or giving unmodified cow's milk can be very dangerous
- contains less sugar (lactose, needed by human infants) than breast milk.

Advantages of bottle-feeding

The advantages of bottle-feeding are as follows.

- It is possible to see exactly how much milk the baby is taking.
- Fathers and other carers can help with the feeding regime, which may give the mother a chance for a good rest, especially at night; she may have more opportunity to go to work or pursue her own interests.
- The baby can be fed anywhere without embarrassment.
- It is less tiring for the mother in the early weeks.

Equipment for bottle feeding

All equipment for bottle-feeding must be thoroughly sterilised following the manufacturer's instructions on the sterilising solution bottle or packet. Equipment must be washed and rinsed before it is sterilised. Do not use salt to clean teats, as this will increase the salt intake of the baby if the salt is not rinsed off properly. Feeds should then be made up according to the guidelines on the modified milk container. The following equipment will be needed:

- bottles (some have disposable plastic liners)
- teats
- bottle covers
- bottle brush
- plastic knife
- plastic jug
- sterilising tank, sterilising fluid or tablets, or steam steriliser.

There are some important points to remember.

- Always wash your hands before and after making up feeds.
- Wipe down the work surface before preparing feeds.
- Rinse the feeding equipment with boiled water after it comes out of the sterilising fluid.
- Always put the water into the bottle or jug before the milk powder.

- *Never*:
  - add an extra scoop of powder for any reason
  - pack the powder too tightly into the scoop
  - give heaped scoops.

  Doing any of these will increase the salt intake. This will make the baby thirsty, so the baby will cry, more food will be given and increase the salt intake further. The baby can quickly become seriously ill.
- Use cooled boiled water to make up feeds.
- Demand feed, rather than time-feed, bottle-fed babies. The primary carer should give the baby most of its feeds to encourage a close bond to develop.
- Never leave a baby propped with a bottle.
- Wind the baby once or twice during a feed; check the size of the hole in the teat: if it is too small the baby will take in air as she sucks hard to get the milk, which will cause wind; if the teat is too large the feed will be taken too quickly and the baby may choke.
- Always use the same brand of baby milk; do not change without the advice or recommendation of the health visitor or doctor.
- Never add baby cereals or other food to the bottle; when the baby is ready for solid feeding, it should be offered on a spoon.

How much milk?

Bottle-fed babies should also be fed on demand and they usually settle into their own individual routine. New babies will require about eight feeds a day – approximately every four hours – but there will be some variations. A general guide to how much to offer babies is 150 ml per kg of body weight per day (24 hours). For example:

- a 3 kg baby will require 450 ml over 24 hours
- a 4 kg baby will require 600 ml over 24 hours
- a 5 kg baby will require 750 ml over 24 hours.

The total is divided by the number of feeds a day to assess how much milk to offer the infant. When a baby drains each bottle, she should be offered more milk.

Colic

Whether breast- or bottle-fed, some babies may experience colic, which is caused by air taken in during feeding or crying. This wind passes through the stomach and becomes trapped in the small intestines, resulting in contractions of the intestines which causes quite extreme pain.

Pain results in inconsolable crying which is very distressing for parents and carers. Colic usually occurs between 2 weeks and 3 months of age. It is commonly known as 'three month colic' because that is the typical duration.

Milk should not be reintroduced into the baby's diet too quickly after a bout of gastro-enteritis. This could result in lactose intolerance and colic.

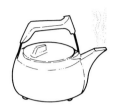

1 Check that the formula has not passed its sell-by date. Read the instructions on the tin. Ensure the tin has been kept in a cool, dry cupboard.

2 Boil some **fresh** water and allow to cool.

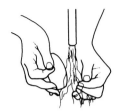

3 Wash hands and nails thoroughly.

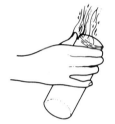

4 Take required equipment from sterilising tank and rinse with cool, boiled water.

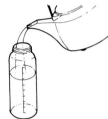

5 Fill bottle, or a jug if making a large quantity, to the required level with water.

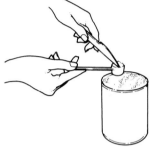

6 Measure the **exact** amount of powder using the scoop provided. Level with a knife. **Do not pack down.**

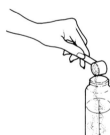

7 Add the powder to the measured water in the bottle or jug.

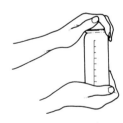

8 Screw cap on bottle and shake, or mix well in the jug and pour into sterilised bottles.

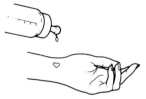

9 If not using immediately, **cool quickly** and store in the fridge. If using immediately, test temperature on the inside of your wrist.

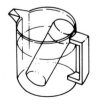

10 Babies will take cold milk but they prefer warm food (as from the breast).If you wish to warm the milk, place bottle in a jug of hot water. **Never keep warm for longer than 45 minutes** to reduce chances of bacteria breeding.

Note Whenever the bottle is left for short periods, or stored in the fridge, cover with the cap provided.

Making up bottle feeds

Signs of colic

The signs of colic are the baby crying, a reddened face, drawing knees up and appearing to be in pain. It is common in the evenings in breast-fed babies. However, some babies are affected by colic in the day and night.

It is unsafe, however, to assume that colic is to blame for all crying – exclude other possible causes. Any concerns should be discussed with the health visitor or doctor.

Care of a baby with colic

- Comfort the baby – pick them up and rub the back to dislodge any trapped wind.
- Lying the baby on the tummy on the carer's lap and rubbing the back usually helps.
- Rocking movements such as those created by car journeys, baby slings and walks in the pram may also help to relieve the pain.
- Some doctors advise breast-feeding mothers to monitor their diet to avoid foods which may exacerbate colic.
- Bottle-fed babies should be winded regularly, with teats checked for hole size and flow of milk – a small hole which does not allow much milk to flow will increase the amount of swallowed air.
- Homeopathic remedies are available from registered homeopathists. The GP may prescribe medicinal drops to be taken before a feed.

✓ Progress check

1. For approximately how long should babies be fed on a milk-only diet?
2. What may influence a mother's decision to breast- or bottle-feed her baby?
3. Why is it generally agreed that 'breast is best'?
4. What is colostrum?
5. List the advantages of breast-feeding.
6. Describe what 'demand feeding' means.
7. What extra care must a breast-feeding mother take of her diet and her health?
8. List the advantages of bottle-feeding.
9. a) Describe the process of sterilising equipment and making up feeds.
   b) How can you calculate how much milk to offer to a bottle-fed baby?
10. a) What may cause colic in a young baby?
    b) How may this condition be treated?

Do this! 17.3

Conduct some research into different brands of infant formula milks and feeding equipment. Visit supermarkets, chemist's shops and mother and baby stores to find out and compare :

- brands of milk available
- cost
- instructions for making up feeds
- health advice for mothers
- accessibility to people whose first language is not English
- availability of toddler milks.

Prepare a report of your findings and draw some conclusions from your research. For example, do you rate one brand or store more highly than another? If so, why? Were the instructions easily understood? How could they be improved? What do you think about toddler milks?

Weaning

weaning
The transition from milk feeds to solid foods

Weaning is a gradual process when the baby begins to take solid foods. This process should not be started before 3 months, and not later than 6 months.

Why is weaning necessary?

Milk alone is not nutritionally adequate for a baby over the age of 6 months. The baby has used the iron stored during pregnancy and must begin to take iron in their diet. Starch and fibre are also necessary for healthy growth and development. Weaning also introduces the baby to new tastes and textures of food.

Babies at around 6 months are ready to learn how to chew food. The muscular movement helps the development of the mouth and jaw, and also the development of speech.

Mealtimes are sociable occasions and babies need to feel part of a wider social group. As weaning progresses, they learn how to use a spoon, fork, feeding beaker and cup. They also begin to learn the social rules in their cultural background associated with eating, if they have good role models; rules such as using a knife and fork, chopsticks, chewing with the mouth closed or sitting at the table until everyone has finished eating.

When to start weaning

Between 3 and 6 months, babies will begin to show signs that milk feeds alone are not satisfying their hunger. There are no strict rules regarding the weight of the baby before weaning. The following are signs that the baby might be ready for weaning:

- still being hungry after a good milk feed
- waking early for feeds
- being miserable and sucking fists soon after feeding (this may also be a sign that the baby is teething)
- not settling to sleep after feeding, crying.

How to wean

As young babies cannot chew, first weaning foods are runny so that the baby can easily suck it from a spoon. Start weaning at the feed at which the baby seems hungriest: this is often the lunchtime feed. Give the baby half their milk feed to take the edge off their immediate hunger, then offer a small amount of baby rice, pureed fruit or vegetables mixed with breast or formula milk to a semi-liquid consistency from a spoon.

The baby should be in a bouncing cradle or similar, but not in the usual feeding position in the carer's arms. There should be a relaxed atmosphere without any stress or distractions which may upset the baby. The carer should sit with the baby throughout the feed and offer their undivided attention. It may take a few days of trying for the baby to take food from the spoon successfully.

Guidelines for weaning

- Never add salt to food, and never sweeten food by adding sugar.
- Do not give very spicy food; avoid chilli, ginger and cloves.
- First foods must be gluten-free, i.e. not containing wheat, rye or barley flour, because research shows that the early introduction of gluten could lead to the development of coeliac disease or other digestive problems in later life.
- Try different tastes and textures gradually – one at a time. This gives the baby the chance to become accustomed to one new food before another is offered. If a baby dislikes a food, do not force them to eat it. Simply try it again in a few days' time. Babies have a natural tendency to prefer sweet foods. This preference will be lessened if they are offered a full range of tastes.
- Gradually increase the amount of solids to a little at breakfast, lunch and tea. Try to use family foods so that the baby experiences their own culture and becomes familiar with the flavour of family dishes.
- As the amount of food increases, reduce the milk feeds. Baby juice or water may be offered in a feeding cup at some feeds. The baby still needs some milk for its nutritional value, and also for the comfort and security of feeding from the breast or bottle.

Cow's milk

After 6 months, babies may be given cow's milk in family dishes. They should not be offered it as a drink until they are over 1 year old. Milk drinks should continue to be modified milk or breast milk.

Iron

By 6 months, the baby's iron stores are low, so foods containing iron must be given. These include:
- liver
- lamb

- beans
- dahl
- green vegetables
- wholemeal bread
- cereals containing iron, for example Weetabix, Readybrek
- eggs, but these should not be offered until 12 months of age; because of the risk of salmonella, they must be hard-boiled and mashed.

Beef products should be avoided because of the risk of BSE.

Weaning stages

Stage 1

Early weaning foods are pureed fruit, pureed vegetables, plain rice cereal, dahl. Milk continues to be the most important food.

Stage 2

The baby will progress from pureed to minced to finely chopped food. Using a hand or electric blender or food processor is helpful to enable babies to enjoy family foods. Milk feeds decrease as more solids are taken. Well-diluted, unsweetened fresh fruit juice or herbal drinks may be offered.

Stage 3

Offer lumpy foods to encourage chewing. The baby may be offered food to hold and chew, such as a piece of toast or apple. A cup may be introduced. Three regular meals should be taken as well as drinks.

Feeding difficulties

Most feeding problems are caused by adults who are unfamiliar with the feeding or weaning process or who have unrealistic expectations of babies and children. Problems may be prevented by following these guidelines.

- Be aware that weaning is a messy business; disapproval will prevent the baby from exploring and experimenting with food.
- Encourage independence by allowing the baby to use their fingers and offering a spoon as soon as the baby can hold one – it will eventually reach the mouth! Offer suitable finger foods too.
- Allow the baby to find eating a pleasurable experience – mixing yogurt and potato may seem revolting to an adult, but if the baby eats this and enjoys it, so be it!
- Babies have not learnt that courses conventionally follow a pattern and may prefer to eat them in a different order. Never start a battle by insisting that one course is finished before the next is offered. When the baby has had enough of one dish, calmly remove it and offer the next.
- Remember that babies will not wilfully starve themselves. They know when they are or are not hungry, so never force a baby to eat anything that they do not eagerly want.

Food allergies

food allergies Reactions to certain foods in the diet

Food allergies can be detected most easily if a baby is offered new foods separately. Symptoms may include:

- vomiting
- diarrhoea
- skin rashes
- wheezing after eating the offending food.

The advice of a doctor should be obtained, and the particular food avoided.

Some babies may have cow's milk intolerance. If the baby is bottle-fed, it may fail to thrive as expected, and should be referred to a paediatrician to confirm the condition. A dietician will give feeding advice and should be consulted before weaning begins.

The allergy may be apparent in a breast-fed baby and the mother may be advised to restrict the cow's milk in her diet. In all cases of cow's milk allergy, re-introduction should be carried out with medical supervision. There are substitute milks available, usually derived from soya beans.

✔ *Progress check*

1 What is weaning?
2 Why is weaning necessary?
3 How may a baby show that it is ready for weaning?
4 Describe the management of introducing the first solids.
5 Which foods are rich in iron?
6 Describe the weaning stages.
7 How can feeding problems be avoided?
8 What are the symptoms of food allergies?

Do this!   *17.4*

1 Make a booklet for parents describing the weaning process.

2 a) Produce a weekly weaning timetable for babies from 4 to 6 months.
   b) Produce a monthly weaning timetable for babies from 7 to 12 months.
   Include in the timetables the timing of meals from first foods to three family meals. Include suggestions for meals and drinks, emphasising home-produced foods.

3 Look at the picture below and make a list of reasons for this baby's unhappiness about mealtimes.

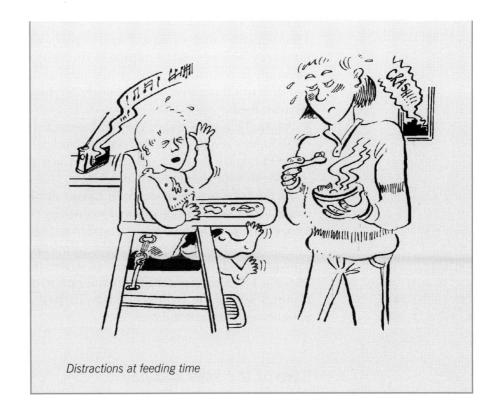

Distractions at feeding time

Routines for care

Babies are completely dependent on an adult to meet all their needs. Although babies' needs are generally the same, the manner in which they are met will differ in the first year. All babies are different – some will sleep well, others will not; some are happy and contented, others not. Caring adults need to be flexible and patient, to accept change and be aware of how and when these changes may occur. The emotional and physical needs of babies and young children can be summarised as follows.

- *Emotional needs* are:
  - continuity and consistency of care
  - physical contact
  - security
  - socialisation
  - stimulation.
- *Physical needs* are:
  - food
  - warmth, shelter, clothing
  - cleanliness
  - rest, sleep, exercise
  - fresh air, sunlight
  - safety and protection from injury and infection
  - medical intervention if necessary.

Babies will eventually settle into a routine that meets their need for food. The regularity of feeding and the urgency with which a baby signals its hunger is the basis of any routine in the early weeks. Feeding the baby on demand, as described earlier, is the most satisfactory method. The baby will develop a pattern of 2–4-hourly feeding and sleeping for periods between feeds.

As the baby gets older, they will sleep for longer at night, although some babies require a night feed or drink well into the second or third year. There are no rules which control how babies behave: they are all individuals with very individual needs.

As the baby begins to sleep for longer at night, they will probably stay awake for longer periods in the day, until by the end of the first year they may only have one long, or two shorter, sleeps during the day. This increasing wakefulness provides the opportunity to develop in all areas, with good care and stimulation (see the table in Chapter 16, pages 298–301). It also gives the carer the opportunity to perform the caring routines which the baby will enjoy if they are treated with affection, patience and understanding.

Care of the skin and hair

Read *Care of the hair, skin and teeth* in Chapter 19, page 371, for information on the structure and functions of the skin and hair.

It is important to give careful attention to caring for a baby's skin and hair, because:
■ the baby is very vulnerable to infection
■ the skin must be able to perform its functions (again, see Chapter 19).
As well as giving attention to keeping adequately clean, this routine care includes frequent observation of the condition of the skin for any rashes or areas of soreness.

Daily care

Babies do not need to be bathed every day. They are not active enough in the early months to require their hair and whole body to be washed more than 2–3 times a week. Some carers prefer to bath the baby every day so that it becomes part of the routine, whether in the morning or evening.

As babies get older and begin to explore the world and investigate their food as they try to put it into their mouths, a daily bath will become an essential way of removing the grime of the day.

Bathtime gives an ideal opportunity to talk and play with the baby. Topping and tailing can, however, be equally pleasurable, and is more reassuring for young babies who can feel insecure when their clothes are removed and they are submerged in water.

Topping and tailing

Topping and tailing involves cleaning the baby's face, hands and bottom.

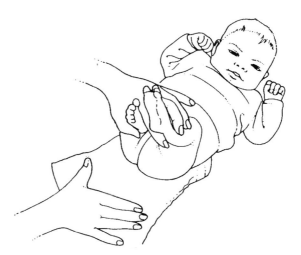

Topping and tailing

Preparation

Collect all the necessary equipment:

- a bowl of warm water
- a separate bowl of cooled, boiled water for the eyes in the first month or so
- cotton wool balls
- baby sponge or flannel
- towel
- change of clothes
- nappies
- creams, if used
- blunt-ended nail scissors.

Method

1. Lie the baby on a towel or changing mat.
2. Remove outer clothing, if it is to be changed.
3. Gently wipe each eye with a separate cotton wool ball, moistened with cooled boiled water, from the inner corner to the outer (nose to ear).
4. Wipe the face, neck and ears with cotton wool balls.
5. Make sure that the baby is dry, especially where the skin rubs together, such as in the neck creases.
6. Clean the hands, using a sponge or flannel. Check that nails are short and that there are no jagged edges that the baby may scratch themself with. Cut them straight across.
7. Remove the nappy and clean the bottom area, using cotton wool or a separate flannel. *Always* wipe from the vulva/scrotum to the anus – front to back direction. If the baby has soiled the nappy, soap is advisable to

clean the area. Wet wipes may be used, but these may sometimes cause soreness.

8 Replace a clean nappy, after the bottom is completely dry.

9 Replace clothing.

Bathing

Bathing should eventually become a 'fun' time for the baby and carer, but there are nevertheless some conditions which are essential.

- The room should be warm – at least 20° C.
- The water should be warm – at body temperature, 37° C.
- Always put the cold water in the bath first.
- Collect all the equipment together before starting the bath.
- Never leave a young child alone in the bath – babies can drown in just 1 cm of water.
- After the bath, ensure that the baby is completely dry, especially in the skin creases, to prevent soreness.

Safety in the bath

As the baby gets older, it may feel more comfortable in a sitting position in the bath. Constant physical support must be given to prevent the baby from sliding under the water, or feeling insecure. Such an experience could put a baby off bathing for a considerable time. A non-slip bath mat is a wise investment for safety. As the baby gets older, standing may seem fun. This should be discouraged, as serious injuries could result from a fall.

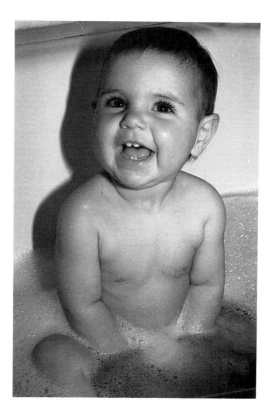

Bath time is fun

Bath time is fun

If the baby is safe in the bath, they will feel secure and begin to enjoy the experience. There are many toys available for the bath, and many can be improvised from objects around the house. Empty washing-up liquid bottles will squirt water, squeezed sponges make a shower. But in the first year a baby is more interested in physical contact and play. Blowing bubbles, tickling, singing songs with actions will all amuse and give pleasure. Hair washing can be fun too. If the baby is accustomed to getting her face wet from an early age, hair washing should be easy. If it proves difficult, leave it for a couple of days. Wipe over the head with a damp flannel and gradually re-introduce the hair-washing gently, using a face shield if necessary. Above all, never let this area become a battle. It is not that important and may create a real fear of water that could hinder future swimming ability.

> ### ✓ Progress check
>
> 1 What are a baby's emotional needs?
> 2 Why do babies settle into different routines?
> 3 Why is it important to give careful attention to caring for a baby's skin and hair?
> 4 How often do babies need to be bathed?
> 5 What is topping and tailing?
> 6 Describe the process of changing a nappy.
> 7 What temperature should the bath water be?
> 8 What is the most reliable method of testing the temperature of the bath water?
> 9 Which important safety precautions should be taken when bathing a baby?
> 10 Why is it important to ensure that bath time is an enjoyable experience?

Non-infectious skin problems

Cradle cap

cradle cap
A scaly, dry crust on the scalp and/or forehead

Cradle cap is a fairly common condition affecting the scalp, especially the area around the anterior fontanelle (soft spot). It is a scaly, greasy or dry crust appearing by about 4 weeks and disappearing by 6 months. It is probably caused by unnecessary fear of rubbing that area of the scalp. Prevention is by washing the hair once or twice a week, and rinsing it very thoroughly. If it becomes unsightly or sore, the crust can be removed by special shampoo or by rubbing olive oil into the scalp, leaving it for 1–2 hours and washing off thoroughly.

heat rash
Pin-point red skin rash

eczema
An irritating dry skin rash often caused by an allergy

nappy rash
Soreness of the skin in the nappy area

Heat rash

Heat rash is caused by over-heating and appears as a red, pin-point rash which may come and go. The treatment is to remove surplus clothing, bath the baby to remove sweat and to apply calamine lotion to reduce the itching and make the baby feel comfortable.

Eczema

Eczema is fairly common in babies, especially if there is a family history of allergies. It begins with areas of dry skin, which may itch and become red, and scaly patches. Scratching will cause the skin to weep and bleed. Cotton scratch mittens should prevent this. The treatment is to avoid perfumed toiletries, use oil such as Oilatum in the bath and an aqueous cream instead of soap. Biological washing powders and some fabric conditioners can irritate the condition, so use a gentle alternative. Cotton clothing is best, and try to prevent the baby scratching if possible. The GP should be consulted if the condition is severe or causing distress.

Nappy rash

Nappy rash usually begins gradually with a reddening of the skin in the nappy area; if this is not treated it will proceed to blistering, spots and raw areas which may bleed. It is extremely uncomfortable for the baby, who will cry in pain when the nappy is changed. Causes of nappy rash are:

- a soiled or wet nappy left on too long – this allows ammonia present in urine to irritate the skin
- concentrated urine (a result of the baby not drinking well)
- an allergy to, for example, washing powder, wet-wipes, baby cream
- infection, for example thrush
- inadequate rinsing of terry nappies
- use of plastic pants, which do not allow the skin to breathe.

Treatment is as follows.
- Remove the nappy.
- Wash the bottom with unperfumed baby soap, rinse and allow to dry thoroughly.
- Let the baby lie on a nappy with the bottom exposed to the air.
- Leave the area free of nappies as often as possible, as contact with fresh air will help the healing process.
- Change the nappy as soon as the baby has wet or soiled it, at least every two hours.
- Do not apply any creams unless the bottom is completely dry; creams can cause nappy rash by sealing dampness in.
- Do not use plastic pants or rubbers.

If there is no improvement, the carer should consult the health visitor or GP.

✅ **Progress check**

1 What may cause cradle cap?
2 How should this condition be treated?
3 How can heat rash be avoided?
4 If heat rash does occur, how should it be treated?
5 List three measures that can be taken to reduce the severity of eczema.
6 List five possible causes of nappy rash.
7 How may this condition be treated?

Nappy care

There are two main types of nappy:

- terry nappies
- disposable nappies.

Muslin nappies may be bought, but are rarely used on the baby's bottom. They are ideal first bibs, or to throw over the shoulder as the baby is winded!

The choice of nappy is based on personal preference. The factors to consider are:

- *cost* – terry nappies involve a larger initial cost (24 will be needed), but are thought to be cheaper in the long term, especially if they are used for a subsequent baby as well. Research shows that this may be misleading, however, as the cost of electricity for washing (and sometimes drying), sterilising solution, washing powder, nappy liners, nappy pins, plastic pants and nappy buckets must also be considered. The cost of disposable nappies may prevent them from being changed as often as they should be
- *time* – disposable nappies certainly take less time generally, but they are bulky and inconvenient to carry. This may be insignificant if the lifestyle is very busy and the carer does not want the inconvenience of washing and drying nappies
- *hygiene* – biological washing powders and other detergents do cause nappy rashes if they are not rinsed out properly.

Both types of nappy are quite adequate if they are used with care. Whichever type is used, babies should be changed 3–4 hourly, at each feeding time, and between if they are awake and uncomfortable. Avoid using nappy creams unless necessary. Clean the baby's bottom with water, baby soap, baby lotion, wet-wipes or baby oil. Make the experience fun, never show disapproval. Talk to the baby and let them enjoy some freedom without the restriction of a nappy.

Case study: Nappy rash

Hamish is 6 months old. He is teething and has had a bout of diarrhoea. He has just completed a course of antibiotics for a chest infection. Hamish has now developed a nappy rash, his bottom and scrotum are red and sore and he cries every time his nappy is changed. His childminder is very gentle with him and washes his bottom carefully at every change and applies a thick layer of petroleum jelly to protect his delicate skin. This is not helping and Hamish's mother notices that his bottom is bleeding slightly.

1 What might have caused Hamish's nappy rash?
2 Why do you think the petroleum jelly was not successful?
3 What treatment would you suggest to help to clear up the condition?

✓ Progress check

1 What different types of nappy are available to parents?
2 What are the advantages and disadvantages of using terry nappies?
3 List the advantages, and possible disadvantages, of using disposable nappies.
4 How should the baby's bottom be cleaned when the nappy is changed?

Think about it

Think of all the ways in which a regular routine can help to meet a baby's emotional needs for security and consistency of care.

Do this! 17.5

Work out the cost of keeping a baby in disposable nappies for one year. Base your calculations on six nappies a day throughout the year. Remember that the baby will require different sizes, which will affect the cost. Some are sold according to age and others according to the weight of the baby, for example newborn, birth to 3 months, 4–8 kg, etc.

Care of black skin

All babies may have dry skin, but it is especially common in black children and should be given special care. The following are general guidelines.

■ Always add oil to the bath water and do not use detergent-based products, as these are drying.
■ Massage the baby after the bath, using baby oil, massage gel or almond oil. This is a wonderful experience for both parties!
■ Observe the baby frequently for signs of dryness and irritation – scaly patches need treating with a moisturising cream.
■ Beware of sunshine – black skin is just as likely to burn as white skin. Always use a sun block on a baby's skin in the sun, and a sun hat.
■ Wash the hair once a week, but massage oil into the scalp daily, as the hair is prone to being brittle and dry.

- Comb the hair with a large-toothed comb.
- Avoid doing tight plaits in the hair as this can pull the hair root out and cause bald patches.

> ✅ **Progress check**
>
> 1 How can a child-care worker try to prevent dry skin in children?
> 2 How can the skin be protected from damage by the sun?
> 3 What special care does black hair need to keep it supple and healthy?

Signs and symptoms of illness

Because young babies cannot say when they feel unwell, or where there is pain, it is very important to be able to recognise the signs of illness. Babies can become seriously ill very quickly, and the advice of a doctor should be obtained whenever there is any concern about a baby's state of health.

Babies usually recover very quickly too, and with the correct treatment can be transformed from misery to smiles in the space of 24–48 hours, or less.

The signs to look out for are as follows:

- *the baby looking pale and lacking energy* (babies with black skin look paler than usual) or *looking flushed and feeling hot*, due to a high temperature
- *loss of appetite* – a baby on milk alone may refuse feeds or take very little; an older baby may refuse solid foods and only want to suck from the breast or bottle
- *vomiting persistently after feeds and in between* – this should not be confused with normal possetting (regurgitation of milk) after feeds. Projectile vomiting in a baby of 4–8 weeks may be a sign of **pyloric stenosis**. This is caused by a thickening of the muscle at the outlet of the stomach to the small intestine. As the baby feeds the stomach fills with milk which cannot pass through the narrowed outlet to the small intestine. The doctor should be consulted urgently
- *diarrhoea* – persistent runny, offensive stools which may be green, yellow or watery should be treated immediately; babies can dehydrate very quickly
- *sunken **anterior fontanelle*** – this is a serious sign of dehydration, perhaps after a period of vomiting and/or diarrhoea or insufficient fluid intake due to loss of appetite.
- *bulging anterior fontanelle* – the 'soft spot' is visible as a pulsating bump on the top of the baby's head, and is caused by increased pressure inside the skull; this requires urgent medical treatment
- *crying constantly and cannot be comforted* – this may occur with any other sign(s) of illness; the cry may be different from any of the usual cries
- ***lethargy*** – the baby lacks energy and may seem to regress (go backwards) in development
- *rash* – if the baby develops a rash and has any other signs of illness,

pyloric stenosis
A thickening of the muscle at the outlet of the stomach to the small intestine – milk cannot pass through the narrowed outlet to the small intestine

anterior fontanelle
A diamond-shaped area of membrane at the front of the baby's head. It closes between 12 and 18 months of age

lethargy
Lacking energy, tired and unresponsive

consult the doctor; a rash alone may be due to heat or allergy. It may be possible to treat this without medical intervention

■ *persistent cough* – coughing is very distressing to a baby and carer; if it does not clear up in a few days, is associated with any other signs of illness or is worse at night, the doctor should be consulted

■ *discharge from the ears, or if the baby pulls at the ears and cries* (especially if there are any other signs of illness) – a doctor should be consulted. Ear infections are common in young children and should be treated promptly to avoid damage to the hearing. Further information on this topic is given in Chapter 23, *Caring for sick children*

■ *changes in the stools or urine* – apart from changes due to diarrhoea (loose, frequent stools) and dehydration (scanty urine output), other changes may be observed. The stools or urine may contain blood or pus, the stools may become bulky and offensive. Stools should be observed for colour, consistency and frequency, and any abnormality recorded and investigated – it may be due to a change in diet. Any concerns should be reported to the doctor, preferably with a sample.

> ### ✓ Progress check
>
> 1 Why is it important for child-care workers to be able to recognise the early signs of illness in a baby?
> 2 What is projectile vomiting a sign of?
> 3 What changes to the anterior fontanelle are serious signs of illness?
> 4 If a baby who is generally well develops a rash, what are the possible causes?
> 5 What changes in the stools and urine of a baby could indicate illness?

Sudden infant death syndrome

sudden infant death syndrome (SIDS)
The unexpected and usually unexplained death of a young baby

Sudden infant death syndrome (SIDS) is the unexpected and usually unexplained death of an infant. It was previously called 'cot death syndrome' because the baby is usually found in the cot after failing to wake for a feed. This may occur between 1 week and 2 years of age, but around 3 months is the most common age. Estimates suggest that 1 in 700 babies are affected, but this figure is falling as parents adopt the recommended practices for cot death prevention.

Causes of sudden infant death syndrome

Research has not isolated a particular cause, but has established that there are some risk factors linked to SIDS:

■ overheating
■ smoking
■ being generally unwell in the few days prior to the death – possibly off feeds and/or snuffly.

SIDS is commoner in:
- winter months
- boys
- premature babies
- low birth-weight babies.

Prevention of sudden infant death syndrome

There are four basic guidelines which, when adopted, reduce the risks of a cot death.
- Put the baby to sleep on their back in the cot, pram or buggy to prevent them from rolling over onto the tummy.
- Do not allow the baby to overheat.
  - 'Feet to foot' in the cot – place the baby at the foot of the cot, with their feet touching the end. This prevents the baby from wriggling down under the covers and over heating, or suffocating.
  - Do not use duvets – use a sheet and layers of blankets instead because these can be adjusted to suit the temperature of the room. The ideal temperature for the baby to sleep in is 18° C.
- Keep the baby out of smoky atmospheres – it is preferable that people do not smoke in the rooms which the baby uses. Parents should stop smoking during the pregnancy.
- The baby should be examined by a doctor if it is unwell in any way. If there is any concern it is better to be safe than sorry.

Support for parents

Parents will go through the stages of grieving – initially feeling shocked and numb, unable to accept what has happened, confusion, anger, guilt and despair (see Book 1, Chapter 16). They may want to talk and should be given every opportunity to do so.

A support network of families who have experienced the same trauma may be available via local voluntary groups. Professional counselling may be required.

There is a slightly increased risk that a second baby may also suffer SIDS and parents will be naturally anxious for the safety of their future children. Care of the Next Infant (CONI) is a programme set up to support parents who have lost an infant – to offer advice, practical help and reassurance.

The Foundation for the Study of Infant Deaths (FSIDS) recommend that parents keep their baby in their bedroom, in a separate cot, for at least the first 6 months.

Each cultural group has their method of child-rearing. In the UK, the rate of SIDS is lower amongst Asians. This may be because most Asian parents keep the baby in the parental bedroom through the night.

> ✓ **Progress check**
>
> 1 Which babies are at most risk of SIDS?
> 2 Between which ages can it occur?
> 3 What steps can be taken to reduce the risks of SIDS?
> 4 What support is available for parents who have experienced a 'cot death'?

Positive health for babies

Babies should be checked regularly by a professional carer to ensure that they are thriving and developing within the average range. This monitoring begins as soon as the baby is born, with the first examination by the midwife. A paediatrician will also examine the baby before they are discharged to go home. If the baby is born at home, the community midwife and GP will be responsible for these checks. The baby will be seen daily for the first ten days by the midwife, who is responsible for her care. The GP should also visit the home to see the baby. When the midwife discharges the mother and baby (usually on the tenth day, if there are no problems), the health visitor will arrange to examine the baby. This 'birth visit' is usually at home. The health visitor will use her professional skills to decide how often the baby needs to be seen.

6-week check

All babies should have a full medical examination at about 6 weeks of age. This may be performed by the GP, community paediatrician or hospital paediatrician.

Hearing test

All babies are offered a hearing test between 6 and 9 months. This is usually performed by the health visitor in the child health clinic. A developmental assessment may be done at this time. (See page 401.)

Child health clinics

Throughout the first year of life, carers are encouraged to attend child health clinics with their baby. Here they can have the baby weighed, discuss progress with the health visitor and see the doctor if necessary. It is also an opportunity to meet other babies of a similar age and stage.

The immunisation programme is also commenced in the first year, at 2, 3 and 4 months. This is another opportunity for the baby to be observed and for a carer to report progress and any difficulties.

Support groups and services

There are often local support groups for parents and carers with young babies. Groups of mothers who have met at relaxation classes may keep in touch and have regular meetings as a form of mutual support. The National Childbirth Trust, the La Leche League and hospital-based postnatal support groups are other alternatives. Gingerbread is a national organisation to help to support lone-parent families. There are probably others in your area.

There should be no need for anyone to sit at home worrying about a baby; there are lots of services and people who are very willing to help. However there may be barriers, such as language, for example, which prevent people from using the services they are entitled to. In areas where there is a high proportion of people who do not speak English as their first language, there should be specialist help available, for example interpreters in clinics, leaflets printed in the relevant language and additional supportive home visiting by specially trained health visitors.

✅ Progress check

1 Which professionals are responsible for the health care of babies?
2 When is the routine screening hearing test performed?
3 What services are available at the child health clinic?
4 What are the benefits of social support groups for mothers?
5 How can mothers whose first language is not English be supported?

Key terms

You need to know what these words and phrases mean. Go back through the chapter to find out.

anterior fontanelle
complementary feeds
cradle cap
demand feeding
eczema
food allergies
heat rash
layette
lethargy
nappy rash
pyloric stenosis
sudden infant death syndrome (SIDS)
weaning

Now try these questions

1 Explain why it is important to observe babies, to monitor their health, in the first year.

2 Describe how a baby's physical needs can be met in the first year of life.

3 What are the signs and symptoms of eczema in young babies?

4 Research the support groups available to families with young children in your area and write a report of your findings.

Part 6: The Physical Care of Children

Caring for children involves meeting all their needs. Part 6 concentrates on children's physical needs beginning with food and nutrition. A well-balanced diet is essential in childhood to ensure healthy growth and development. Child carers must be familiar with the components of a healthy diet so that they can provide the essential nutrients to all the children in their care. Knowledge of special dietary requirements and how to provide for them will show respect for children's culture, religion and individual needs.

Promoting physical development requires detailed knowledge of the stages of development and access to a range of activities to provide stimulation. Disabled and able-bodied children require support and encouragement from their carers in a positive atmosphere where their triumphs are celebrated.

All child-care workers have an important role in preventing the spread of infection and disease in children. By scrupulous attention to personal hygiene and high standards of care in the workplace, children can be protected from illness. Care of the skin, hair and teeth enhances children's natural defences to infection and boosts self-esteem.

Child carers should be able to provide children with appropriate clothing and footwear, which allows room for easy movement and promotes independence with accessible fasteners.

Knowing how environmental factors may affect children should help child-care workers to understand the need for providing settings which promote and support children's health and development. It will also increase awareness about strategies for modifying the environment to promote good health and safety for children.

18 Food and nutrition

This chapter includes:

- **Digestion**
- **The nutrients in food and drink**
- **A balanced diet**
- **Diets of different groups**
- **The social and educational role of food**
- **Problems with food**
- **Food safety**

Good nutrition is essential for general good health and well-being. We need food for four main reasons:

- to provide energy and warmth
- to enable growth, repair and replacement of tissues
- to help fight disease
- to maintain the proper functioning of body systems.

The food we eat each day makes up our diet and contains the nutrients we need. Before these nutrients can be used, the food must be digested by the body. Digestion is the process that breaks down food into smaller components that the body can absorb and use.

Inadequate dietary intake is still the most common cause of failure to thrive. Good eating habits begin at an early age and child-care workers need to ensure that children establish healthy eating patterns which will promote normal growth and development.

You may find it helpful to read this chapter in conjunction with:

▶ **Book 2, Chapter 17**   Physical needs in the first year

Digestion

digestion
The process of breaking down food so that it can be absorbed and used by the body

Digestion of food takes place in the alimentary canal which is a long muscular tube made up of the:

- mouth
- oesophagus (gullet)
- stomach
- small intestine
- large intestine
- rectum
- anus.

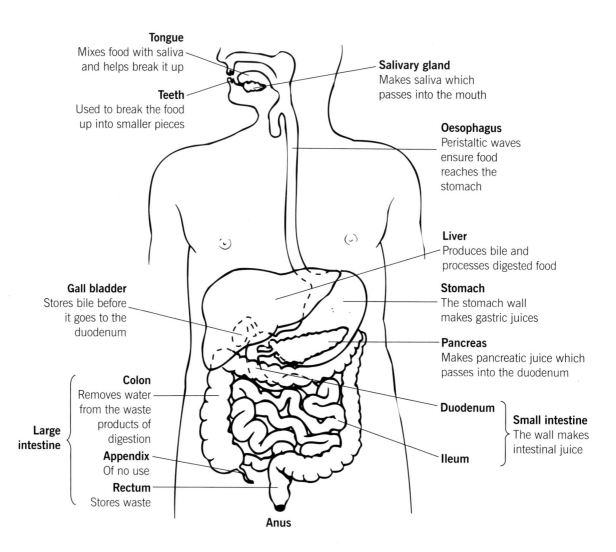

Tongue
Mixes food with saliva and helps break it up

Teeth
Used to break the food up into smaller pieces

Salivary gland
Makes saliva which passes into the mouth

Oesophagus
Peristaltic waves ensure food reaches the stomach

Liver
Produces bile and processes digested food

Gall bladder
Stores bile before it goes to the duodenum

Stomach
The stomach wall makes gastric juices

Pancreas
Makes pancreatic juice which passes into the duodenum

Colon
Removes water from the waste products of digestion

Large intestine

Appendix
Of no use

Rectum
Stores waste

Duodenum

Ileum

Small intestine
The wall makes intestinal juice

Anus

The alimentary canal and the process of digestion

The process of digestion

In the mouth

The food is chewed to break it up into small pieces. At the same time it is mixed with saliva. **Enzymes** in the saliva start to work on the food. The food is then swallowed and passes down the oesophagus into the stomach.

> **enzyme**
> A substance that helps to digest food

In the stomach

Food is churned up and mixed with the gastric juices that continue the process of changing and digesting the food.

In the small intestine

Digestive juices containing enzymes from the pancreas, gall bladder and intestine are mixed with the food and further digestion takes place. The components of the digested food are absorbed into the body through the walls of the small intestine.

In the large intestine

Materials remaining after absorption in the small intestine are mainly water and fibre. Water is absorbed in the large intestine and the remaining fibre, bacteria and some water form the waste products that pass into the rectum and out of the body via the anus.

✅ *Progress check*

1 Define digestion.
2 What are the different parts that make up the alimentary canal?
3 What do the digestive juices contain?

The nutrients in food and drink

nutrient
A substance that provides essential nourishment

To be healthy, the body needs a combination of different **nutrients**. These nutrients are:

- protein
- fat
- carbohydrate
- vitamins
- minerals
- water
- fibre.

Protein, fat, carbohydrates and water are present in the foods we eat and drink in large quantities. Vitamins and minerals are only present in small quantities, so it is much more common for those to be lacking in a child's diet.

Protein

Protein foods are essential for:

- growth of the body
- repair of the body.

complete protein
A protein containing all the essential amino acids; also called first-class proteins

Protein foods are divided into **complete proteins** (first-class proteins) and **incomplete proteins** (second-class proteins). Sources of complete protein come from animal sources and include:

- meat
- fish
- chicken
- cheese
- milk and milk products.

incomplete protein
A protein containing some essential amino acids; also called second-class proteins

Sources of incomplete proteins come from vegetable sources and include:

- nuts and seeds
- pulses (for example, black beans, chick peas, lentils, soya beans, kidney beans)
- cereals (rice, cornmeal, oats) and cereal-based foods (such as bread, pasta, chapattis, noodles).

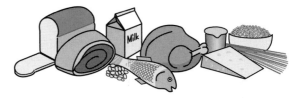

Some sources of protein

amino acid
A part of protein

Protein foods are made up of **amino acids**. There are ten essential amino acids. Complete protein foods contain all of them; incomplete protein foods contain some. If protein in the diet is wholly restricted to vegetable sources, care will need to be taken that a variety of vegetable proteins are used. This will ensure that all ten essential amino acids are included in the diet.

Carbohydrates

Carbohydrate foods are divided into starches and sugars, which provide energy for the body. Sources of starch include:

- cereals
- beans
- lentils
- potatoes
- plantain
- pasta
- yams.

Sources of sugar include:

- sugar from cane or beet
- fruit and vegetables
- honey
- milk.

Carbohydrates are broken down into glucose before the body can use them. Sugars are quickly converted and give a quick source of energy; starches take longer to convert to glucose so they provide a steadier longer-lasting supply of energy. That is why marathon runners eat large quantities of pasta the night before they race.

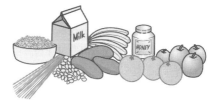

Some sources of carbohydrate

saturated fats
Solid at room temperature and come mainly from animal fats

unsaturated fats
Liquid at room temperature and come mainly from vegetable and fish oils

Fats

Fats provide energy for the body and contain essential vitamins. They also make food more pleasant to eat and aid its passage through the digestive tract. Fats are divided into **saturated fats** and **unsaturated fats**. Sources of saturated fat include:

- butter

- cheese
- milk
- lard
- meat
- palm oil.

Sources of unsaturated fat include:

- fish oil
- olive oil
- sunflower oil
- corn oil
- peanut oil.

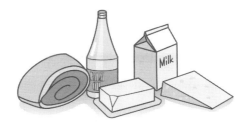

Some sources of fat

Vitamins and minerals

> **fat-soluble vitamin**
> A vitamin that can be stored by the body, so it need not be included in the diet every day

Vitamins and minerals are only present in small quantities in the foods we eat, but they are essential for growth, development and normal functioning of the body.

The tables below show the main vitamins and minerals, which foods contain them and their main functions in the body.

The main vitamins

Vitamin	Food source	Function	Notes
A	Butter, cheese, eggs, carrots, tomatoes	Promotes healthy skin, good vision	**Fat-soluble**, can be stored in the liver; deficiency causes skin infections, problems with vision
B group	Liver, meat, fish, green vegetables, beans, eggs	Healthy working of muscles and nerves; forming haemoglobin	Water-soluble, not stored in the body, so regular supply needed; deficiency results in muscle wasting, anaemia
C	Fruits and fruit juices, especially orange, blackcurrant, pineapple; green vegetables	For healthy tissue, promotes healing	Water-soluble, daily supply needed; deficiency means less resistance to infection; extreme deficiency results in scurvy
D	Oily fish, cod liver oil, egg yolk; added to margarine, milk	Growth and maintenance of bones and teeth	Fat-soluble, can be stored by the body; can be produced by the body as a result of sunlight on the skin; deficiency results in bones failing to harden and dental decay
E	Vegetable oils, cereals, egg yolk	Protects cells from damage	Fat-soluble, can be stored by the body
K	Green vegetables, liver	Needed for normal blood clotting	Fat-soluble, can be stored in the body

The main minerals

Mineral	Food source	Function	Notes
Calcium	Cheese, eggs, fish, milk yoghurt	Essential for growth of bones and teeth	Works with vitamin D and phosphorus; deficiency means risk of bones failing to harden (rickets) and dental caries
Fluoride	Occurs naturally in water, or may be added artificially to water supply	Combines with calcium to make tooth enamel more resistant to decay	There are different points of view about adding fluoride to the water supply
Iodine	Water, sea foods, added to salt, vegetables	Needed for proper working of the thyroid gland	Deficiency results in enlarged thyroid gland in adults, cretinism in babies
Iron	Meat, green vegetables, eggs, liver, red meat	Needed for formation of haemoglobin in red blood cells	Deficiency means there is anaemia causing lack of energy, breathlessness; vitamin C helps the absorption of iron
Sodium chloride	Table salt, bread, meat, fish	Needed for formation of cell fluids, blood plasma, sweat, tears	Salt should not be added to any food prepared for babies: their kidneys cannot eliminate excess salt as adult kidneys do; excess salt is harmful in an infant diet

Other essential trace minerals include:
- potassium
- phosphorus
- magnesium
- sulphur
- manganese
- zinc.

A well-balanced diet which includes a variety of foods will provide all the vitamins and minerals required for the efficient functioning of the body. It is only when diet becomes restricted in illness or because of food shortages or poor choice of foods that shortages of essential vitamins and minerals will occur.

Fibre

Fibre in the form of cellulose is found in the fibrous part of plants. It provides the body with bulk or roughage. Fibre has no nutritional value, as it cannot be broken down and used by the body. It is, however, an important part of a healthy diet. Fibre adds bulk to food and stimulates the muscles of the intestine, encouraging the body to eliminate the waste products left after digestion of food.

Water

Water is a vital component of diet. It contains some minerals, but its role in maintaining a healthy fluid balance in the cells and blood stream is crucial to survival.

✓ *Progress check*

1 Name two sources of complete protein.
2 Name two sources of incomplete protein.
3 Why are starches a more valuable source of carbohydrate than sugars?
4 What are the essential differences between saturated and unsaturated fat?
5 What is the advantage of a vitamin being fat-soluble?
6 What is the function of:
  a) vitamin C?
  b) vitamin D?
  c) vitamin K?
  d) iron?
  e) calcium?
7 Which vitamin helps the absorption of iron?
8 Why is excess salt harmful in an infant diet?
9 What is the essential function of water in the diet?
10 What is the essential function of fibre in the diet?

A balanced diet

A balanced diet means an intake of food which provides the nutrients that the body needs in the right quantities. There are many nutrients that the body is able to store (fat-soluble vitamins are an example of this) so nutrients can be taken over several days to form the right balance.

A diet which includes a selection of foods is likely to be nutritious. Different combinations of vitamins are found in different foods, so a varied selection of foods will ensure an adequate supply of all the vitamins needed. Offering a variety of foods gives children an opportunity to choose foods they like. It also encourages them to explore other tastes and to try new foods and recipes.

Proportions of nutrients

Children are growing all the time, so they need large amounts of protein to help the formation of bone and muscle. They are also using a lot of energy, so they need carbohydrate in the form of starches that they can use during the day to sustain their activities. In addition, they will need adequate supplies of vitamins and minerals.

Suggested daily intakes are as follows:

- two portions of meat or other protein foods, such as nuts and pulses
- two portions of protein from dairy products (for vegans substitute two other protein foods from plant sources)
- four portions of cereal foods
- five portions of fruit and vegetables
- six glasses of fluid, especially water.

> **calorie**
> A unit of energy

Although children are small in size they need a considerable amount of food. The table below shows the number of **calories** recommended for children and adults. The energy value of food is measured in calories: a medium egg, for example, is about 75 calories. Comparing the requirements of children and adults gives some idea of portion size. A child of 2 or 3 needs roughly half the amount of food, in terms of calories, of an adult.

The required number of calories for children and adults

Age range	Energy requirements in calories
0–1 year	800
1–2 years	1,200
2–3 years	1,400
3–5 years	1,600
5–7 years	1,800
7–9 years	2,100
Women	2,200–2,500
Men	2,600–3,600

Once children are weaned, they can eat the same food as adults. More information about early infant feeding and weaning can be found in Chapter 17.

✔ *Progress check*

1 What is the best way to provide a balanced diet?
2 How many portions of protein should be included in a child's daily intake?
3 What is the advantage of a fat-soluble vitamin?
4 What is the calorie requirement of a 2-year-old?
5 How many portions of fruit and vegetables should a child have each day?

Diets of different groups

Each region or country has developed its own local diet over many years. Diets have evolved based on available foods, which in turn depends on climate, geography and agricultural patterns, as well as social factors such as religion, culture, class and lifestyle. Each diet contains a balance of essential nutrients.

When people migrate, they take their diet with them and generally wish to recreate it as a familiar feature of their way of life. The psychological importance of familiar food should never be overlooked.

Religious aspects of food

For some people, food has a spiritual significance. Certain foods may be prohibited and these prohibitions form a part of their daily lives.

Adhering to religious food restrictions should not be taken as being faddy about food. Respecting an individual's culture and religious choices is part of respecting that individual as a whole. Talking to parents and carers about food requirements is important for child-care workers, especially when caring for a child from a cultural or religious background different from your own.

Religious restrictions may affect the diets of Hindus, Sikhs, Muslims, Jews, Rastafarians and Seventh Day Adventists. Members of other groups may also have dietary restrictions. People are individuals and will vary in what they eat and what restrictions they observe; you should be aware of this when discussing diet with parents or carers.

- Many devout Hindus are vegetarian. The cow is sacred to Hindus and eating beef is strictly forbidden. Alcohol is also forbidden.
- Sikhism began as an offshoot of Hinduism. Some Sikhs have similar dietary restrictions to Hindus. Few Sikhs eat beef and drinking alcohol is not approved.
- Muslim dietary restrictions are laid down by the Holy Qur'an and are regarded as the direct command of God. Muslims may not eat pork or pork products and alcohol is strictly prohibited. Other meat may be eaten provided it is *halal* (permitted). Healthy adult Muslims fast during the month of Ramadan.
- Jews may not eat pork or pork products, shellfish, and any fish without fins or scales. All meat eaten must have been killed in a special way so as to be *kosher* (fit). Milk and meat may not be used together in cooking.
- Most Rastafarians are vegetarian, but some may eat meat, except pork. No products of the vine, such as wine, grapes, currants or raisins are eaten. Some Rastafarians will only eat food cooked in vegetable oil. Whole foods are preferred.
- Seventh Day Adventists do not eat any pork or pork products.

Other dietary restrictions

- Vegetarians do not eat meat and restrict their intake of other animal products in different ways.
- Vegans do not eat any animal products at all. A vegan diet needs careful balancing if it is followed by children, to ensure that they get the right nutrients to sustain normal growth.

It is not possible to make blanket statements about the diets of different groups, only to suggest possibilities and factors which may be important and which child-care workers may find useful when discussing food and diets with carers.

It is also very important to take account of these points when preparing activities involving food. If you are setting up a baking activity, for example, it would be best to make sure that you use vegetable fats, as these are generally more acceptable. Many more people today are moving towards a vegetarian diet or a diet that restricts the intake of animal products.

Progress check

What dietary restrictions *may* be followed by:
a) vegans?
b) Muslims?
c) Rastafarians?
d) Jews?
e) vegetarians?
f) Sikhs?

The social and educational role of food

Children like to take part in cooking and food preparation at home and in nurseries. These activities can create learning opportunities and enhance developmental skills.

Physical development

Gross motor skills are developed through mixing and beating. Manipulative skills are improved by cutting and stirring. Hand–eye co-ordination is improved by pouring, spooning out and weighing ingredients.

Cognitive development

Scientific concepts are learnt by seeing the effects of heat and cold on food. Mathematical skills are developed by counting, sorting and grading utensils, laying the table for the correct number of people and weighing and measuring the ingredients. Children can be encouraged to plan and make decisions about what they will eat.

Language development

Conversation and discussion can be encouraged at mealtimes. Adult interaction will promote and extend vocabulary. Children and adults can share their ideas and experiences of the day.

Emotional development

Eating food is often a comfort, and sharing and preparing food for others provides pleasure. Helping to prepare a meal for themselves and others will give children a sense of achievement.

Social development

Children can learn the skills of feeding independently. They can share with others and learn about appropriate behaviour at mealtimes.

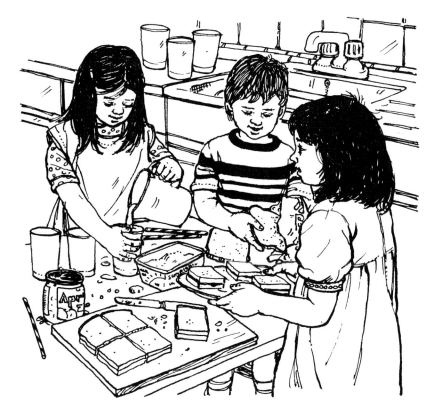

Mealtimes are a good opportunity for families and other groups to exchange their news and ideas.

Problems with food

Food allergy and food intolerance have received a lot of publicity. Only a small number of reactions to food are true allergic responses, involving the immune responses of the body.

Food intolerance

Food intolerance is a condition in which there are specific adverse effects after eating a specific food. This may be caused by an allergic response or an enzyme deficiency. The removal of foods from a child's diet must be carried out with medical supervision. If the suspected food source is a major source of nutrients, for example milk, then alternatives must be included to make good any deficiency. Conditions such as PKU and coeliac disease require very specialised diets. There is more information about these conditions in Book 1, Chapter 18.

Food refusal

Toddler food refusal is common. If the child is of normal body weight and height, is thriving and no medical condition is identified by the doctor, then carers should be reassured. It is important that mealtimes should not become a battleground. The child should be offered food at mealtimes and allowed to eat according to appetite. Any remaining food should be removed without fuss. The next meal is offered at the usual time and no snacks or 'junk food' given between meals. It is important that the child participates in family meals rather than eating in isolation. Allow the child to feed himself and don't fuss about any mess if he is just learning to do this. The child should see eating as a pleasurable and sociable experience and be encouraged to enjoy mealtimes with the family or in other groups.

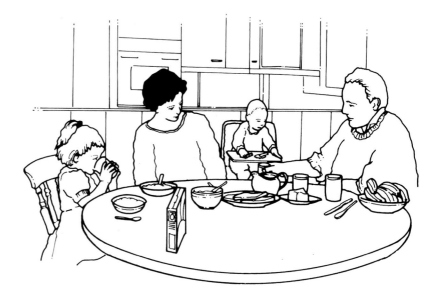

Eating should be a sociable experience, with the family or other groups

Case study: Food refusal

Joanna is a nanny who looks after Joshua, who is 2 years 6 months old and Anna who is 6 months old, each day while their parents are at work. Joshua is a lively, happy little boy who knows Joanna well, as she was his nanny before Anna was born.

Joanna has continued to care for him and also his sister when their mother returned to work four weeks ago. Joshua seems well and healthy but for the last week or two he has been refusing to eat his meals. He has become very upset and on one occasion threw his plate onto the floor when Joanna insisted that he eat his dinner. As his nanny, Joanna has decided that she must take some action.

1 What should Joanna do first?
2 What steps should Joanna then take to try to re-establish Joshua's previous good eating patterns?

Food additives

Additives are added to food to:
- preserve it for longer
- prevent contamination
- aid processing
- enhance colour and flavour
- replace nutrients lost in processing.

Care should be taken with children's diet because:
- they often eat more foods with additives, for example drinks and sweets
- they are smaller and the amount they take is, therefore, greater in proportion to their size.

To reduce additives in the diet:
- use fresh foods as often as you can
- make your own pies, cakes, soups, etc.
- avoid highly processed foods
- look at the labels: the ingredients are listed.

Case study: Labels on food

Anne is a childminder who looks after Holly, who is 4, and Emma, who is 2, every day. Anne is out shopping at the supermarket, as she needs to give lunch to Holly and Emma today. Holly's family are vegetarian and Emma is allergic to food colourings. Anne has brought home a tin of baked beans from the supermarket that will be part of the girls' lunch. This is a copy of the nutritional information on the label.

Baked beans		
Nutritional information		
Typical values	**Amount per 100 g**	**Amount per serving 150 g**
Energy	75 cal.	113 cal.
Protein	4.7 g	7.1 g
Carbohydrate	13.6 g	20.4 g
Fat	0.2 g	0.3 g
Fibre	3.7 g	5.6 g
Sodium	0.5 g	0.7 g
No artificial colourings		

1 What does the label tell you about the content of the food?
2 Will Anne be able to give the food to Holly?
3 Will Anne be able to give the food to Emma?

E numbers

Permitted food additives are given a number. If the number has been approved by the European Union (EU), as well as the UK, there is an E in front of the number – an **E number**. A category name such as

E number
A number given to an additive approved by the European Union

'preservative' must come before the additive number to tell you why it has been included, for example preservative E200.

Food additives and behaviour

Some children may have erratic behaviour after taking, for example, orange squash or coloured sweets, and behaviour improves when these colourings are avoided. Avoiding additives need not affect the nutritional value of the diet, but any regime which leads to a nutritionally inadequate diet should not be followed. Hyperactivity can only be diagnosed by a paediatrician. Dietary manipulation, for example elimination diets, must be prescribed by a paediatrician and supervised by a dietician. Behaviour and hyperactivity problems are, however, rarely caused solely by food additives.

Food and poverty

Research has shown that food is one of the first things people cut back on when they are short of money. This can have a serious effect on the nutritional quality of the diet of families managing on a low income.

There may be other problems which contribute to this: cooking facilities may be limited, or impossible if, for example, the family live in bed and breakfast accommodation and much of the food eaten has to be brought in ready cooked. Fuel costs for cooking will also be an important consideration if money is tight. Shopping around for food to get the best bargain or selection may not be possible if bus fares are needed or food has to be carried a long way.

In these circumstances, knowing about food and the nutrients which are essential to provide an adequate diet is very important. Help needs to be concentrated on achieving an adequate diet within the budget and ability of the family. Knowing which cheaper foods contain the essential nutrients will enable sensible advice to be offered.

> ✅ **Progress check**
>
> 1 How can you know that a food additive has been approved by the European Union?
> 2 What are the main reasons for including additives in food?
> 3 Describe two examples of food intolerance.
> 4 What strategies would you use to deal with food refusal?

Food safety

Food is essential to good health and survival, but it has to be looked after to avoid contamination with harmful bacteria that could cause food poisoning. Since January 1991 there have been stricter laws about storage and handling of food in shops and restaurants. These laws help to keep food safer and cleaner. Once food has been bought, it must be stored safely and prepared hygienically in order to prevent food poisoning.

Buying food

- Check the 'use by' dates.
- Take chilled and frozen food straight home and use an insulated bag.
- Make sure you buy from a shop where cooked and raw foods are kept and handled separately.

Storage at home

- Put chilled and frozen foods into the fridge or freezer as quickly as possible.
- The coldest part of the fridge must be between 0 and 5° C, and the freezer temperature below 18° C: use a fridge thermometer to check the temperature.
- Keep raw meat and fish in separate containers in the fridge and store them carefully on the bottom shelf so that they do not touch or drip onto other food.

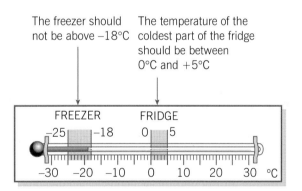

Temperatures for home storage in the fridge or freezer

In the kitchen

- Always wash your hands well before touching food.
- Cover any cuts with a waterproof dressing.
- Wear an apron and tie hair back when preparing food.
- Avoid touching your nose and mouth, or coughing and sneezing in the food preparation area.
- Kitchen cloths and sponges should be disinfected and renewed frequently.
- Disinfect all work surfaces regularly and especially before preparing food.

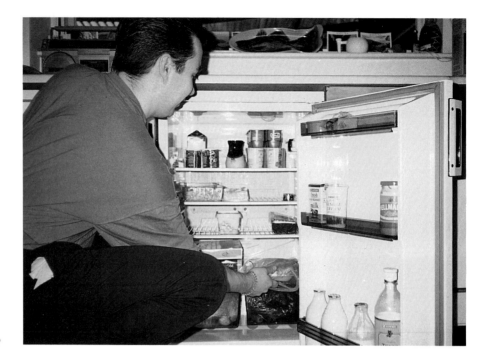

Store raw meat and fish on the bottom shelf of the fridge

Cooking

The following guidelines should always be followed when preparing and cooking food.

- Defrost food thoroughly before cooking.
- Make sure all food is thoroughly cooked – chicken and meat need special care, and must be cooked through to the centre.
- Prepare raw meat separately – use a separate board and knife.
- Cooked food should be cooled quickly and then refrigerated or frozen.
- Cover any food standing in the kitchen.
- Eggs should be thoroughly cooked before eating. For babies and small children, cook the eggs until the white and yolk are solid.
- Cooked food should only be reheated once – reheat until piping hot all the way through.
- Reheat cooked chilled meals properly.
- Pregnant women and anyone with a low resistance to infection should not eat pâté, nor soft cheeses of the Brie or Camembert type.

Children are particularly vulnerable to infection, so it is important to make sure that food is prepared and handled safely. It is also vital that children learn the basic rules about handling food. Always make sure that they wash their hands before eating. If children prepare food as part of a learning activity, the food safety rules should always be followed. Children need to understand why this is important, so that they develop important life skills.

Progress check

1 What are the basic rules of food handling?
2 If you buy chilled or frozen food, what is the best way to transport it?
3 What temperature should the coldest part of the fridge be?
4 Where should you store raw meat and fish?

Do this! 18.1

1 Write an activity plan that will involve a group of 5–6-year-olds preparing
and serving food. Your plan should be:
- appropriate to the children's level of development and have clear
learning outcomes
- consistent with maintaining health and safety
- encouraging respect for dietary and cultural differences.

2 Here is part of a label from a pot of yoghurt:

Values	Amount/100 g
Energy	97 k cal
Protein	5.7 g
Carbohydrate	17.2 g
Fat	0.9 g
Sodium	0.1 g

What information does this give you about the nutritional value of the
food?

3 Link each food in the table below with the vitamins and minerals it
contains.

Vitamin/mineral	Food
B group	Egg
A	Vegetable oil
C	Carrot
D	Liver
Calcium	Cabbage
Iron	Cheese
E	Pineapple
K	Green vegetables
Fluoride	Milk
Sodium chloride	Water

Key terms

You need to know what these words and phrases mean. Go back through the chapter to find out.

amino acid

calorie

complete protein

digestion

E number

fat-soluble vitamin

incomplete protein

nutrient

saturated fat

unsaturated fat

Now try these questions

1 What are the essential nutrients in a balanced diet? Give examples of foods containing these nutrients.

2 What would you include in a day's menu for a 3-year-old? Show how you have ensured a balanced diet.

3 How would you make mealtimes a pleasureable experience for a 4-year-old?

4 What are the important points to bear in mind to ensure that food is safe to eat?

5 What influences might poverty have on a child's diet?

19 Physical care

This chapter includes:
- **Promoting physical development**
- **Exercise**
- **Rest and sleep**
- **Toilet training**
- **Hygiene: care of the hair, skin and teeth**
- **Clothing and footwear**

All child-care workers recognise that each child is different and that meeting individual needs is the basis of providing for equality of opportunity. This chapter concentrates on some important aspects of the physical care of young children and highlights the particular care they require to promote good health and development.

You may find it helpful to read this chapter in conjunction with:

▶ **Book 1, Chapter 3**   Physical development
▶ **Book 2, Chapter 17**   Physical needs in the first year

Promoting physical development

Babies and young children need a safe yet stimulating environment if they are to grow and develop to their full potential. They need space and encouragement to develop new skills, and the opportunity to practise and perfect their technique.

A positive atmosphere in which adults praise children's efforts and recognise their achievements will encourage trust and progress. This is why all child-care workers need a thorough knowledge of child development. With this information, they can provide the correct environment for the child to progress at their own individual pace.

Age 1–4

The toddler stage

Many babies are mobile by the time they reach their first birthday. This new-found freedom of movement is exciting and should be encouraged, but there is always an element of risk. Babies have no concept of danger and need a watchful adult to ensure their safety. They will fall often, until they can anticipate dangers and avoid obstacles in their path. Their great need to explore and investigate the world should not be prevented, but encouraged in an environment that is safe. They have a desire to find out about everything around them, and an adult who can see the world from the child's point of view will enable this discovery. A safe environment to investigate could include containers with safe, but interesting, contents and not random emptying of drawers. A 'safe' cupboard full of exciting things that may be changed frequently will add to the thrill of discovery and learning.

As the child gets older and their gross motor development progresses, they can run easily, sometimes falling, but less often now. Climbing stairs, jumping, riding a tricycle, gradually beginning to use the pedals are among their achievements.

To stimulate development, carers need to provide:

- space
- opportunity
- freedom to learn from experience
- reassurance
- praise
- access to some equipment.

Age 4–7

The skills learned in the first two years will be perfected as childhood progresses. The hesitant and wobbly runner at 18 months will become the sprinter from 4–7 years. The toddler climbing forwards into a chair will eventually perform increasingly hair-raising stunts on climbing apparatus. Skills are being advanced daily and the need to be given the opportunity to practise continues, for example from riding a tricycle, propelling it with the feet, to riding a bicycle without stabilisers, manoeuvring it around obstacles and using the brakes effectively and safely.

When the child has perfected the basic skills of walking, running, climbing, their future physical development will depend on the

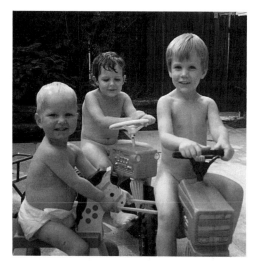

...from propelling 3-wheelers with the feet...

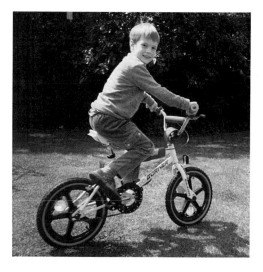

...to controlling a bicycle without stabilisers

opportunities that are made available to them. Ice-skating, gymnastics, judo, horse-riding and ballet-dancing are some of the activities children may enjoy if they are available to them.

Some physical activities may have an element of cost and it may be expensive to provide lessons, but an increasing number of children do participate in them. Some charitable organisations provide funding for children who are skilled in sport, but whose families cannot afford the cost involved in training.

These activities are not a necessary factor in healthy physical development and available opportunities will depend partly on where the child lives and partly on the financial circumstances of their family. For example, a child living in a snowy country may ski, or a child brought up on a farm may ride a horse. The present interests and hobbies of parents or carers may also have an influence on the type of activity offered to a child.

More commonplace activities are swimming, riding a bicycle and football, but they will all require practice. This will increase confidence, which in turn will encourage progression. As children get better at a particular skill, their self-esteem will increase. An interested adult who encourages them to repeat a skill, without forcefulness or disappointment if they do not succeed immediately, will help this process.

Not all children enjoy physical activity or exertion. As they get older and develop other interests, like reading, they may prefer not to take part in outdoor pursuits. Gentle encouragement should be used, but without putting undue pressure on the child to participate. Seeing other children's fun and enjoyment will be more of an incentive than a nagging adult.

Physical development at nursery and infant school

At nursery and infant school, the curriculum includes the opportunity for physical pursuits of a wide variety. At nursery, outdoor play with tricycles, prams, trolleys, large building blocks, dens, tyres and climbing frames may create an environment for imaginative physical activity. Using music to encourage movement by using the body to interpret the sounds may motivate activity. Group activities may encourage children who lack confidence in themselves.

At infant school, opportunities for exercise should include:

- PE, apparatus, dance, music and movement
- football, rounders, throwing and catching, team games, group activities, swimming.

Rainbows, Beavers and other clubs for children will provide the opportunity for physical pursuits. Non-stereotypical activities should be encouraged, such as girls playing football, boys using skipping ropes.

Children with disabilities

When caring for disabled children, it is vital to remember that every child is a unique individual with specific needs, which will depend on their own abilities and capacity for independence.

Disabled children may not achieve the level of physical competence expected for their age group, so emphasis must be on an individual programme of stimulation which will enable the child to progress at their own pace within the usual sequence of development. They may spend longer at each stage before progressing to the next. Their present developmental achievements must be compared with their past achievements, so that progress can be assessed and improvement recognised.

Remember that disabled children are children first. Their special/individual needs must be viewed positively as additional needs to those shared with 'average' children. Each achievement should be encouraged and praised so that they develop a high self-esteem. Make the child believe that they are important and are not being compared with other more able children, peers or siblings. Children with disabilities may become frustrated if they cannot achieve a skill quickly, and will require additional, sometimes specialist, help. Adapting the environment to suit their individual needs will help their progress.

Providing a safe environment

Children are the responsibility of the adults who are caring for them. This is often the parents but it may be a nanny, a childminder or playgroup or nursery staff. In the absence of the primary carer, the child is their responsibility. It is of prime importance to keep the child safe and in doing so, prevent accidents.

An accident is something that happens that is not anticipated or foreseen. This definition is certainly misleading, as it gives the impression that accidents are not preventable, but most accidents that occur to children could be prevented with care and thought. (The topic of safety is covered more fully in Chapter 20.)

Fresh air

All children need regular exposure to fresh air and preferably an opportunity to play outside. If conditions are not suitable for outdoor play – if it is foggy or raining heavily – the indoor play area should be well ventilated to provide fresh air and to prevent a build-up of carbon dioxide.

The benefits of fresh air are that:

- it contains oxygen (released by plants); breathing in oxygen gives energy and stimulates exercise
- it contains fewer germs than air indoors; germs are killed by the ultra-violet rays in sunshine
- exposure to sunlight causes the skin to produce vitamin D.

✅ *Progress check*

1 How can children be encouraged to progress in physical skills?
2 Which safety factors should be considered when providing the opportunities for physical development for a toddler?
3 What type of environment must carers provide to stimulate physical development?
4 What facilities for physical play should be available in a nursery?
5 How can physical skills affect self-esteem?
6 How can disabled children be encouraged in physical development?
7 What are the benefits of fresh air?

Exercise

Exercise is a necessary and natural part of life for everyone. It is especially important for young children who need to develop and perfect physical skills.

All physical exercise strengthens muscles, from a young baby kicking on the floor to a 7-year-old playing football. Encouraging exercise from an early age will lay the foundations for a life-long healthy exercise habit.

It is generally believed that many children do not get enough exercise and will be at increased risk of heart disease and/or other health problems later in life.

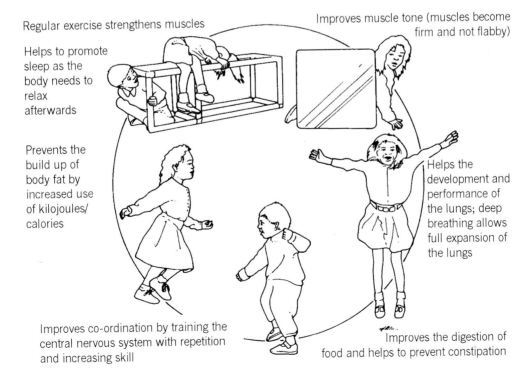

Regular exercise strengthens muscles

Improves muscle tone (muscles become firm and not flabby)

Helps to promote sleep as the body needs to relax afterwards

Prevents the build up of body fat by increased use of kilojoules/calories

Helps the development and performance of the lungs; deep breathing allows full expansion of the lungs

Improves co-ordination by training the central nervous system with repetition and increasing skill

Improves the digestion of food and helps to prevent constipation

The benefits of exercise

✓ **Progress check**

1 Why is exercise important?
2 What are the benefits of regular exercise?
3 What illnesses are children at increased risk of developing if they do not get enough exercise?

Think about it

1 Think about why children may not get enough exercise.
2 Think about what sort of exercise is required to maintain good health.

Do this! 19.1

1 Write a report describing how you think that children can be encouraged to take more exercise.

2 a) Research playground games – ask older friends and relatives what sort of games they played at school. What sort of physical exercise did children have:
 ■ 20 years ago?
 ■ 30 years ago?
 ■ 40 years ago?
 ■ 50 years ago?
 ■ 60 years ago?
 Ask people you know. Elderly relatives usually love to talk about their childhood antics!
 b) Compare these activities with evidence from:
 ■ your own experience
 ■ observing children that you know.

3 Research and investigate exercise programmes at your local or placement nursery or infant school. Do you think that they are adequate?

Rest and sleep

Rest is necessary after physical exercise, and children will know when to stop their vigorous activity as they begin to feel tired.

The benefits of rest are:
■ to allow tissues to recover
■ the heart rate will fall
■ to allow oxygen to be replaced
■ for body temperature to drop
■ to allow the central nervous system (CNS) to relax
■ to take in food if required
■ to prevent muscles from aching and becoming stiff after heavy exercise.

Children should exercise regularly to promote their strength, suppleness and stamina, but they must be allowed to rest – this may be relaxation, sleep or just a change of occupation. One of the values of relaxing or of quiet areas in nursery and school is in providing children with the opportunity to rest and recharge their batteries. A book corner, story time, a home corner, soft cushions, relaxing activities can be provided at nursery and at home. Children need not be challenged all the time; it is sometimes useful for them to be given toys or activities that are relatively easy and do not require deep concentration to complete.

Sleep

Everyone needs sleep but everyone has different requirements. The sleep needs of children will depend on their age and stage of development, the amount of exercise taken and also their own personal needs.

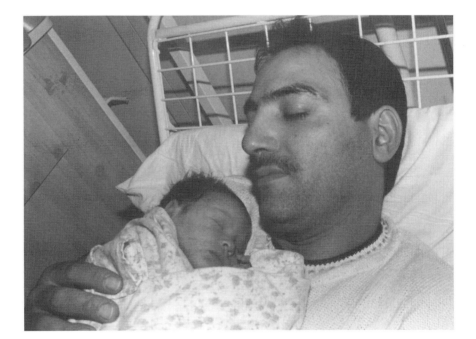

Everyone needs sleep

deep relaxing sleep (DRS)
Periods of unconsciousness during the sleep cycle

rapid eye movements (REM)
Periods of dream sleep

Sleep is a special kind of rest which allows the body to rest and recuperate physically and mentally. There are two kinds of sleep:
- **deep relaxing sleep (DRS)**
- **rapid eye movement sleep (REM),** or dream sleep.

It is generally believed that babies do not dream, but they do have periods of REM, probably when their brains are making sense of all the external stimuli received during the day. Periods of DRS and REM alternate during the sleep period. It is important that periods of REM are completed to awake refreshed. Children who are woken during this period of sleep may be drowsy, disorientated or confused.

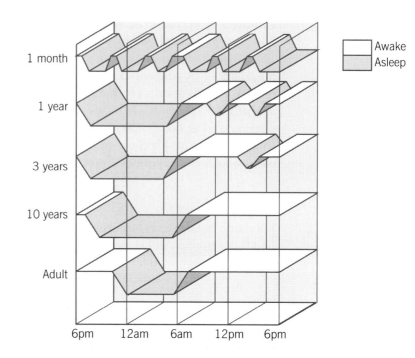

Graph of sleep needs

Sleep routines

Babies and children need varying amounts of sleep. Some babies may seem to sleep and feed for the first few months, while others sleep very little. Toddlers vary too. Some need a nap morning and afternoon, others need one of these or neither.

Some children wake often at night even after settling late. There is little that can be done apart from following a sensible routine. This will involve

- patience
- not stimulating the child, remaining quiet, calm, not encouraging interaction
- remaining upstairs (do not take the child to where there is any activity)
- encouraging daily exercise
- trying to reduce stress or worries
- being prepared to use the carer's bed – this may resolve waking in the night.

Bedtime routine

Social and cultural expectations of children may include letting them stay up later at night. As long as the child is given the opportunity for an adequate amount of sleep, it should not create a difficulty.

When children need to be at nursery or infant school by 8.45–9 in the morning, their bedtime must be early enough to allow for sufficient sleep. Children who share bedrooms or who live in bed and breakfast accommodation may have more distractions and difficulties sleeping, and these may be difficult to overcome.

For successful settling to bed at night, it is important to have a regular **bedtime routine**. The same process each night helps the child to feel

bedtime routine
A consistent approach to putting children to bed which encourages sleep by increasing security

secure and comfortable and so aids sleep. Children need a period of relaxation before going to sleep, and should never be threatened with bed as a form of punishment. This can result in difficulties at bedtime. A suggested routine is as follows:

- a family meal at 5–6 p.m., about two hours before bedtime – this is a chance to talk about the day's events. Babies and toddlers enjoy this social occasion too
- playtime – with siblings and carers; this is time for individual attention
- bathtime – fun, play, relaxation, learning hygiene routines; talking about worries, experiences; this should be one-to-one if possible
- offer a drink if required
- storytime – preferably in bed, after saying goodnight to other family members and cleaning the teeth; storytime should be an opportunity for a cuddle, and to snuggle up in bed preparing to sleep
- sleep, in a comfortable, warm bed with the light out or night light on if the child requests it.

Avoid loud noises coming from conversations or the TV which might distract from sleep. This is not always possible and will depend on the housing situation.

Using a familiar routine and reassurance that carers are nearby may encourage children who are unwilling to go to bed to settle more willingly.

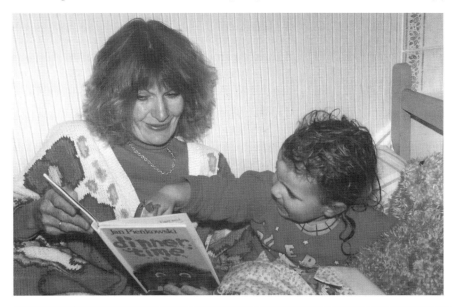

Storytime should be an opportunity for a cuddle, and to snuggle up in bed preparing to sleep

✓ Progress check

1 What are the benefits of rest?
2 What sort activities should be available for children to enable them to rest during a busy day?
3 What factors influence the sleep needs of children?
4 What are the two types of sleep called?
5 How can children be encouraged to have a sensible sleep routine?

> **Do this!**   19.2
>
> **1** Observe a child over a morning and/or an afternoon session in your placement. Note their patterns of vigorous activity and rest. Evaluate the observation by interpreting the value of the activities the child has taken part in, and by assessing their individual need for exercise and rest.
>
> **2** Do a snapshot observation in your placement with the purpose of assessing the value of the whole range of activities on offer to the children. Look at:
>
> - whether the available activities give children the opportunity for energetic exercise
> - whether the available activities give children the opportunity to rest and 'recharge their batteries'
> - the number of children participating in the various vigorous and restful activities.
>
> Comment on your findings and the children's general activity level. Are there any other activities which could be provided to increase the amount of exercise taken?

Toilet training

toilet training
Teaching young children the socially acceptable means of emptying the bladder and bowels into a potty and/or toilet

There are many different theories about **toilet training** – about when and how to train babies and children in the use of the potty and the toilet. Some people report that their children were 'trained' before the first birthday. These are the exception and not the rule! There are wide variations in this area of development, as in all others.

A child will only become reliably clean and dry by the age of 2 to 3 years, at whatever age the potty is introduced. There does not seem to be any point in rushing this skill. It is much more easily achieved if it is left until the child is 2 years at least, unless they show an interest earlier.

General guidelines

- The child must be aware of the need to use the toilet or potty. The central nervous system (CNS) must be sufficiently developed for the message that the bowel or bladder is full to be understood by the brain. A baby of 12–18 months may know when they are soiled or wet, but are not yet able to anticipate it.
- They must have sufficient language to tell their carer, verbally or with actions, that they need to go.
- Too much pressure at an early age can put the child off the idea completely and create a 'battleground'.
- Wait until the child is ready.
- Make training fun! Carers should be relaxed and not show displeasure or disapproval about accidents which will certainly happen. The child may be more upset than the adult and deserves understanding.

- Provide good role models. Seeing other children or adults use the toilet will help the child to understand the process.
- In theory, bowel control comes first: the child may recognise the sensation of a full bowel before that of a full bladder. However, most carers report that children are dry earlier than they are clean. This may be because children urinate more often than they have their bowels open, so have more practice.
- Have a potty lying around for a long time before it is used. Then it will become familiar and children can sit on it as part of their play.
- Watch for signs of a bowel movement and offer the potty, but do not force it. If it is successful then congratulate the child and show them how pleased you are.
- Training is easier in warm weather when children can run around without nappies or pants. They can become aware of what is happening when they urinate or have their bowels open.

Bedwetting

enuresis
Involuntary bedwetting during sleep

Bedwetting (**enuresis**) is often a hereditary tendency and is particularly common in boys. If it begins after a long dry period, it may be due to an infection of the urinary tract or to a stressful event, for example a new baby, moving house or school or the death of a relative or friend. Regression in this area may also be caused by illness.

Children usually become dry at night of their own accord. Accidents are common and should be treated with understanding and not displeasure. There is no need for concern about occasional accidents unless the child is upset. Seeing a sympathetic doctor or health visitor should help.

Soiling

encopresis
Deliberate soiling into the pants, onto the floor or other area after bowel control has been established

Soiling (**encopresis**) may be caused by an objection to using the potty or toilet that grows to an aversion, and the child withholds the motion until they can relieve themselves elsewhere. Soiling may be due to an emotional disturbance, or it may cause one. Children with this difficulty need very sensitive treatment. It can be resolved, often with the help of the health visitor and/or GP.

Think about it

Think about what advice you would offer to a parent who approached you with concerns about toilet training.

✓ Progress check

1 What signs may indicate that a child is ready to be toilet trained?
2 At approximately what age are children reliably clean and dry during the day?
3 What is enuresis?
4 What factors may contribute to enuresis?
5 What is encopresis?

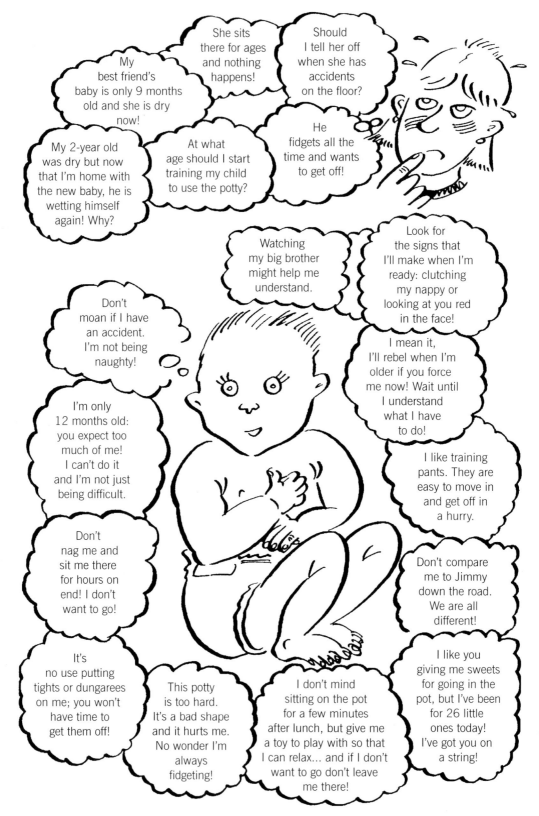

Toilet training: two points of view

> ### *Do this!* 19.3
>
> Make a wall display for a day nursery giving general guidelines in a visually interesting way for toilet training. The display must be eye-catching to encourage parents or carers to read it.

> ### Case study: *Successful toilet training*
>
> Jeremy is just 2 years old and shows no interest in using a potty. His mother, Jane, has left the potty lying around during Jeremy's second year and he is very familiar with it – he always wants to sit on it before he gets into the bath, but has not used it at all! He tells his mother when he has passed urine or had his bowels open in his nappy. Jane is not concerned – she has decided to try and train Jeremy during the family camping holiday. She explains to Jeremy that he can stop wearing nappies in the day time while they are on holiday and that she will take the potty everywhere with them. On the beach, Jeremy wees in the sand frequently for the first few days and begins to tell his parents when he is about to do so! They encourage him to use the potty and when he does they clap and congratulate him on his clever achievement. Jeremy begins to ask for the potty and despite the occasional 'accident' he is out of nappies by the time the holiday ends.
>
> 1 Why was a holiday 'training' such a success?
> 2 How do you think his parent's attitude helped Jeremy in this process?

Hygiene: care of the hair, skin and teeth

Read the section *Care of the skin*, Chapter 17, page 326.

hygiene
The study of the principles of health

All children need adult help and supervision in their personal **hygiene** requirements. Good standards of hygiene in childhood are important because they:

- help to prevent disease
- increase self-esteem and social acceptance
- prepare children for life by teaching them how to care for themselves.

To understand the importance of hygiene, it is valuable to understand the functions of the skin and hair. The structure of the skin is shown in the diagram on page 372.

Functions of the skin

The skin performs the following functions:

- *protection*
  - of underlying organs
  - against germs entering the body

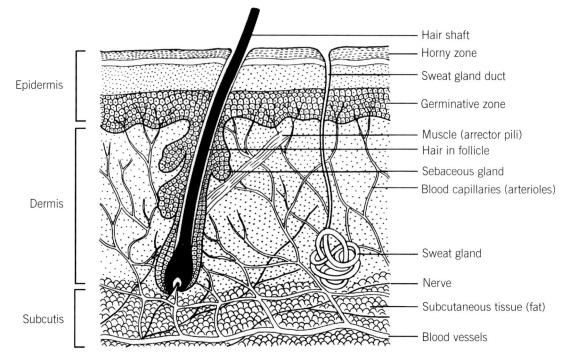

Epidermis

Dermis

Subcutis

Hair shaft
Horny zone
Sweat gland duct
Germinative zone
Muscle (arrector pili)
Hair in follicle
Sebaceous gland
Blood capillaries (arterioles)
Sweat gland
Nerve
Subcutaneous tissue (fat)
Blood vessels

The structure of the skin

> **sebum**
> An oily substance which lubricates the skin, it is produced by the sebaceous glands and secreted through the hair shaft

> **sweat**
> Liquid produced in the sweat glands and secreted through the pores onto the surface of the skin

- *sensation* – the skin is the organ of touch, and conveys sensations of hot, cold, soft, hard, etc.
- *secretion of **sebum***, an oily substance, which:
  - lubricates the hair
  - keeps the skin supple and waterproof
  - protects the skin from moisture and heat
- *the manufacture of vitamin D*, from exposure to ultra violet rays from the sun; vitamin D which is necessary for healthy bone growth. (Black children may need a supplement in the winter as their skin does not easily make vitamin D.)
- *sweat* – the skin excretes sweat and this:
  - gets rid of some waste products
  - helps to regulate the temperature when the body is hot.

Guidelines for good hygiene

Because the skin has so many important functions and because it is the first part of the body to come into contact with the environment, it must be cared for adequately. This does not mean obsessive cleaning of the skin – too much cleaning can be as harmful as too little because it may make the skin dry and sore and also washes away sebum, which protects it.

- Wash the face and hands in the morning and before meals.
- Wash hands after going to the toilet and after messy play.
- Keep the nails short by cutting them straight across. This will prevent dirt collecting under them.

- A daily bath or shower is necessary with young children who play outside and become dirty, hot and sweaty. Dry them thoroughly, especially between the toes and in the skin creases to prevent soreness and cracking.
- Observe the skin for rashes and soreness. If treatment is prescribed it must be followed.
- Black skin needs moisturising. Putting oil in the bath water and massaging almond oil or coconut butter into the skin afterwards helps to prevent dryness.
- If a child does not require a daily bath, a thorough wash is good enough. Remember to encourage children to wash their bottoms *after* the face, neck, hands and feet.
- Hair only needs to be washed once or twice a week unless it is full of food or the residue of messy play! Avoid using a hairdryer every time the hair is washed as this can damage the hair.
- Rinse shampoo out thoroughly in clean water. Conditioners may be useful for hair that is difficult to comb.
- Black curly hair needs hair oil applying daily to prevent dryness and hair breakage.
- Skin needs protecting from the sun to prevent burning and the associated risks of cancer. Use a sunblock or high factor sun cream and monitor the length of time in the sun. Black skin needs the same protection as pale skin.

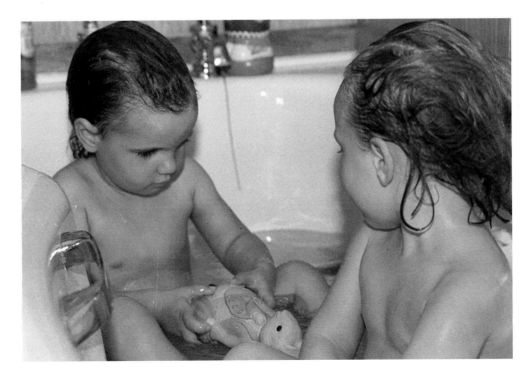

A daily bath is necessary for active toddlers playing outside

> ## Case study: Unexpected sunburn
>
> Ashley, aged 4 years, is an energetic child who loves to play outside in all weathers. In the summer his childminder often takes the children to a local outdoor paddling pool where they have a picnic on the grass next to the water – there is a playground nearby where the children also play. She always makes sure that the children are protected by using creams, hats and t-shirts when the sun is shining. One warm but overcast day in May she takes them to the park for a picnic, not expecting them to use the pool. Ashley insists on stripping down to his underpants for a paddle and proceeds to spend two and a half hours playing in the water. On arriving home he complains that his shoulders and back hurt. When she looks at them the child minder sees that Ashley's black skin is dark and swollen.
>
> 1 What is the cause of Ashley's discomfort?
> 2 How could this have been prevented?

The benefits of good hygiene

- Clear, glowing skin and shiny hair are a sign of good health.
- The child looks attractive and feels well, and develops a positive self-image.
- Washing is a tonic; children feel healthy as a result.
- Infection is prevented (it can spread from child to child from dirty hands and nails).
- Health is maintained.
- Good habits give a pattern for life.
- It allows the skin to perform its functions.
- It treats skin problems, for example eczema, sweat rash; itchy, sore skin can prevent sleep and make the child irritable and restless. This may affect all-round development.

Teeth

Teeth may appear at any time during the first two years of life. It is usually expected that they will begin to erupt during the first year but this is not necessarily so. They usually come through in the same order as shown in the illustration opposite, but variations may occur. The first 20 teeth are called the **milk teeth**, and they will usually be complete by the age of 3 years. From 5–6 years, these teeth begin to fall out as the adult teeth come through. There are 32 permanent teeth, and the care they are given in childhood will help them to last a lifetime.

> **milk teeth**
> The first 20 (deciduous) teeth

Care of the teeth

Provide a soft toothbrush for a baby to use and become familiar with. It is not necessary for babies to have teeth to begin oral (mouth) hygiene. They will enjoy playing with the brush, and as they get older, will put it in their mouths to suck it and to rub their gums. Give them the opportunity to watch adults

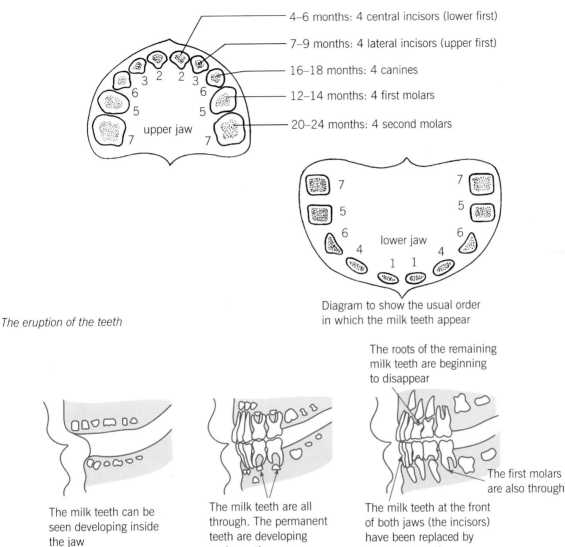

4–6 months: 4 central incisors (lower first)

7–9 months: 4 lateral incisors (upper first)

16–18 months: 4 canines

12–14 months: 4 first molars

20–24 months: 4 second molars

upper jaw

lower jaw

Diagram to show the usual order
in which the milk teeth appear

The eruption of the teeth

The roots of the remaining
milk teeth are beginning
to disappear

The first molars
are also through

The milk teeth can be
seen developing inside
the jaw

The milk teeth are all
through. The permanent
teeth are developing
underneath

The milk teeth at the front
of both jaws (the incisors)
have been replaced by
permanent teeth

Development of the teeth

and siblings clean their teeth. When the first tooth does appear, try to clean it gently with a small, soft brush. If the baby objects, do not force them to have the tooth or teeth cleaned – make it a game and increase their confidence. Teach older children how to clean their teeth. A dental hygienist will be able to offer professional assistance – the dentist will arrange this. Ensure that cleaning the teeth becomes a habit: in the morning after breakfast and after the last drink or snack before bed. Cleaning the teeth after meals should be encouraged, but this may not always be possible.

Diet

Encourage healthy teeth and prevent decay by providing a healthy diet that is high in calcium and vitamins and low in sugar. Avoid giving sweet drinks to babies and children, especially in a bottle or soother; this coats the gums and teeth in sugar and encourages the formation of acid which dissolves the enamel on the teeth. Sugar can penetrate the gum and cause decay before the teeth come through. This is common in babies and children who are frequently offered sweet drinks.

Children will probably demand sweets. Give them after a meal and then encourage them to clean their teeth. Do not offer sweets and sugary snacks between meals, as this will encourage decay. If you do need to feed a child between meals, provide food that needs to be chewed and improves the health of the gums and teeth, like apples, carrots and bread.

Fluoride

fluoride
A mineral which helps to prevent dental decay

Fluoride in the water supply has been proven to strengthen the enamel on the teeth, and so prevent decay. In areas where the fluoride content is low, drops can be given daily in drinks. Fluoride toothpaste also helps to prevent decay.

The dentist

Visit the dentist regularly. A baby who attends with an adult, and then has their own appointments, will feel more confident about the procedure. Prepare children for their dental appointments by explaining what will happen and participating in role play. Never pass on any adult feelings of terror, fear or anxiety about the dentist.

Encouraging independence in hygiene

There are several ways in which carers can encourage a child to develop independence in personal hygiene.

- Provide positive role models.
- Establish caring routines that encourage cleanliness from early babyhood.
- Make hygiene fun: use toys in the bath, cups and containers, sinkers and floaters.
- Provide the child with their own flannel, toothbrush, hairbrush, etc. that they have chosen themselves.
- Allow the child to wash themselves and participate at bath time. Let them brush their hair with a soft brush and comb with rounded teeth.
- Provide a step so that they can reach the basin to wash and clean teeth.
- Make haircuts fun too: some barbers and hairdressers specialise in children's hair.

> ### ✓ Progress check
>
> 1 What are the functions of the skin?
> 2 What particular care should be given to black skin?
> 3 What are the benefits of good hygiene?
> 4 How can independence be encouraged in hygiene routines?
> 5 How many milk teeth are there?
> 6 How can healthy teeth be encouraged?

Do this!   *19.4*

Plan a hygiene routine for a young child that includes all aspects of care related to the child's needs and development. Include the following:
- encouraging independence during bathing and dressing
- sleeping requirements
- opportunity for rest and exercise
- stimulation
- safety factors
- awareness of the needs of the family.

Think about it

How can you make care of the skin, teeth and hair fun? Remember how you were taught to take responsibility for your own personal hygiene. You may want to use some of the ways that were successful with you, or you may decide to adopt an entirely different approach with the children you care for.

Clothing and footwear

Toddlers and children work hard at their play, and this will mean that they get dirty. Although they are often washed for their health and comfort they will soon be dirty again. The attraction of a muddy puddle, digging soil and exploring the sandpit will see to that! This is all natural and should be encouraged. Children should not be pressurised into keeping clean or the spontaneity and excitement of play will be lost.

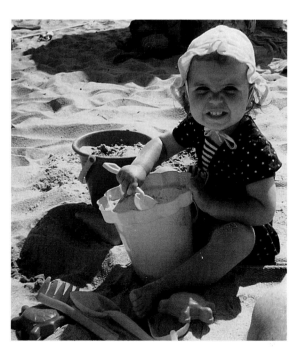

Toddlers will inevitably get dirty when they play

Clothing

Clothing must be comfortable and loose enough for easy movement but fitted well enough to prevent loose material from catching and hindering movements. It should be easily washable; children do get dirty. This should be expected and not disapproved of.

Clothes should have fasteners that a child can reasonably manage, for example large buttons, toggles, velcro and zips.

Underwear

- Cotton is preferable, to absorb sweat and increase comfort.
- When babies are in nappies, all-in-one vests prevent cold spots.

General clothing

- Trousers or shorts are best for both sexes when a child is crawling and falling. Dresses often get in the way of active play.
- Stretch track-suits are ideal.
- Dungarees, except when the child is learning to use the toilet, as they are difficult to remove and replace.
- T-shirts, cotton jumpers.
- Add extra, light layers when it is cold.

Coats

- A showerproof, colourful anorak with a hood is warm and easily washed. Extra underlayers can be added when the weather is very cold.
- Waterproof trousers and wellingtons enable happy puddle splashing.

Pyjamas

Use all-in-one suits without feet, with correctly sized socks.

Footwear

The bones of the feet develop from cartilage, and are very soft and vulnerable to deformity if they are pushed into badly fitting shoes or socks. A child may not complain of pain because the cartilage will mould into the shape of the shoe.

Shoes should not be worn unless it is absolutely necessary, and not indoors. Walking barefoot in the house is preferable, partly because babies and children use the toes to balance, and floors can be like skating rinks for a baby or child wearing socks alone. If floors are cold or damp, socks with non-slip soles can be worn. Shoes are not necessary until a child will be walking outside, when they protect the feet and preserve warmth.

Feet grow two or three sizes each year until the age of 4. The primary carer is responsible for making sure that footwear fits correctly. This should be done by regularly checking the growth of the feet. They must be checked every three months by an expert trained in children's shoe fitting. Both the length and width are important.

Shoes should:

■ protect the feet
■ have no rough areas to rub or chafe the feet
■ have room for growth
■ have an adjustable fastener, for example a buckle or velcro
■ be flexible and allow free movement
■ fit around the heel
■ support the foot and prevent it from sliding forwards.

Socks must be of a size to correspond to the size of the shoe. Stretch socks should be avoided.

✓ Progress check

1 What type of clothing is most suitable for a toddler?
2 When are shoes necessary?
3 On average, how many sizes do feet grow in a year until the age of 4 years?
4 How often should children's feet be measured by an expert?
5 What are the qualities of a good pair of shoes?

Do this!   19.5

Plan a suitable wardrobe for a child between 1–4 years. Take into account the seasons, the child's age and stage of development, laundering, etc. Give reasons for your choices of clothing, including their advantages.

Key terms

You need to know what these words and phrases mean. Go back through the chapter to find out.

bedtime routine
deep relaxing sleep (DRS)
encopresis
enuresis
fluoride
hygiene
milk teeth
rapid eye movements (REM)
sebum
sweat
toilet training

Now try these questions

1 How can a child-care worker actively promote physical development?
2 Explain why equal opportunities is important when providing physical care for children.
3 Why is it important for child-care establishments to provide a variety of activities which offer the children opportunities for exercise and rest?
4 What positive steps can parents and carers take to ensure a happy transition from nappies to toilet?
5 How can children be encouraged to develop independence in hygiene routines?

20 Safety

This chapter includes:

- **Anticipating accidents**
- **Preventing accidents**
- **Safety at home**
- **Outdoor safety**
- **Workplace safety policies and procedures**
- **Outings with children**

Child-care workers have a fundamental responsibility to keep the children in their care safe. A stimulating and exciting environment must also incorporate vital safety elements to protect children. Hazardous and dangerous experiences should be anticipated and avoided. The presence of a watchful and vigilant carer at home, in the child-care establishment, on outings and when travelling from place to place is essential if accidents and unintentional injuries to children are to be prevented.

You may find it helpful to read this chapter in conjunction with:

▶ **Book 2, Chapter 24**   Responding to emergencies

Anticipating accidents

Children are born with no awareness of danger. They are totally dependent on their carers for protection and survival. Carers need a sound knowledge of child development to be able to anticipate when an **accident** may occur due to a child's increasing physical skills or curiosity. For example, a baby of 4 to 5 months may seem quite safe lying on the sofa, until the day they can roll over and off onto the floor. Or the young baby sitting on a carer's knee as they drink a cup of tea may seem to have no interest or curiosity about the cup or its contents until the day their co-ordination allows them to grab the cup and scald themselves.

Babies and children are constantly changing. It may be surprising when they do things for the first time, but their increasing abilities should be expected. Carers should anticipate and avoid dangerous situations. Children have a right to this level of care.

> **accident**
> An unexpected and unforeseen event

Protecting from accidents

Babies and toddlers cannot remember what they have been told from one moment to the next. Saying 'No!' as they crawl towards the open fire may stop their progress for a moment, but they will soon be off again. They are not being naughty or disobedient. They are naturally curious and need to investigate. They have lots of energy and will keep trying until they succeed. This is usually encouraged by adults, so babies will be confused and upset when they are discouraged from an unsafe situation, for example trying to pull at that tempting wire hanging from the kitchen worktop, emptying kitchen cupboards, or grabbing a pan handle when it is on the hob. The adult carer must try to make all situations safe, while leaving children space to explore.

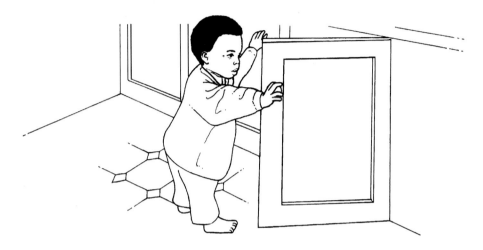

Children love to explore

As children get older and their memory develops, their awareness of what is dangerous increases. They will begin to remember what *hot* feels like, that it hurts, and they will avoid touching the oven door or radiator. They are beginning to protect themselves. As they mature they may begin to protect other, younger toddlers, giving them some of the benefit of their own experience.

It is still necessary to provide a balance between protecting the child from danger yet allowing them the space and opportunity to explore and develop at their own pace to their full potential. Achieving this balance will require an adult to provide a safe environment for exploration. The home, the nursery, the car, the school, the playground must be as child-safe as possible. A watchful adult presence is always necessary.

Accidents

Unintentional injuries (accidents) are the greatest cause of death in children over 1 year old. Most accidents happen at home, and 1–4-year-olds are most at risk. Look at the following statistics.

■ Three children die every day as the result of an accident.

■ 120,000 children are admitted to hospital every year as the result of accidents.

■ 3,000,000 children attend casualty departments for accidental injuries every year.

Think about it

Why should 1–4-year-olds be most vulnerable at home? Think about their development and write down as many dangerous situations as you can, that may be encountered at home.

- One in 5 children needs medical treatment after an accident every year.

The causes of unintentional injuries are directly related to:

- the developmental age/stage of the child
- the child's changing perception of danger
- the degree of exposure to different hazards at various ages.

Social class can affect the chances of an accident occurring – some injuries are up to six times more common in the poorest areas compared to the most affluent.

Attitudes to child care can also affect this, for example:

- how much independence children are allowed
- supervision travelling to and from school
- opportunities to play safely outdoors – children may be allowed to play on the street and to cross the road before they are old enough to judge traffic safely.

Common factors in accidents

All carers are human, and there may be times when they are less vigilant than others, but when caring for children constant awareness is essential. Children may take more risks when adults are distracted, or when they have seen other children do dangerous things. Accidents may occur in the following situations.

Stress

When adults or children are worried or anxious, they may be less alert or cautious. Carelessness creates dangerous situations.

Haste

When late for school or an appointment, anyone may take less care in keeping safe; we may, for example, rush across the road.

Tiredness

Tiredness makes everyone less alert. Adults may be pleased that children are quietly playing which allows them to rest. They may be unaware that the garden gate is open, or that the children have wandered onto the balcony of the flat.

Remember that when children are unusually quiet in their play, they have probably found something which fascinates them. Check that they are not playing with a dangerous object or in a potentially dangerous situation.

Under-protection

Children who are not supervised by caring adults are more likely to have accidents. They have not been made aware of dangers and are allowed to play in hazardous situations.

Over-protection

Children who are so protected that they are not allowed to explore are less likely to be aware of danger when they are left alone. They may be determined to do something usually disallowed.

Think about it

Why do you think children who live in poverty are more vulnerable to unintentional injuries?

Progress check

1 Why is it important for adults to be aware of safety when working with young children?
2 How can attitudes to child care influence the accident statistics?
3 What is the greatest cause of death in children over 1 year of age?
4 When are accidents most likely to happen?
5 How can adult tiredness increase the risk of accidents to children in their care?
6 Give four general ways that adults can prevent accidents.
7 Where do most accidents take place?

Preventing accidents

The successful prevention of accidents depends largely upon the following.

Role models

Think about it

Think of as many ways as you can of being a good safety role model to a child.

The most important way of reducing risk is by setting a good example to children. Children copy adult actions so adults have a responsibility to teach them how to be safe in, for example crossing the road, wearing a seat belt, closing the door.

Modifying the environment

Make sure that the home, and other areas used by children, are as safe as possible, while still allowing them to become independent and learn for themselves

Education

Children need to be educated about safety. Many national campaigns, for example Play it Safe, Green Cross Code, Stranger Danger, have aimed at increasing awareness of safety issues. Children can be taught how to avoid dangers and how to cope if a hazardous situation occurs. Adults too need educating in these areas: this means child-care workers, teachers, parents, health professionals and those who design environment areas such as shopping centres, parks or roads.

Product safety

All equipment should be safe for use with children and preferably approved for safety and display, for example, the BSI kitemark, European standards markings, the BEAB Mark of Safety (see page 307).

Legislation

safety legislation
Laws which are created to prevent accidents and promote safety

Pressure on local and national government may encourage them to make and enforce **safety legislation** which supports the prevention of accidents and the promotion of safety.

> ### ✔ Progress check
>
> 1 How can the child-care environment be modified to make it as safe as possible for a child?
> 2 Which national campaigns have helped to increase awareness about safety issues?
> 3 How can adults ensure the safety of products which they buy for children?

Safety at home

> ### Do this!   20.1
>
> Before reading this section, look around your home room by room, include the garage, garden shed and garden.
> a) Make a list of all the potentially dangerous items.
> b) Make a list of all the accidents that could occur if a young child lived with you.
> c) How could you prevent these accidents from occurring?

Everyone is relaxed at home, and may feel safe because they are at home. This is clearly not true. It is interesting to note that most home accidents occur during the summer months, especially in July. Children most at risk are those between 1 and 4 years old, because they are mobile and want to explore, but they cannot yet anticipate danger. Accident figures indicate that boys are more at risk than girls. Causes and ways of preventing home accidents are given below.

Fire

House fire is the commonest cause of death by fire. Death usually results from inhaling poisonous fumes given off from furniture. The risk of fire must be reduced because:

■ a child could cause a house fire
■ children may burn themselves, even if they do not cause a house fire.

Prevention

- Reduce the source of fire, for example do not leave matches in children's reach, restrict smoking, use a fireguard (it is illegal to leave a child under 12 in a room with an open fire), avoid using chip pans, store petrol and other **flammable** (burnable) materials correctly.
- Reduce the risk of materials such as nightwear and soft furnishings catching fire by ensuring that children wear nightclothes made from low-flammable material and by ensuring that any soft furnishings are made with fire-retardant fabric and foam – modern furnishings should have labels stating this (old furnishings are a particular fire risk).
- Restrict the possible spread of fire by the use of fire doors (which should always be kept closed), fire extinguishers and fire blankets.
- The use of an early warning system such as a smoke alarm will give the extra minutes needed to escape from a fire. All houses should have at least one, especially if children live there.

> **flammable**
> Material which burns easily

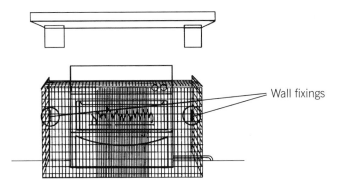

Wall fixings

A fireguard correctly fitted

Falls

Half of all domestic accidents involving children are due to falls. Twenty children die each year after falling. Toddlers are most in danger. Some dangerous situations are:

- a baby in a baby bouncer or carrycot placed on a high surface such as a table or bed.
- the baby himself placed on a high surface
- toddlers in a house with unguarded stairs, open unprotected windows, balconies or bunk beds.

Prevention

- Never leave babies unattended on a high surface; lie them on the floor instead.
- Use stairgates at the top and bottom of stairs, to prevent babies and toddlers from entering the kitchen unattended, or getting out of the back or front door.
- Teach children to use the stairs safely, how to crawl up and down with supervision. This will increase their confidence and reduce fear. It should help to prevent a fall if the stairs are accidentally left

unguarded. Ensure that banister rails are close enough to prevent a young child climbing through.

■ Use childproof window locks or latches.
■ Move furniture away from windows so that children will not be so tempted to climb up.
■ Avoid baby walkers. These are very dangerous and cause many accidents. Babies do not need them; they will learn to walk when they are ready.
■ Use reins in the pram, pushchair and supermarket trolley.
■ Place garden climbing equipment on safe surfaces such as grass or wood chippings.

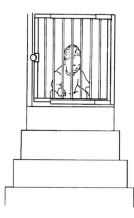

Always use a stairgate

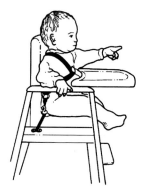

Children must be safely strapped into highchairs

Burns and scalds

Burns and scalds occur most commonly to babies and toddlers. The causes may be:

■ the bathwater too hot
■ hot drink spilling onto the child
■ pulling the kettle flex
■ hot fat from cooking or chip pan
■ contact burns from fires, radiators, irons, etc.
■ playing with matches.

Prevention

■ Use a playpen if you are cooking and prevent toddlers entering the kitchen with a safety gate.
■ Use a coiled kettle flex.
■ Use a cooker-guard and turn pan handles inwards.
■ Do not keep matches where a child can find them. They should be safely locked away.
■ Use non-flammable clothing.
■ Teach children the dangers of fire.

■ Keep children away from bonfires and fireworks, except at safe, public displays.
■ Put cold water in the bath first.

Choking

Each year, 50–60 children die as the result of a choking accident. It is the largest cause of accidental death in children under 1 year. At 6 months, babies can grasp objects and put them in their mouths to explore them. Small objects such as marbles, Lego, peanuts, sweets, buttons, bottle and pen tops must be kept out of their reach.

Prevention

It is the responsibility of the carer to remove all potentially dangerous items from the child's reach.

■ Dummies must meet safety standards with holes in the flange, in case it is drawn to the back of the throat.
■ Never leave small items lying around at home.
■ Do not use toys with small parts that are unsuitable for young children.
■ Do not give the child peanuts, nor have them available.
■ Do not allow the child to play when they are eating.

Suffocation

suffocation
Stopping respiration

Suffocation occurs when the airways are covered and the passage of air to the lungs is obstructed. Hanging and strangulation will also cut off the air supply.

Prevention

■ Some household items are dangerous for babies and young children:
  – plastic bags
  – cords around the necks of clothing
  – pillows.
■ Never prop feed a baby (i.e. do not prop the bottle so that the baby sucks without being held).
■ Make sure that there are no jagged edges on the cot or pram which could trap the clothing and strangle the baby as he moves.
■ Do not use babynests, unless the baby is actually being carried in one.
■ Avoid using quilts with young babies under 1 year.
■ Warn older children of the dangers of ropes, strings, and dangerous places such as old fridges, freezers, cupboards that could trap them inside.

Cuts

Cuts are usually caused by ordinary items such as glass, sharp knives or tin cans; there are also dangers from items such as gardening equipment, or broken windscreens, windows, etc.

Prevention

- Keep knives out of reach.
- Use plastic drinking cups and bottles.
- Use safety glass in doors or cover glass with safety film.
- Put stickers on large glass areas such as patio doors, so that it is obvious when they are closed; it is much safer to board up low-level glazing such as this.

Electricity and electrocution

The most likely cause of electrocution in the home is toddlers sticking objects into electrical sockets. Electrical equipment in a bathroom can cause death and it is against the law to have any sockets there other than those for shavers or electric toothbrushes. Faulty electrical appliances are lethal.

Prevention

- Use safety sockets, to prevent investigation with small fingers or objects.
- Use circuit breakers, which will instantly cut off the electricity supply when there is a short circuit.
- Switch sockets off when not in use.
- Do not use a hair dryer or any other electrical equipment in the bathroom.
- Check all electrical equipment for safety, for example check for worn flexes.

Case study: Promoting home safety

'Safety First' is a voluntary organisation which was created by parents living in a deprived area of a Midlands city, with the aim of reducing the number of accidents involving children in their area. The Children's Accident and Emergency Department at the city's hospital conducted a 'Geography of Accidents' study, which showed that 30 per cent of all accidental injuries presented in casualty involved children who lived in their postcodes. With the co-operation of the local council and the health authority, the group have successfully applied for a grant from the European Social Fund (ESF). They have also been allocated some financing from a manufacturer of home safety equipment. Parent volunteers visit families with children under 5 who live in the area, and offer them the opportunity to purchase safety equipment (stairgates, window locks, cooker guards, socket covers, smoke alarms and fireguards) at 50 per cent of the retail price. Because the volunteers are local and understand the particular difficulties faced by the families, they are generally well accepted. Families who are dependent upon social security benefits are given the necessary equipment free of charge.

1 Why are socket covers, smoke alarms and fire guards important safety items?

2 What other forms of support (apart from safety equipment) could be offered to families in the interests of child safety?

3 Do you think that this type of community action should be encouraged? If so why do you think it is important?

Poisoning

About 2,000 children each year are admitted to hospital after taking a poisonous substance. Those most at risk are between the ages of 2 and 3. They are exploring the environment, but cannot yet distinguish tastes. At this age, there may be easy access to poisons, such as adult medicines, bleach or cleaning fluids. There may also be dares from other children.

Prevention

- Use child-resistant containers.
- Close all containers after use.
- Store medicines in a high, preferably locked cupboard. If there is no lock, use a child-proof latch.
- Put child-resistant locks on all cupboards.
- Do not store dangerous substances in the cupboard under the sink. Find a safer storage area.
- Keep chemicals in their original containers. Do not store them in old drink bottles or jam jars that may look attractive to young children.
- Prevent children eating berries or seeds from the garden or park.

Think about it

Try to see the world from a child's viewpoint. Crawling on the kitchen floor will help you to see the hazards that may look so interesting to a child.

Remember these dangers and modify the environment to remove all avoidable dangers.

✓ Progress check

1 How can fires be prevented?
2 Which children are most at risk of falling?
3 What may cause burns and scalds?
4 How can the home be adapted to reduce the risk of burns?
5 How can choking accidents be prevented?

Do this! 20.2

a) Research the occurrence of accidents at home to children who attend your placement.
b) With the permission of your placement supervisor, send a questionnaire home with the children.
c) Display the results visually to show the age at which accidents have occurred and the scene of the accident. This could be part of a display about safety.

Outdoor safety

Play areas

Children should be supervised by a responsible 'watchful' adult during outdoor play who should:

■ encourage co-operative play
■ discourage aggression
■ ensure climbing equipment is sited on suitable soft landing surfaces with space around it
■ lock all external gates and ensure that children cannot leave the play area unsupervised
■ remove potential hazards, for example broken equipment, sharp edges, dangerous litter
■ ensure that play equipment is appropriate for the age group
■ allow children to return to indoor play area at will
■ provide areas for alternative play, for example wheeled toys, ball play, obstacle course, etc.

Road safety

Children are at risk on the road as pedestrians and as passengers in motor vehicles. Child-care workers can help to ensure their safety as pedestrians by:

■ setting a good example when crossing the road
■ discouraging parents from allowing children under 8 years to cross roads alone
■ only allowing children to leave their establishment with a responsible adult who is known to them
■ ensuring the adult:child ratio is within the prescribed limit when going out on trips and visits
■ having and using a crossing patrol outside schools
■ talking to children about road safety and teaching them the Green Cross Code. The Tufty Club may generate interest in road safety for young children
■ discouraging children from using roads and pavements as play areas.

Do this! 20.3

1 Complete a project about road safety. Include research about the incidence of accidents involving children as pedestrians and as car passengers. Suggest methods of ensuring the safety of children on the roads.

2 Prepare a topic within your placement to increase awareness about road safety. You could invite speakers in to talk to the children about various aspects of safety, and/or arrange suitable visits.

Workplace safety policies and procedures

General conduct

Most establishments have clear safety rules for children's conduct which make it clear what is expected of them and encourage children to behave in a sensible and responsible manner, for example walking and not running along corridors, keeping to the left on corridors and stairs, not shouting, fighting or bullying, etc.

Stringent safety precautions are also required, for example space to move around the building and classrooms safely, doors with safety catches, non-slip surfaces, safety glass, safe gym equipment.

Security in establishments

Many child-care establishments have introduced stringent security measures in recent years. These may include locked doors when the children are inside the building and name badges for all staff and students. Door entry phones and bells give the staff the opportunity to enquire about the nature of the business of any visitors before allowing them to enter the building. It is always advisable to make an appointment before visiting a child-care establishment to show respect for the establishment's security policies. Staff are always with the children during outdoor play times to ensure their individual and group safety.

Home times

Child-care workers must be vigilant to ensure that children are collected by adults who are known to them. Parents should inform staff about who will be collecting the child if they cannot do so themselves. It is preferable for children to remain inside the building to await collection at home time. Every establishment should have a procedure for collecting children.

Emergency procedures

All establishments should have:
- written emergency procedures
- staff who have been trained in first aid
- first aid equipment
- an accident book for accurate recording of all incidents requiring first aid
- regular review of incidents of accidents to highlight areas of concern
- planned programme of accident prevention.

✔ **Progress check**

1 How can children's safety be ensured at home times?
2 Which emergency procedures should be in place in all child-care establishments?
3 How can accidents be prevented in child-care establishments?

> ### Do this! 20.4
>
> Look at your child-care placement and try to assess its safety from a child's point of view. Are there any improvements which could be made? Are home-time procedures always followed?

> ### Case study: Safety on the roads
>
> Josie is a childminder who looks after three children under the age of 5 years during the day. She always pays great attention to safety and her home is regularly inspected by an officer from the Under Eights Unit at the local social services department. The officer notes the safety equipment and its use, for example a fireguard and a stairgate.
>
> Josie also collects three children from infant school and takes them home with her until their parents finish work and are able to collect them. Walking with six children is an enormous responsibility and, although Josie does not have to cross any busy roads, she is very aware of the children's safety on the pavement and when crossing minor road junctions. The two youngest are strapped into the double buggy and George, aged 4, walks holding onto the buggy. After school Sadie, aged 5, holds onto the other side of the buggy. Naomi and Kylie, both aged 7, walk together in front of Josie and the other children. They are not allowed to rush off alone, but walk at a steady pace that George and Sadie can keep up with. They stop at kerbs so that the whole goup can cross the road together.
>
> 1 Josie uses a stairgate and fireguard. What other safety measures should she take to protect the children in her home?
> 2 How does she ensure the children's safety on the journey to and from school?
> 3 Can you think of any other safety measures that Josie could take to protect the children on the pavement and road?

> ### ✓ Progress check
>
> 1 What can a child-care worker do to ensure children's safety during outdoor play?
> 2 Which children should not be allowed to cross the road without an adult?

Outings with children

Child-care workers must be able to plan appropriate outings for children and to ensure their safety at all times. Choosing an outing that is consistent with the age/stage of development of the children must include an awareness of the statutory requirements and the safety issues involved.

The following factors are of paramount importance when considering taking children on an outing:

- safety
- appropriate clothing
- food/refreshments
- necessary equipment
- involving parents.

Planning an outing

An outing is any trip away from the usual care and education setting. It can range from a visit to the shops to a whole day away. With thorough planning, it will be an enjoyable and educational experience for the children. The benefits of outings are wide-ranging because they give children the opportunity to:

- benefit from new and unfamiliar experiences
- learn about the environment generally or a specific area
- follow up an interest or educational topic
- meet new people.

Choosing where to go

It may be a straightforward process to decide on where to take the children – there may be a local venue which has been visited successfully by previous groups of children from your setting. However when planning any trip remember to consider the following.

- *The age and stage of development of the children* There are differences in physical capabilities between average children from 1–7 years, as well as variations in concentration levels and intellectual skills. Choose a destination which meets the needs of all the age groups you are taking. Think about what you want the children to learn (learning outcomes) from the trip, whether it is a trip to the library or a day at a farm.
- *Adult help* A general guide for ratios on trips away from the setting is:

    1 adult to 1 child 0–2 years
    1 adult to 2 children 2–5 years
    1 adult to 5 children 5–8 years.

    It is essential to arrange to have a higher adult:child ratio on any outing away from the establishment because of the increased risks due to traffic, a new environment with no physical boundaries, a different routine for the day and the extra people needed to carry any equipment, for example first aid box, picnic/snacks/educational resources, etc.
- *Distance of the destination* This can mean the difference between a morning, afternoon or whole day trip. It is vital to make sure that the time spent at the venue will be of value. Children do not like spending a disproportionate amount of time travelling.
- *Cost* If there is an entry fee or travelling costs, it may not be open to all children in the establishment if some families cannot afford to pay. Check whether there is enough funding to cater for all the children.

■ *Transport* Is the venue within walking distance? If not, can people offer lifts? Do they have child restraints in their cars?

Is there an establishment minibus? Are drivers insured?

If arranging transport with an outside organisation, make sure that:
- they are insured
- the vehicle is large enough to seat everyone – adults and children
- there are sufficient child restraints, booster seats, seat belts, etc.
- the vehicles are safe.

Stages in the planning process

1 Research into the destination, for example opening times and accessibility for children. It may be possible to visit to find out. Are there toilet facilities? Picnic areas? Refreshments? First aid provision?

2 Prepare a timetable for the day. Everyone will need to know times of departure and arrival. Ensure that your programme is practical and that there is enough time to do everything that you have planned for.

3 Plan to take all the necessary equipment with you, for example the first aid kit, labels for the children, camera, money, audio tapes for the journey, and ask children to bring items with them, for example a packed lunch, wet weather wear, pencils/paper.

4 Consult parents. It is necessary to get written consent from parents to go on any trip away from the establishment? They will need to know about the cost, the day's programme, transport arrangements, special requirements – lunch, clothing, etc. A letter home with a consent slip is the best way to achieve this.

✔ Progress check

1 What are the benefits of taking children on outings?
2 Why do you need to provide a higher adult/child ratio on outings?
3 What are the stages in the planning process for an outing?
4 Which important safety issues are involved in arranging transport for an outing?

Key terms

You need to know what these words and phrases mean. Go back through the chapter to find out.

accidents
flammable
safety legislation
suffocation

Now try these questions

1 How can adults protect children from unintentional injuries in the home?

2 What can a child-care worker do in an establishment to keep the children safe?

3 What is the role of the child-care worker in organising an outing for children?

4 Explain why children under 1 year of age are most at risk of choking and how this can be prevented.

Part 7: Health and Sickness

Child health services are introduced, and the role of the child-care worker in screening and surveillance is described.

Child-care workers need to know about the types of micro-organisms which cause disease and how they are transmitted. Children are vulnerable to infections, so people who work with them must be familiar with the signs and symptoms of a range of illnesses. They also should be able to distinguish between minor problems and those which require immediate attention.

Child-care workers are responsible for reporting their concerns about changes in the child's physical condition and/or behaviour promptly and sensitively to the child's parent or main carer. The values of record-keeping are reinforced so that child-care workers can keep parents accurately informed about their child and give correct details to medical staff.

All child carers will be expected to care for ill children at some time in their careers. Knowing the general and specific needs of ill children, and how to provide for them, enables carers to supply the necessary nurturing environment. Preparing all children for hospital is important because many children are admitted to hospital without warning as the result of accidents or sudden illness. Providing play opportunities in hospital and an insight into the effects of hospitalisation on development is also included.

Chapter 24 does not replace a recognised first aid course and all prospective child-care workers are strongly recommended to complete a first aid training.

21 Child health promotion

This chapter includes:

- ■ Health promotion and education
- ■ Child health surveillance
- ■ Screening for hearing impairment
- ■ Screening for visual defects
- ■ The Guthrie test
- ■ Immunisation

Child health promotion includes:

- ■ promoting a healthy lifestyle by encouraging the positive aspects of improving and maintaining health
- ■ child health surveillance – a programme of care to monitor children's health and prevent illness
- ■ health education – an ongoing programme of education and information for parents, carers, and children about all aspects of child health, accident prevention, growth and development
- ■ screening – the examination of children to detect specific conditions/impairments.

You may find it helpful to read this chapter in conjunction with:

- ▶ **Book 1, Chapter 1**   Physical growth
- ▶ **Book 1, Chapter 18**   Conditions and impairments
- ▶ **Book 2, Chapter 22**   Illnesses and ailments

Health promotion and education

There are many important factors involved in maintaining children's health and keeping them safe from illness. Child-care workers can have an impact on the health of the children in their care by providing routines and activities and education that increase adults' and children's awareness of the importance of good health and ways of keeping healthy.

It is important that health topics and activities are part of the planned programme for children. It is often possible to link these successfully with other areas of the curriculum. For example, topic work about 'Ourselves' will cover aspects of Knowledge and Understanding of the World in the Desirable Outcomes curriculum (see Chapter 6, page 86), while helping children to understand how their body works.

Health issues should be part of the daily routines and reminders and explanations about health and hygiene will reinforce healthy life skills.

Child-care workers should work in ways that will promote children's self-esteem so that they can feel good about themselves, develop independence and form positive relationships. This will have a positive effect on their health and well-being.

Child-care workers should provide children with positive role models. For example, children who see their carers smoke are more likely to go on to smoke themselves. Smoking should be positively discouraged in child-care settings.

The child-care environment should be safe. The staff and children should be aware of safety issues at all times and child-care workers should use all available opportunities to raise children's awareness and understanding of safety and keeping themselves safe.

Providing healthy choices at mealtimes and discussing food with children will enhance their understanding of the importance of a healthy diet and its influences on good health.

Health-related activities

Many activities can be offered to children to raise their awareness of and promote good health. They must be appropriate for the developmental stage of the child and be interesting and stimulating. They may also be successfully linked with children's learning in other areas of the curriculum.

Activities could include:

- *imaginative play* – setting up the imaginative play area as a health centre, dental surgery, hospital, shop, cafe

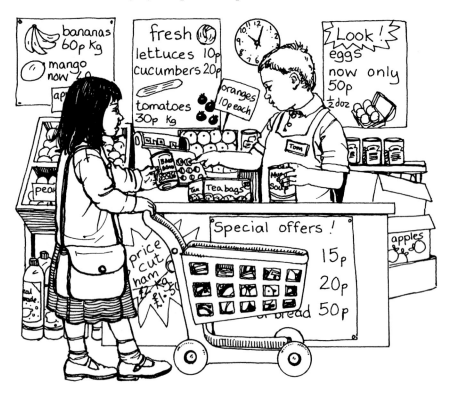

Activities such as this can be related to health promotion and to other areas of the curriculum (healthy eating, mathematics and language and literacy)

- *visits to places of interest* – to food shops, farms, gardens where vegetables and fruit are grown
- *visitors* – the health visitor, school nurse, road crossing patrol, dentist
- *daily routines* – hygiene routines, safety routines
- *books and stories* – books in child-care settings should present health issues positively; story and group time can be used for discussion
- *games* – board games created with a health aspect in mind
- *displays and interest tables* – displays can be created to convey particular health messages. Children's work can contribute to displays, for example, their writing, drawing and paintings about health topics
- *demonstrations* – of hand washing, hairbrushing, crossing the road safely.

> ### ✓ *Progress check*
>
> List five activities related to health topics that would be suitable for each of the following age groups:
> a) 1–3 years   b) 3–5 years   c) 5–7 years.

Child health surveillance

Child health surveillance is a system of reviewing a child's progress. These reviews are carried out at certain ages in the child's life. Programmes with regular reviews at fixed ages safeguard children from slipping through the net, especially when families move home frequently and change doctors and **health visitors**. In many areas of the country the child health record is held by the main carer of the child in the form of a book. This book, the child health record, has spaces that can be filled in by the parent or carer and other people who care for the child. These may be:

health visitor
A trained nurse who specialises in child health promotion

- health visitors
- family doctors
- child health clinic staff
- hospital emergency department staff
- hospital outpatient staff
- school health team
- dentists.

In this way information can be shared and is easily available to all those caring for the child. Parents or carers have an ongoing record to which they can refer.

Principles of child health surveillance

There are certain principles that underpin the effective use of a child health surveillance programme. Child health surveillance should be:

- carried out in partnership with the parents or carers. They are the experts and the best people to identify health, developmental and behavioural problems in their own children

- a positive experience for parents or carers
- a learning experience for the parents or carers, the child and the health professional; it should involve exchanging information
- an opportunity to provide guidance on child health topics and health promotion
- a continuous and flexible process; as well as fixed assessments there should be opportunities for other reviews as required by each child
- carried out by observation and talking with the parents or carers; tests and examinations should complement the process
- based on good communication and teamwork.

The professionals involved

Most child health surveillance is carried out in the child's own home or at the child health clinic. Clinics are held in health centres, GPs' premises or in other convenient places, like church halls. The professionals most concerned with child health surveillance are health visitors and doctors. Health visitors are trained nurses who have undertaken further training in midwifery and health visiting. The doctors have a special interest in child health and could be the child's GP. Each of these professionals is responsible for part of the child health surveillance programme; they work as a team with the parents or carers. The general practitioner and the health visitor are part of the **primary health care team**.

> **primary health care team**
> A group of professionals who are concerned with the delivery of first-line health care and health promotion

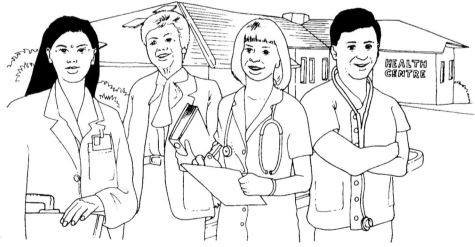

The primary health care team

The child health surveillance programme

Assessment of the developmental progress of the child is part of each review.

Birth review

The birth review is normally carried out before discharge from hospital, or by the family doctor if the birth is at home. The birth review includes:

- measurements – weight and head circumference are recorded on a percentile chart

- Guthrie test to exclude phenylketonuria (see page 408)
- hip examination to detect any congenital dislocation or instability of the hip (see Book 1, Chapter 18)
- general examination to exclude congenital conditions or acquired disease.

Health promotion topics covered at this review include advice on feeding, safety and car transport.

10 to 14 days review

The 10 to 14 days review is usually carried out by the health visitor at the child's home and includes:

- review, with the parent or carer, of progress and development since the birth
- general examination
- hip examination repeat
- measurements – head circumference and weight are recorded on the percentile chart.

Health promotion topics covered at this review include feeding, immunisations, further health reviews and safety.

6-week review

The 6-week review is usually carried out by the doctor at the child health clinic and includes:

- review, with carer, of progress and development from 2 weeks
- physical examination
- measurements – weight and head circumference are recorded on the percentile chart
- hip examination repeat.

Health promotion topics covered at this review include feeding and safety.

3 to 4 months review

There is another hip examination for any signs of disability or instability.

6 to 9 months review

The review at 6 to 9 months is usually carried out by the health visitor at home or at the clinic and includes:

- review, with parent or carer, of progress and development from 6 weeks
- measurements – weight and head circumference are recorded on the percentile chart
- hip examination
- hearing test, using a distraction test (see page 404)
- observation of visual behaviour
- check for **undescended testicles** – in males the testes, which are in the body before birth, should come down into the scrotum (see the diagram in Book 1, page 15).

Health promotion topics covered at this review include safety, use of fireguards, stairgates, car seats and dangers of glass doors.

undescended testicles
When the testes remain located in the body instead of coming down into the scrotum

18 to 24 months review

The review at 18 to 24 months includes:

■ review, with parent or carer, of development and progress from 9 months
■ measurements – weight is recorded on the percentile chart
■ language development is checked (see Book 1, Chapter 8)
■ vision test.

Health promotion topics covered at this review include accident prevention, water safety (for example, ponds), safe storage of medicines and other dangerous fluids, and kitchen safety.

Heart check

Between 1 and 3 years, all children should have a heart check by the doctor.

Testicular examination

Between 1 and 3 years all males should have their testes checked again to make sure both of them have come down into the scrotum.

3 years to 3 years 6 months review

The review at 3 years includes:

■ review of progress and development with parent or carer, especially of language development
■ measurements – height is recorded on the percentile chart

Health promotion topics covered at this review include road and car safety.

At this stage the doctor and health visitor will review the records with the parents or carers and discuss the need for further regular reviews.

School entry review

The school entry review is undertaken by the school nurse and doctor. The review involves:

■ review, with parent or carer, of progress and development
■ measurement of height and weight
■ vision test
■ hearing test
■ immunisation booster (see *The immunisation programme*, page 409).

Health promotion topics covered at this review include road safety and stranger danger.

8 years appraisal

This appraisal is carried out by the school nurse and involves:

■ review of progress and development
■ measurement of height and weight
■ vision test.

Health promotion topics covered at this review include road safety, stranger danger, dental health, diet and exercise.

✓ *Progress check*

1 Who writes in the child health record?
2 Who are the best people to identify health and developmental problems?
3 How are reviews carried out?
4 Which professionals are most involved in child health surveillance?
5 What measurements are recorded in the first year?
6 Where are the measurements recorded?
7 What is the starting point of each review?
8 What does the hip examination detect?
9 What is the testicular examination for?
10 When should all children have a heart check?

Think about it

1 Think of all the benefits of child health surveillance.
2 Think of the benefits of a parent-held child health record.
3 What do you think 'slipping through the net' means in terms of child health surveillance? How might this happen? How might it be prevented?

Do this! 21.1

1 Find out if parent-held child health records are in use in your area. Try to see one.

2 Look for a diagram of the hip joint (for example, Book 1, Chapter 18) and copy it into your notes. Find out more about congenital dislocation of the hip.

3 Find a diagram of the male reproductive organs and make sure you know where the testes are normally located.

4 Find out about the members of the primary health care team. Who are they and what are their roles?

5 Look back at the health promotion topics suggested at each review. Can you add to these? Make sure that your additions are appropriate to the age and stage of development.

6 If you can, try to arrange to go with a parent or carer and their child to a child health surveillance review.

Screening for hearing impairment

Parents or carers will often recognise that their child has a hearing loss. Child-care workers should listen carefully to these concerns and refer the child for further investigation. There are special tests that are done as part of the child health surveillance programme, but tests can, and should, be done at any time if a hearing problem is suspected. There is more information about deafness in Book 1, Chapter 18.

Neonatal screening

Parents or carers will know whether their child is responding to sounds. Responses to loud sounds at this age include:

- stiffening
- blinking
- the Moro reflex
- crying.

The baby may respond to quieter, prolonged sounds by becoming still and quiet. There are methods of testing the hearing of **neonates**, but these are not tests that are done routinely on every newborn baby. Tests include:

- auditory response cradle (ARC)
- otoacoustic emissions (OAE)
- brainstem evoked response audiometry (BSERA).

These are complex tests and are not routine. They are usually used if there is some reason to suspect a hearing problem.

> **neonate**
> A newborn baby

Distraction test: 6 to 9 months

The best age for screening hearing in the first year of life is at about 7 months old. All babies should have their hearing tested at this age. Developmentally, the baby must be able to sit and have good head control. The **distraction test** needs two people as well as the carer: one to observe and one to test.

The baby sits on the carer's lap facing the observer. The observer holds the baby's attention with a soundless toy. When the observer has engaged the baby's attention, the toy is withdrawn and the tester makes the stimulus sound at ear level. The baby should turn, search for and find the source of the sound. This is called **localising**. Both ears must be tested with a range of quiet sounds, both high- and low-pitched.

> **distraction test**
> A hearing test carried out at about 7 months

> **localising**
> Searching for and locating the source of a sound

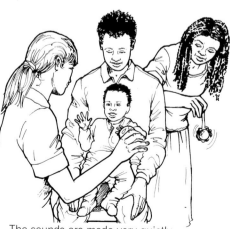
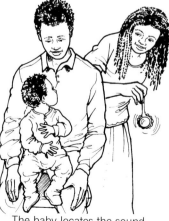

A distraction hearing test   The sounds are made very quietly   The baby locates the sound

Stimulus sounds include:

■ rattles – there are specialised rattles, such as Manchester and Nuffield rattles
■ voice – low-pitched sound such as *oo*, high-pitched sound such as *ss*, quiet conversation using the baby's name.

There are many reasons, such as illness or tiredness, why a baby might not respond to a hearing test. If the baby does not respond to all of the test, it is repeated after 2 to 4 weeks. Further failure to respond needs referral for a full audiological assessment.

Tests for older children: 2 to 5 years

As children develop, it becomes possible to use tests that need the child's co-operation. Examples of these are the Go game and the speech discrimination test

Go game

In this game test, the child is asked to post a brick into a box when they hear the word 'Go'. An experienced tester can vary the pitch and sound level of the voice and each ear can be tested separately.

Speech discrimination test

This test is more difficult than the Go game and the child's co-operation and understanding are needed. The child is presented with a selection of toys. These toys are specially selected to test the child's ability to hear different consonants, for example p, g, d, hard c, s, m, f, b. After naming the toys in a normal voice with the tester, the child is asked in a quiet voice to identify each of the toys, for example 'Show me the duck'; 'Give the brick to Mummy'. Again, each ear is tested though the range.

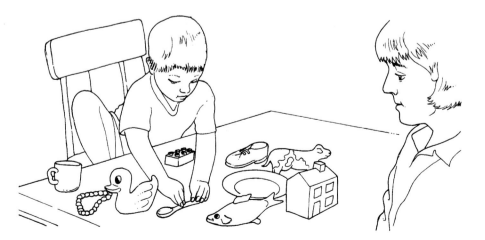

The speech discrimination test

Pure tone audiometry (from 5 years)

audiometry
A method of testing hearing using sound produced by a machine called an audiometer

For pure tone **audiometry**, the child puts on earphones and listens for the tone produced by the audiometer. The tones are given at different pitch and intensity. Each ear is tested separately. This is a lengthy and complicated test.

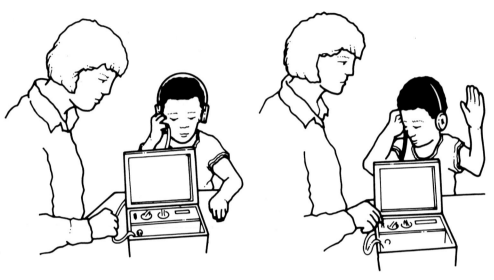

Audiometry: using an audiometer to measure hearing

Sweep audiometry

Sweep audiometry is a less complicated method of pure tone audiometry, where a range of selected frequencies is tested. This test is usually performed at around the time of school entry.

✓ **Progress check**

1 What is the best age to test a child's hearing using a distraction test?
2 Name two other tests which can be used to test hearing.
3 What does localising a sound mean?
4 What sort of sounds are used to test hearing?
5 Why is it important to have two people involved in the distraction hearing test?

Do this!   **21.2**

Devise a checklist showing some of the signs to look for, in the first year, that will indicate that a baby's hearing is developing normally.

Case study: A hearing test

Jade is 8 months old and has come to the health centre with Dulcie, her mother, for her routine hearing test. Ruth, her health visitor, talks to Dulcie about Jade's development and Dulcie tells her that Jade is vocalising and making sounds with two syllables. Ruth observes Jade and notes that she is sitting up unsupported and has good head control. Jade sits on her mother's knee and faces Colin, another health visitor, who is helping Ruth with the tests. Colin plays with Jade for a while and keeps her attention. Meanwhile Ruth makes a very quiet sound level with Jade's ear and about 1 metre away. Jade immediately turns to find the sound, sees Ruth and smiles broadly. Ruth praises her and then encourages her to return her attention to Colin. Ruth continues the test in this way using different sounds including high and low pitched sounds. Jade quickly responds to all the sounds and Ruth is satisfied with the test and she tells Dulcie that Jade is hearing normally.

1 Between what ages is it best to test the hearing of a baby under 1?
2 Why did Ruth check with Jade's mother about her development?
3 Why are two people needed for the hearing test?
4 Why did Ruth wait for Jade to turn to the sounds?
5 What is the term used to describe this?

Screening for visual impairment

In many instances, visual defects are first detected by parents or carers. The child-care worker should be sure to listen carefully to any concerns expressed and refer the child for further investigation to the GP or health clinic. Some of the general signs that will indicate that a baby's vision is developing normally are as follows.

- *At birth*, the baby will look briefly at the mother's face.
- *At 1 month*, the baby will watch the carer's face intently while being fed and follow the carer's face as it moves from side to side.
- *At 3 months*, the baby will follow a dangling toy held in front of his face; he starts to look at his own fingers.
- *At 6 months*, the baby can see across a room and can see small objects like a smartie.
- *At 9 months*, the baby can recognise toys across a room and see small crumbs on the floor and try to pick them up.

If a child does not seem to be doing these things, it is important that further tests on vision are carried out.

In addition to general observation of the child's progress, there are routine checks on children's vision which are part of the child health surveillance programme.

- *At birth and 6 weeks*, the doctor will examine the eyes for any signs of abnormality, in particular any evidence of cataract, a condition where the lens of the eye is not transparent.

■ *Between 6 weeks and 6 months*, the doctor and health visitor will look for any sign of a squint, a condition where the eyes do not work together properly and the baby seems not to look straight at you. There are special tests used to identify a squint: the corneal reflection test and the cover test.

■ *Between 2 and 5 years* By this age children are able to co-operate with vision testing. Distance vision can be assessed using single letters with a letter matching chart. The child looks at the letter being held up by the tester, then points to the matching letter on her chart. Older children will be able to name the letters. Each eye must be tested separately from a distance of 3 metres.

■ *Pre-school* Routine screening of vision is usually carried out at school entry and at three-yearly intervals.

■ *Colour vision defects* Screening for colour vision impairment is usually recommended at the beginning of secondary school.

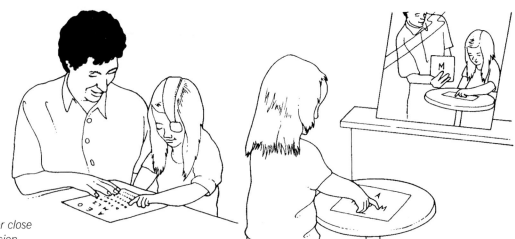

Vision testing for close and distance vision

✓ Progress check

1 What are the general signs that vision is developing normally at:
  a) birth?
  b) 3 months?
  c) 9 months?
2 What is a squint?
3 What might lead you to suspect that a baby of 6 weeks was not able to see?

The Guthrie test

The Guthrie test is a screening test to detect phenylketonuria (PKU is an inherited condition which affects the baby's ability to metabolise part of protein foods (see Book 1, Chapter 18, page 334). Other conditions such as hypothyroidism (a condition in which the thyroid gland is not working properly) and cystic fibrosis (an inherited condition) may also be detected. The test is carried out when the baby is about 6 days old and has been taking milk feeds for several days. Blood is collected from a heel prick to cover four circles on a specially prepared card that is then sent to the laboratory. Early treatment of PKU gives the child a good chance of developing normally.

> ### ✓ *Progress check*
>
> 1 When is the Guthrie test carried out?
> 2 What feeds must the baby have had before the test can be done?
> 3 What does the Guthrie test detect?

Immunisation

Immunisation is the use of vaccine to protect people from disease. You will need to read Chapter 22, *Illnesses and ailments* to find out more about how the body remembers and recognises infections so that people become immune to diseases.

Vaccines used in immunisations contain either small parts of the viruses or bacteria that cause the disease, or very small amounts of the chemicals (toxins) they produce. These have been treated to make sure that they do not cause the disease, but are still capable of stimulating the body to make antibodies. In this way, the body will be able to defend itself against future infections. Vaccines provide most children with effective and long-lasting protection. Some immunisations need topping up and **boosters** may be needed as the child gets older.

Immunisation protects children from serious diseases. It also protects other children by preventing diseases being passed on.

booster
An additional dose of a vaccine given after the initial dose

The immunisation programme

Advice and guidance on immunisation is part of the programme of child health promotion. Doctors and health visitors will advise parents or carers about immunisations and discuss any worries they may have about their child. More information about each of the diseases and their treatment is given in Chapter 22.

The booster MMR

Since October 1996 all children having their pre-school booster against diphtheria, tetanus and polio are also offered a booster dose of measles, mumps and rubella. A booster is needed because around 5–10 per cent of children remain unprotected after their first MMR immunisation. A second dose will offer protection to those children and boost the immunity of the others.

The immunisation programme

Age	Vaccine	Method
2 months	Hib (haemophilus influenzae type b meningitis)	1 injection
	Diphtheria, tetanus, pertussis (whooping cough) (DTP)	1 injection
	Polio	By mouth
3 months	Hib	1 injection
	DTP	1 injection
	Polio	By mouth
4 months	Hib	1 injection
	DTP	1 injection
	Polio	By mouth
12–15 months	Measles, mumps and rubella (MMR)	1 injection
3–5 years (school entry)	Diphtheria, tetanus	1 injection
	MMR	1 injection
	Polio	By mouth
Girls 10–14 years	Rubella	if not previously given at 12-15 months 1 injection
Girls/boys 10–14 years (sometimes shortly after birth)	Tuberculosis	1 injection (BCG)
School leavers 15–19 years	Diphtheria, tetanus	1 injection
	Polio	Booster by mouth

Side-effects after immunisation

After immunisation some children may be unwell, have a fever or be irritable for a while. Sometimes the skin becomes red and swollen around the place where the injection was given, or a small lump appears. If the child does develop a fever after being immunised, keep them cool and give plenty to drink. The doctor or health visitor may advise a dose of paracetamol syrup, but always check first to make sure the right dose is given. Any red or swollen area around the injection site should gradually disappear. If there are any other worrying symptoms such as a high temperature or a convulsion, consult the doctor immediately.

Side-effects of the DTP triple immunisation

Side-effects after having the DTP (diphtheria, tetanus, pertussis – whooping cough) immunisation are mild. The baby may become miserable, fretful and slightly feverish in the 24 hours after the injection. Some children may have a convulsion (fit) after the DTP immunisation. It is the whooping cough part of the triple vaccine that often worries parents and carers. There have been questions about the safety of the vaccine and the possibility of brain damage. New research has not found a link between the vaccine and permanent brain damage.

Side-effects of the Hib (haemophilus influenzae type b) immunisation

About one baby in ten will have some redness or swelling at the site of the injection. The swelling goes down very quickly and has usually disappeared after a day or so.

Side-effects of the measles, mumps and rubella (MMR) immunisation

Some children develop a mild fever and a rash about seven to ten days after the immunisation. This usually lasts for a day or two. A few children get a mild form of mumps about three weeks after their immunisation. These are all mild symptoms and are not infectious to other children or pregnant women. A few children may have more serious reactions such as a convulsion or encephalitis (inflammation of the brain) but this is very rare. Recently, the MMR vaccine has been linked to incidences of autism and bowel disorders in children, but research has *not* found conclusive evidence to support this.

Side-effects of the polio immunisation

The polio vaccine is a live virus given by mouth. The virus is passed through the digestive tract and into a dirty nappy. It is very important, therefore, for care workers to wash their hands carefully after changing nappies to avoid becoming infected. Child-care workers need to check that their own polio immunisation is up-to-date.

Immunisation protects children from serious diseases. It also protects other children by preventing diseases being passed on.

Child-care workers will benefit from keeping their own immunisations up-to-date. Immunisations requiring boosters are polio and tetanus. Child-care workers could also be protected against hepatitis.

✔ Progress check

1 Give two reasons why it is important for children to be immunised.
2 Describe the most common mild reactions to an immunisation.
3 Describe the more serious side-effects.
4 Which vaccine is given by mouth?
5 If a baby has had the polio vaccine, what special precautions should the carer take?
6 What is contained in the triple vaccine?

Do this!   21.3

Write a page outlining what you would say to a parent or carer who is unsure about the value of immunisations.

Key terms

You need to know what these words and phrases mean. Go back through the chapter to find out.

audiometry
booster
distraction test
health visitor
localising
neonate
primary health care team
undescended testicles

Now try these questions

1 Why is it important for children to be immunised?

2 Why is it important to detect any hearing loss that a child might have, as early as possible?

3 What is the value of a programme of child health surveillance?

4 Why is health promotion an important part of the role of a child-care worker?

5 In what ways can child-care workers contribute to children's awareness of the importance of keeping safe and healthy?

22 Childhood illnesses and ailments

This chapter includes:
- **Disease transmission**
- **Immunity**
- **Infectious diseases**
- **Common childhood illnesses**
- **Infestations**

Children have illnesses and infections that are passed very easily from one child to another. Understanding how diseases are spread will help child-care workers to prevent children in their care from being infected and from passing that infection on to others. As children grow up, they develop their own immunity to disease. Many children will develop natural immunity, but they will also benefit from a programme of immunisation that will protect them by giving immunity to diseases. Infectious diseases that affect children in childhood can have lasting consequences. It is important to know how to recognise these diseases, the likely treatment and care required.

You may find it helpful to read this chapter in conjunction with:

▶ **Book 2, Chapter 21**   Child health promotion

Disease transmission

Disease is a condition that arises when something goes wrong with the normal working of the body. As a result the child becomes ill. Signs that a child is ill and has a disease include:
- raised temperature
- headache
- sore throat
- rashes on the skin
- diarrhoea.

Other possible signs of illness are a lot of crying, being irritable, behaviour that is unusual. Possible signs of illness are always more worrying and significant in a baby or very young child.

Organisms that cause disease are called **pathogens**. The most important pathogens are bacteria, viruses and some fungi. The everyday name for pathogens is *germs*. Pathogens get into the body mainly through the mouth and nose and sometimes through cuts on the skin. Once they are inside the body, they multiply very rapidly. This is called the

pathogen
Germs such as bacteria and viruses

incubation period
The time from when pathogens enter the body until the first signs of infection appear

toxin
A poisonous substance produced by pathogens

incubation period and can last for days or weeks depending on the type of pathogen. Although the person is infected during the incubation period, they only begin to feel ill and have signs of the infection towards the end of the incubation period.

Pathogens work in different ways when they infect the body. Some attack and destroy body cells, others produce poisonous substances in the bloodstream called **toxins**. The intense activity of the pathogens produces a lot of heat; so one of the signs of infection by pathogens is that the child's temperature goes up.

How diseases spread

The ways in which diseases are spread are by:
- droplets of moisture in the air
- touch
- food and water
- animals
- cuts and scratches.

Droplets in the air

When you cough, sneeze, talk and sing, tiny droplets of moisture come out of your nose or mouth. If you have a disease, these droplets will be swarming with pathogens. If these infected droplets are breathed in by another person, the disease can be spread to them. Colds (caused by viruses) spread rapidly in this way.

Touch

It is possible to catch some infectious diseases by touching an infected person, or by touching towels or other things used by that person. The skin disease impetigo (caused by bacteria) is spread in this way. Another skin disease, athlete's foot (caused by a fungus) can be picked up from the floors of changing rooms and showers.

Food and water

The urine and faeces of an infected person will contain pathogens. Drinking water may be contaminated if sewage gets into it. Food and drinks can be contaminated if they are prepared or handled by a person with dirty hands, or if the food preparation area is dirty. This is why hand-washing after visiting the lavatory and before handling food is so important. Food poisoning (caused by bacteria) easily spreads in this way, especially in places where lots of children play and eat together, such as nurseries.

Animals

Pathogens are brought on to food by animals like flies, rats, mice and cockroaches. Animals that suck blood spread other diseases; an example of this is malaria, which is spread by mosquitoes.

Cuts and scratches

Pathogens can enter the body through a cut or other injuries to the skin. Examples of these are the tetanus bacteria and the hepatitis virus.

> ✔ *Progress check*
>
> 1 What are the signs of disease?
> 2 What are pathogens?
> 3 Give some examples of pathogens.
> 4 Explain briefly the different ways that diseases are spread.
> 5 What are toxins?

Immunity

When pathogens do enter, the body does not just sit back and let them take over. White blood cells work to try to destroy the invading bacteria or viruses. The white cells identify the invading pathogens as a foreign substance and begin to make **antibodies**. Antibodies make the pathogens clump together so that the white cells can destroy them by absorbing them – this process is called **phagocytosis**.

antibody
A substance made by white cells to attack pathogens

phagocytosis
The process by which white cells absorb pathogens and destroy them

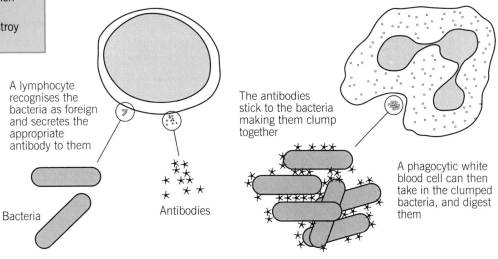

A lymphocyte recognises the bacteria as foreign and secretes the appropriate antibody to them

Bacteria

Antibodies

The antibodies stick to the bacteria making them clump together

A phagocytic white blood cell can then take in the clumped bacteria, and digest them

Phagocytosis: how white cells destroy bacteria

It will take some time for the white cells to make enough antibodies. This may give the pathogen enough time to multiply so that the child shows signs of having the disease. Eventually, however, the white cells make enough antibodies to destroy the pathogens and the child recovers from the illness. If the same pathogen attacks again some time later, the white cells recognise it and can quickly make large quantities of antibody so that

immunity
The presence of antibodies which protect the body against infectious disease

the pathogen is destroyed before it has chance to multiply – **immunity** has been created; the child is now immune to that pathogen and the disease it causes.

Active immunity

Having a disease and recovering from it is one way of becoming immune to it. This is called **active immunity**, because the white cells make the antibodies against the pathogens causing the disease. Active immunity is also acquired by having an immunisation with a **vaccine**. Vaccines contain killed or weakened forms of the pathogens that cause the particular disease. The BCG vaccine for tuberculosis, for example, contains bacteria that have been weakened. When they are injected into the body, they are too weak to multiply, but the white cells can identify them as foreign cells and begin to make antibodies to overcome them. Immunity to the disease is then acquired because the body has learnt to recognise that pathogen and can make the antibody required to combat it.

active immunity
The body's ability to resist a disease that has been acquired by having the disease or by having a specific immunisation

vaccine
A preparation used to stimulate the production of antibodies and provide immunity against one or several diseases

Passive immunity

Another type of immunity is called **passive immunity**. Here the antibody is put into the body ready-made. Passive immunisation can be given by injecting a serum that contains antibodies into the body, but this not done very often. The most common example of passive immunity is when breast-fed babies acquire immunity to diseases because there are antibodies in breast milk that are passed to the baby from the mother. Passive immunity does not last indefinitely, because the antibodies gradually disappear from the blood. Active immunity lasts much longer because the white cells have learnt to make the antibody and can do this if the pathogen enters the body on future occasions.

passive immunity
The body's ability to resist a disease, acquired from antibodies given directly into the body, for example the antibodies passed on in breast milk

> ### ✓ Progress check
>
> 1 What is an antibody?
> 2 Which cells in the body destroy pathogens?
> 3 What is phagocytosis?
> 4 How is active immunity acquired?
> 5 How is passive immunity acquired?

Infectious diseases

The table on pages 417–19 lists some of the diseases child-care workers are likely to meet.

Meningitis and septicaemia

Meningitis is an inflammation of the lining of the brain. It is a rare but very serious illness. There are two main types of bacterial meningitis in

Infectious childhood diseases

Disease	Incubation period	Signs to look for	Care
Chicken pox: viral infection	14–16 days	Begins with general signs of feeling unwell, maybe a slight temperature; spots appear first on the chest and back and then spread; red at first but become fluid filled blisters; they eventually dry off into scabs which drop off; spots come in successive crops and are very itchy	Give plenty to drink, keep the child as comfortable as possible, with baths, loose comfortable clothes and calamine lotion to ease the itching; prevent scratching as this may leave scars
Diphtheria: bacterial infection	2–6 days	General signs of being unwell, difficulty with breathing; classic sign of diphtheria is white membrane forming across the throat and restricting the airway; toxins produced by the bacteria can damage the heart and brain	Requires prompt medical treatment with antibiotics and admission to hospital
Gastroenteritis: bacterial or viral infection spread by direct contact or eating infected food or water	Very variable: 1–14 days; viruses affect more quickly	Child is generally unwell, with severe vomiting and diarrhoea; babies and young children quickly show signs of dehydration, with dry mouth and skin, decreased urine output; anterior fontanelle (Book 1, pages 7–8) in small babies sinks down	Call the doctor, initial treatment in hospital may be necessary; keep the child cool and comfortable; give drinks of water very regularly; oral rehydration solutions may also be given
Measles: viral infection	7–12 days	Begins with signs of bad cold and cough; child gradually becomes more unwell and miserable with raised temperature and sore eyes; before rash appears on the skin white spots can be seen inside the mouth (Kopliks spots); when rash appears spots are red and rash is blotchy; rash usually starts behind the ears and quickly spreads downwards to rest of the body	Child may be very unwell; call the doctor; in addition to any medical treatment, give rest and plenty of fluids; eyes may need special attention and gentle bathing; keep mouth clean and moist; watch for signs of ear infection
Meningitis: inflammation of the membrane covering the brain; can be caused by bacterial or viral infection *If meningitis is suspected, it is important to get medical help as quickly as possible*	2–10 days	Important to recognise meningitis early as it develops very rapidly; usually begins with high temperature, headache, vomiting, confusion, irritability; later signs may develop, pain and stiffness in the neck, dislike of the light	Get medical help early; treatment and care in hospital will be required See Meningitis and septicaemia, pages 416 and 420–1

(Continued)

Infectious childhood diseases (continued)

Disease	Incubation period	Signs to look for	Care
Mumps: viral infection	14–21 days	Generally unwell; pain and tenderness around the ear and jaw, uncomfortable to chew; swelling starts under jaw and up by the ear, usually on one side of the face, followed (though not always) by the other	Keep the child comfortable and give plenty to drink; doctor may advise analgesic (such as paracetamol) to ease soreness; rest is necessary as rare complication in boys is inflammation of the testes
Poliomyelitis (polio): viral infection which attacks the nervous system causing muscle paralysis; a water-borne infection	5–21 days	Becoming suddenly unwell, with headache, stiffness in the neck and back, followed by loss of movement and paralysis; maybe difficulty with breathing	Initial hospital care, followed by rest and rehabilitation
Rubella (German measles): viral infection	14–21 days	Begins like a mild cold, but often child does not feel unwell; rash appears first on the face, then spreads to the body; spots are flat and only last for about 24 hours; glands in the back of the neck may be swollen	Children with rubella often do not feel unwell; give plenty to drink; if a pregnant woman gets rubella, there is a risk of damage to her baby; keep the child away from anyone who is pregnant or likely to be; if the child was with anyone who is pregnant before you knew about the illness let them know; any pregnant woman who has had any contact with rubella should see her doctor urgently
Scarlet fever: bacterial infection	2–6 days	Begins with child suddenly feeling unwell, with sore throat, temperature, feeling sick; tongue looks very red, cheeks are flushed, throat looks red and sore, with white patches; rash starts on the face and spreads to the body	Make sure child rests and drinks plenty; doctor may prescribe antibiotics; observe for complications, such as ear and kidney infections
Tetanus: bacterial infection; bacteria found in soil, dirt and dust, enter the body through cuts, scratches and other wounds	4–21 days	Tetanus attacks the nervous system, causing painful muscle spasms; muscles in the neck tighten and the jaw locks	Any cuts, etc. must be properly cleaned; immunisation kept up-to-date; immediate hospital treatment needed for suspected tetanus
Tuberculosis (TB): bacterial infection	28–42 days	Persistent coughing, weight loss, further investigation shows lung damage	Initial period of treatment in hospital may be required; specific antibiotics given, rest and good quality diet essential

Infectious childhood diseases (continued)

Disease	Incubation period	Signs to look for	Care
Whooping cough (pertussis): bacterial infection	7–14 days	Begins like cough and cold; cough usually gets worse; after about 2 weeks coughing bouts start; long bouts of coughing and choking are exhausting and frightening, as coughing can go on for so long that child finds it hard to breathe and may be sick; sometimes there is a whooping noise as child draws in breath after coughing; coughing bouts can continue for several weeks	Call doctor who may prescribe antibiotics; child will need lots of support and reassurance, especially during coughing bouts; encourage child to drink plenty; may be necessary to give food and drink after coughing bouts, especially if child is being sick; possible complications: convulsions, bronchitis, hernias, ear infections, pneumonia and brain damage

Note Rashes look different on different people. The colour of the spots may vary and on black skin rashes can be less easy to see. If you are doubtful, check with the doctor, especially if the child is showing other signs of illness. Some infectious diseases can be prevented by immunisation (see Chapter 21)

the UK. They are named after the pathogens (germs) that cause the infections. The two types are:

■ meningococcal
■ pneumococcal.

Septicaemia is a form of blood poisoning that may be caused by the same pathogens (germs) that cause meningitis. Septicaemia is very serious and must be treated straightaway; it is the more life-threatening consequence of meningococcal infection. The pathogen enters the body through the throat (droplet infection) and travels though the blood stream. In some cases, the pathogens multiply in the blood stream and cause blood poisoning.

Meningitis and septicaemia occur most commonly in:

■ babies
■ children
■ teenagers.

In children under 4 the most common type of meningitis used to be haemophilus influenzae type b (Hib.) This pathogen could also cause septicaemia. Immunisation against Hib infection is now part of the routine childhood immunisation programme (see Chapter 21, page 410) and, as a result, Hib has virtually disappeared.

Recognising meningitis

Meningitis is not easy to recognise at first because the symptoms are similar to those of flu. Symptoms may not all appear at the same time, and they may be different in babies, children and adults.

Symptoms in babies
■ A high pitched moaning cry
■ Difficult to wake
■ Refusing to feed
■ Vomiting
■ Pale or blotchy skin
■ Red or purple spots that do not fade under pressure. *Do the glass test* (see below)

Symptoms in older children and adults
■ Red or purple spots that do not fade under pressure. *Do the glass test*
■ Stiffness in the neck
■ Drowsiness or confusion
■ Severe headache
■ Vomiting
■ High temperature
■ Dislike of bright light

The glass test
Press the side of a glass firmly against the rash. You will be able to see if the rash fades and loses colour under the pressure. ***If it doesn't change colour, contact the doctor immediately.***

Symptoms of septicaemia

- A rash that may be small spots or large blotchy bruise like spots
- Pale clammy skin
- Joint and limb pains
- High temperature

Note that the rash will be more difficult to see on a dark skin. The rash may develop very quickly in a matter of hours – the spots can grow to red or purple bruises.

If you suspect meningitis or septicaemia, call the doctor immediately.

Treatment

Bacterial meningitis and septicaemia are treated with antibiotics, which are also given to the immediate family and any close contacts.

Case study: Recognising early signs and symptoms of an illness

David had been playing happily all morning at playgroup. His dad had fetched him at lunch time because this was the afternoon that his mum went to work. David ate all his lunch and went off to play in the garden with his friend, Andrew. David's dad took the paper into the garden to read so that he could keep an eye on the children. They had not been playing long before David came over and said he felt 'funny and his tummy hurt'. David's dad took him inside and made him sit in the cool, but he was immediately sick and said he felt much worse. David's Dad put him to rest in bed and went to telephone Andrew's mum to ask her to come and take him home. When she arrived, they went in to look at David and they were alarmed to find that he was much worse – he looked hot and sweaty, his neck hurt and he had a purple rash on his tummy.

1 What action should David's dad take now?
2 What illness are David's symptoms a sign of?
3 Who else should consult the doctor?

Progress check

1 Name two waterborne infections.
2 a) What are the signs of measles?
   b) What are the complications of measles?
3 a) If a child in your care has rubella, what is the important thing you must do as well as caring for the child?
   b) Why is rubella particularly dangerous to pregnant women?
4 Describe a chickenpox rash.
5 Where is the tetanus bacteria found?
6 What are the possible complications of whooping cough?

7 What are the signs of meningitis in:
a) a baby?
b) an older child?
8 Describe the glass test.
9 What are the symptoms of septicaemia?
10 What are the two pathogens that cause meningitis and septicaemia?

Common childhood illnesses

Colds

Viruses cause colds, and children get many colds because there are many different cold viruses and young children are infected with each virus for the first time. As they grow up they build up immunity and get fewer colds. Viruses, not bacteria, cause colds, so antibiotics will not help. There are things you can do to help the child breathe more easily: keep the nose clear and use a menthol rub or decongestant capsule especially at night. Make sure the child has plenty to drink, and give light, easily swallowed food. Don't fuss if a child does not want to eat for a while, just give plenty to drink.

Coughs

A virus causes most coughs, like colds. If a cough persists or the chest sounds congested, a doctor should be consulted. Most coughs are the body's way of clearing mucus from the back of the throat, or from the air passages in the lungs. The cough, therefore, serves a useful purpose and should be soothed rather than stopped. Honey and orange or lemon in warm water or a bought cough mixture will help. If you use a bought cough mixture, check that it is suitable for the age of the child and stick to the recommended dose. Do not combine cough mixtures with other medicines, such as paracetamol, without advice from a doctor.

Diarrhoea

stools
Faeces, the product of digested food

Young babies' **stools** are normally soft and yellow, and some babies will soil nearly every nappy. If you notice the stools becoming very watery and frequent, with other signs of illness, consult the doctor. Young babies who get diarrhoea can lose a lot of fluid very quickly, especially if they are vomiting as well. This can be very serious. Call the doctor and, in the meantime, give as much cooled, boiled water as you can. Use a teaspoon if the baby is reluctant to suck and try to give some water every few minutes. Diarrhoea in older children is not so worrying, but maintain the fluid intake. If the diarrhoea persists for more than two or three days, consult the doctor.

Ear infections

Ear infections often follow a cold. The child may be generally unwell, pull or rub the ears or there may be a discharge from the ear. There may be a raised temperature. The child may complain of pain, but small babies will just cry and seem unwell or uncomfortable. If you suspect an ear infection, it is important that it is treated promptly by the doctor to prevent any permanent damage to the hearing. Ear infections especially of the middle ear (**otitis media**) are quite common. These infections will often temporarily affect the hearing of a child and this can then affect their ability to participate at nursery and school. Repeated infections of the middle ear where infected material builds up in the middle ear (sometimes called **glue ear**) can result in long-term problems with hearing.

> **otitis media**
> An infection of the middle ear

> **glue ear**
> Where infected material builds up in the middle ear following repeated infections

Sore throat

Like colds, sore throats are caused by viruses. The throat may be dry and sore a day or so before the cold starts. Sometimes a sore throat is caused by tonsillitis, and the throat is red and sore with white patches on the tonsils, which are enlarged. The child may find it hard to swallow and have a raised temperature with swollen glands under the jaw. If there is a raised temperature, consult the doctor who may suggest giving paracetamol. Meanwhile, give plenty of clear drinks, soft food to eat and keep the child warm and comfortable.

Bronchitis

Infection and inflammation of the main airway cause **bronchitis** (chest infection). The child will have a persistent chesty cough and may cough up green or yellow phlegm. There may noisy breathing, a raised temperature and the child feels very unwell. Consult the doctor as soon as possible, who may give antibiotics. Meanwhile, allow the child to rest quietly. Sitting well propped up will help breathing. Give paracetamol to reduce the temperature and plenty of warm soothing drinks such as honey and lemon. It may help to moisten the atmosphere by putting a damp towel on the radiator. This could help to loosen phlegm in the airways so that coughing becomes easier. Some children are prone to repeated attacks of bronchitis.

> **bronchitis**
> A chest infection caused by infection of the main airway

Temperatures

As you know from studying this chapter, a raised temperature of 38° C or above, is a sign that pathogens have entered the body and are multiplying. Children, especially babies, can develop high temperatures very quickly. If a baby has a raised temperature and/or other signs of illness, always consult the doctor as soon as possible. With older children, contact the doctor if the temperature remains high or if the child has other signs of illness. It is important to bring the temperature down to avoid any complications. Do not wrap a baby up; take off a layer of clothing and let older children wear light clothes. Keep the room cool and fan the child if possible. Give plenty of cool drinks, little and often. Give paracetamol to help lower the temperature, but consult the doctor first if the baby is less than 3 months old.

Febrile convulsions

| **febrile convulsion** |
| A fit or seizure that occurs as a result of a raised body temperature |

Febrile convulsions are fits that occur as the direct result of a raised temperature. They usually occur in babies and younger children between the ages of 6 months and 5 years.

Signs of a febrile convulsion are:

- loss of consciousness
- stiffness of the body
- twitching movements of the body
- the eyes may roll back
- may wet or soil themselves.

It is important to act effectively and quickly.

- Stay with the child and protect them from injury or falling.
- Get medical aid.
- Put the child in the recovery position when the convulsions have stopped.
- When the child regains consciousness, continue to try to reduce the temperature.

See also Chapter 24, page 453.

Thrush

Thrush is a fungal infection that forms white patches in the mouth, usually on the tongue and the inside of the cheeks and lips. If you try to rub off the fungus, it leaves a red sore patch. A baby may also have a sore bottom because the thrush has infected the skin in the nappy area. Consult the doctor who will give the specific anti-fungal treatment to clear up the infection. Thrush is often spread from one child to another because feeding equipment is not properly sterilised and handled. It can also be passed on from an infected adult. It is very important that all feeding equipment is thoroughly cleaned and properly sterilised before use. Effective hygiene practices in kitchens where feeds are prepared and good personal hygiene routines by child-care workers will prevent the spread of thrush.

Vomiting

All babies will bring up some milk from time to time. If the baby is vomiting often or violently and/or there are other signs of illness, contact the doctor. Babies can lose a lot of fluid if they vomit frequently. Maintain the fluid intake, but stop giving milk and give clear fluids as often as possible. Oral rehydration fluids may also be given and may be advised by a doctor.

✅ *Progress check*

1 List all the signs you can think of that would indicate that the child has an infection.
2 Why is it important to act quickly if a baby has diarrhoea?
3 Why do children get repeated colds?
4 What does a raised temperature indicate?
5 How is thrush spread?

Think about it

1 Think of all the situations in the day when a child might be at risk of getting an infection.
2 Think of all the general safeguards that people use to protect themselves from infection.

Do this! 22.1

You are a nanny looking after a child of 5 who has measles. Write a plan of care for one day.

Infestations

parasite
Lives on and obtains its food from humans

Parasites obtain their food from humans and are likely to affect all children at some time. Common parasites which infest children include:

- fleas
- head lice
- ringworm
- scabies
- threadworms.

Fleas

Fleas are small insects. They cannot fly, but jump from one person to another. The type of flea that feeds on human blood lives in clothing next to the skin. When it bites to suck blood, it leaves red marks which itch and swell up. Fleas lay their eggs in furniture and clothing to be near to humans, their source of food. The insect bites can be treated with antiseptics or calamine lotion to stop itching and swelling. To get rid of fleas, it is important to get rid of the eggs as well as the live insects. Insecticide powder can be applied to clothes and bedding. Cleanliness is very important; regular washing of clothes and bedding will get rid of the eggs. Sometimes children are sensitive to fleas that normally live on cats and dogs. Animals need to be treated regularly to prevent this problem.

Head lice

Head lice are small insects that live in human hair, near to the scalp, where they can easily bite the skin and feed on blood. Many children get head lice; they catch them by coming into contact with someone who is already infested. When heads and hair touch, the lice simply walk from one head to another. Children are vulnerable because they work and play with their heads close together. The lice lay eggs, called nits, close to the scalp and cement the eggs firmly to the hair. Nits look like specks of dandruff, but when you try to remove them they are firmly attached to the hair. The first sign of head lice is usually an itchy scalp.

If a child has head lice, the condition must be treated straight away. Treatment is an insecticide lotion available from the chemist, clinic or doctor. Follow the instructions carefully and treat the whole household. The lotion kills the lice and nits, but the nits are not washed off. To remove dead nits you need to use a plastic tooth comb which is obtainable from the chemist. Some head lice are becoming resistant to these lotions and there has been concern about the safe use of the lotions; so treatment is relying more on natural methods.

Fine tooth-combing is the preferred natural method of treatment and should be done every two to three days. Wet the hair and apply a little conditioner, comb the hair from root to tip, over a piece of white paper, paying particular attention to the areas behind the ears and in the nape of the neck. Lice will fall out of the hair and will easily be seen on the paper.

Oils like tea-tree oil and eucalyptus oil have some effect when dealing with head lice.

The most effective way of preventing and discouraging head lice is to:
- inspect the hair regularly
- comb the hair thoroughly at least twice a day and always after school or nursery – this injures the lice so that they don't lay eggs
- wash brushes and combs regularly in hot soapy water.

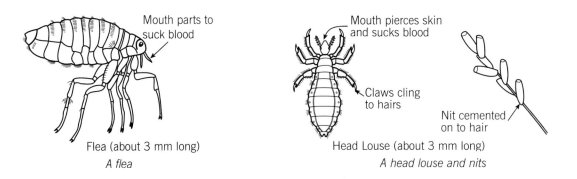

Mouth parts to suck blood

Flea (about 3 mm long)
A flea

Mouth pierces skin and sucks blood

Claws cling to hairs

Nit cemented on to hair

Head Louse (about 3 mm long)
A head louse and nits

Ringworm

Ringworm is a fungus which can be caught from animals. It is seen as a raised red circle with a white scaly centre. It is very itchy. Ringworm patches can occur on the body and on the scalp. Contact the doctor who will prescribe the specific treatment, usually an antibiotic cream.

Case study: Coping with head lice

Aaron is 5 years old and started at his local infant school a few months ago. The school has sent home a letter to parents and carers informing them that there are problems with infestations of head lice and that children in school have been affected. When Aaron returns home from school, his mother Marcia decides to look carefully at his hair. She finds a few live head lice. Marcia comes to you for advice.

1 How would you advise Marcia to treat Aaron's hair now?
2 How would you advise her to care for Aaron's hair in the future to try to prevent further infestations?

Scabies

Scabies is caused by a tiny mite, *sarcoptes scabiei*, that burrows under the skin, causing intense itching. The mites spend their lives feeding on the skin and laying their eggs. It may be possible to see the burrows, or red raised spots which are very itchy. Scratching may cause redness and infection. Scabies is mostly seen on the hands between the fingers, on the wrists and sometimes in the armpit and groin. Scratching and scratch marks may draw attention to the presence of scabies in a child. The mites crawl from one person to another and several family members may be affected. If there is severe itching and soreness the doctor may prescribe a specific treatment such, as an anti-histamine cream. Otherwise calamine lotion or a mild antiseptic cream will soothe the itching. The doctor will prescribe a lotion to kill the mites and eggs; it will be necessary to treat all the affected members of the family. All the bedding and clothing will need to be washed and all family members treated.

Threadworms

Threadworms are small white worms that look like pieces of cotton. They live in the bowel and can be seen in the stools. Threadworms come out of the bowel at night to lay their eggs around the bottom. This causes itching and when the child scratches, the eggs are transferred to the fingers and under the nails. Later, the child will lick their fingers and eggs are swallowed, to hatch and develop in the bowel, perpetuating the cycle. Constant itching and scratching may cause a very sore bottom and disturb the child's sleep. The doctor will prescribe the specific anti-worm treatment. Everyone in the household needs to be treated, keep their nails short and wash their hands well after using the lavatory and before eating. At night, close fitting pyjamas may help to stop the child scratching. All bedding, night clothes and pants need to be washed and changed regularly.

Progress check

1 How can you discourage headlice?
2 How is ring worm caught?
3 What signs might lead you to suspect that a child has scabies?
4 Where are threadworms seen?
5 What are nits?

Do this! 22.2

1 Look at the ways in which disease can be transmitted. Suggest and describe three hygiene routines that will help to prevent infection.

2 Plan an activity which will help children aged 5 and over to learn how infection is spread.

3 Plan a display that you could put in the parents' and carers' area to give information about head lice.

4 Design a leaflet for parents giving information about headlice. If you have access to one, use a computer to produce your leaflet

Key terms

You need to know what these words and phrases mean. Go back through the chapter to find out.

active immunity
antibody
bronchitis
febrile convulsion
glue ear
immunity
incubation period
otitis media
parasite
passive immunity
pathogen
phagocytosis
stools
toxin
vaccine

Now try these questions

1 In what different ways are diseases spread?

2 Describe how immunity is acquired. What are the different types of immunity?

3 Describe the care you would provide at home for a child of 2 years old who has a chest infection.

4 How would you advise a mother to treat a child who has head lice? What further advice would you give about preventing infestations of head lice?

5 What hygiene routines should be established in a child-care setting to help prevent the spread of infection?

6 Describe meningitis and septicaemia. What are the signs and symptoms of meningitis and septicaemia?

23 Caring for sick children

This chapter includes:

- **Caring for sick children at home**
- **Caring for sick children in the work setting**
- **Children in hospital**
- **Children with life-threatening and terminal illness**

Children, like adults, suffer a range of illnesses. Sick children are often cared for at home, as it is better for the child to be in familiar surroundings and with their primary carers. Children usually go into hospital for short stays for specific treatment and are sent home as soon as possible.

You may find it helpful to read this chapter in conjunction with:

▶ **Book 2, Chapter 22**   Childhood illnesses and ailments

Caring for sick children at home

Babies and children need to be with their main carer when they are ill. Unless the doctor suggests that the child stays in bed, they may feel less isolated if they come downstairs. Here they can see and hear what is going on and a bed could be made up, for rest, on the settee. Some children may need the quiet and comfort of bed and in this case the carer and other adults should try to spend much of the time as possible with them.

Physical care

The child should be kept clean and comfortable. Change their clothes frequently and make sure they are loose and made of absorbent material. If the child is staying in bed, give an all-over wash if a bath is not possible. Straighten up the bed, smooth the sheets and pillows, wash the hands and face and comb the hair at regular intervals.

Food and drink

Drinking is important. Having plenty of fluids during illness will help recovery and prevent dehydration, especially if the temperature is raised, so it is vital to encourage a child to drink as much as possible. Offering a variety of drinks may encourage an unwilling child to drink more. Appetite may be affected by illness, so do not worry about food for the first day or so unless it is wanted; after this, try to find ways of making food tempting. Offering favourite foods and serving small appetising portions will help to encourage a reluctant child to eat.

Room temperature

Make sure the room is kept warm and well-ventilated (not too hot) day and night.

Medicines

The following points are important to note in the giving of medicines.

- Only give medicines prescribed or advised by the child's doctor.
- Medicines need to be given at the right time and in the right **dose** (quantity); check the instructions on the label each time the medicine is given.
- If a course of medicine is prescribed, it is very important to finish the full course. This must be done even if the child seems to be better, so that the full benefit is obtained.
- When a medicine is prescribed, ask about any possible side-effects. If you think the child is reacting badly to a medicine (for example, with a rash or diarrhoea), stop giving it and tell the doctor.
- Never use medicines prescribed for someone else.
- Aspirin should not be given to children. There is a risk of Reye's disease which causes damage to the liver.
- Keep all medicines in a locked cupboard if possible.
- Do not keep prescribed or out-of-date medicines.

> **dose**
> The prescribed amount of medicine to be taken

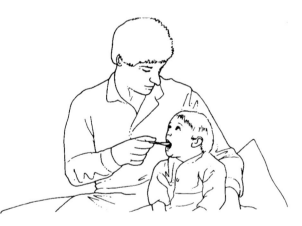

Giving medicine

Taking a temperature

Thermometers that you hold on the child's forehead show the skin temperature, not body temperature; to take an accurate temperature it is best to use a mercury thermometer.

First shake down the mercury in the thermometer. Hold the child on your knee and tuck the thermometer under the armpit next to the skin. Leave the thermometer there for about three minutes; it might help to read a story while you do this.

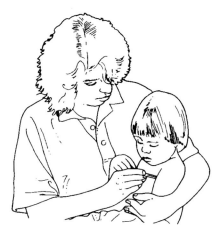

Taking a temperature under the arm

A normal temperature taken under the tongue is 37° C; taken under the arm, it is 36.4° C.

Activities

A carer should give time for games, stories, company and comforting the sick child. Children will need activities that are not too difficult or needing lots of concentration. They may like to return to activities and games that they enjoyed when they were younger.

Sick children are easily tired and need plenty of rest. They may not manage to concentrate for long and may want you to do things for them that they did quite capably when they were well.

✓ Progress check

1 When giving medicines to children, what two important things should be checked?
2 What is a normal temperature taken under the arm?
3 What is a normal temperature taken under the tongue?
4 Why is it important to finish the full course of a medicine that the doctor has prescribed?
5 If a sick child has no appetite, what is the best thing to do?

Do this! 23.1

Write a plan of care for one day for a child aged 3 who is recovering from a severe stomach upset.

Caring for sick children in the work setting

When a child is taken ill outside the home environment, it is important to report any concerns to the appropriate people so that the illness can be properly diagnosed. At a nursery, school or playgroup, the illness should be reported to a senior staff member who will follow the workplace policy and decide whether to contact the child's parents/carers. A childminder or nanny should contact the parents direct.

It is important to keep a record of the symptoms, noting how they first appeared and how they have progressed, as this information may need to be passed on to a doctor and the parents. When caring for a child who is unwell at school or nursery you will need to:

- give practical help, for example take a temperature, help if the child is vomiting, provide a quiet place for them to lie down
- provide reassurance and stay with the child
- tell the child what you are doing, for example contacting a parent
- relax your normal expectations of the child – a child who is feeling ill will not be able to concentrate and may be very miserable and distressed and want their parent or carer.

What to report to a doctor if a child is ill

It is very important to have a clear history of the child's illness so that you can give accurate information to the child's parent/carer or to a doctor. These are the important things to record:

- when you first noticed that something was wrong and suspected that the child was ill
- what the symptoms were
- what action you took, for example taking a temperature, taking steps to cool a child, arranging for the child to rest.
- how the symptoms have progressed since you fist noticed them
- the child's behaviour and what they told you about how they were feeling.

Working with parents

If a child is ill, parents will need information and reassurance. The child-care worker can help parents by:

- informing them promptly if there are concerns about a child
- remaining calm
- giving parents accurate information about their child
- reassuring parents that appropriate steps have been taken
- showing understanding of parents' concerns
- offering support and practical help where possible.

The parents of other children may need to know if another child in the setting has an infectious disease, so that they can take steps to ensure their child's health and well-being. This information will need to be given while ensuring confidentiality, so it is important not to name children in these circumstances.

Information needed about each child in your care

Child-care workers need to keep information about each child to enable contact to be made in the case of an emergency. Records should include:

- child's full name and date of birth
- child's full address and telephone number
- names and addresses of child's parents/carers
- emergency contact telephone numbers
- telephone numbers for the child's GP and health visitor and other agencies, if applicable, such as a social worker.

All the records should be regularly updated and child-care workers should stress the importance of parents/carers informing them of any changes.

Giving medicines

There are occasions when children will be taking medicines and the child-care worker could be giving these medicines. Each child-care establishment will have its own policy about giving medicines to children in its care. Child-care workers should always follow this policy.

These are the important points to remember when giving medicines to any child in your care.

- Follow the policy of your establishment.
- Get the parents'/carers' written consent.
- Only give medicines advised or prescribed by the child's GP or hospital doctor.
- Follow the instructions for dosage and frequency carefully.
- Store medicine safely in a locked cupboard.
- Keep a record of all the medicines given, include the date, time and dose.

✅ Progress check

1 What important points should you check when giving medicines to children?
2 What facts should you report to a doctor about a child who is ill?
3 What information is needed about a child for emergency contact purposes?
4 How can you help parents when their child is ill?

Case study: Feeling ill at nursery

Leroy is 3 years old and comes to the nursery on three days each week while his parents are working. He has been coming to nursery for two months now and has settled in happily. He is very sociable and loves to play with the nursery nurses and with the other children. Leroy came into nursery this morning his usual bright cheerful self, but as the morning went on

Sandra, the nursery nurse in charge of his group, noticed that he was sitting alone looking miserable. She tried to involve him in the activities, but he was reluctant to join in and became tearful. When Sandra went to comfort him, she noticed he was hot and decided to take his temperature. Leroy's temperature was raised and Sandra noticed that he had a flat, red rash on his face and body.

1 What should Sandra do now?
2 What information should Sandra record?
3 What should Sandra tell Leroy's mother?

Children in hospital

Preparation for hospital

A large number of children have to go into hospital at some stage in their lives; many go into hospital as emergency admissions so it is important that all children get to know about hospitals. Children often see ambulances and play with toy ones and this will give an opportunity to talk about hospitals. You may pass the hospital in the car or on the bus and can point out the building. There are lots of books about hospitals that you can look at and read with children.

In child-care settings the imaginative play area can be used to give opportunities for hospital play or play about doctors and clinics, children can handle toy medical equipment and dress up in uniforms. Role-play will enable them to try out the situation in a protected environment. Do not wait until the child is going to be admitted before making them familiar with hospitals. This familiarity will help if a child does have to go in to hospital with little or no warning.

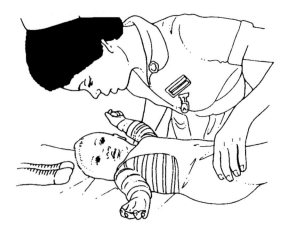

A large number of children have to go into hospital at some stage in their lives

Planned admissions

Despite general preparation, the prospect of hospital admission can be frightening for the child and the parents or carers. Planned admissions have the advantage of contact with doctors and nurses in the out-patients department. Visits to the ward may be arranged before admission. A hospital booklet especially for children is an important source of information. It may contain pictures of children or a familiar toy such as a teddy participating in hospital activities. It will also have pictures of things that a child is likely to see, like a thermometer or stethoscope.

Preparing at home

At home the child can be helped to understand what will happen by playing at hospitals. A few days before admission, the child should be told clearly and honestly what will happen. Any questions should be answered as truthfully as possible in a way that the child can understand. The child should be assured that parents or carers will be able to arrange to stay overnight and visit whenever possible. How much a child can be told or will understand will depend on their age. Older children may enjoy packing and unpacking their case, choosing favourite toys to bring into hospital, especially if they have a cuddly or toy which they like to hold. Any special name for these things should be mentioned to the ward staff.

Case study: Emergency admission

Jamie is 5 and has been admitted to hospital as an emergency with bad stomach pains and being very sick. Jamie's GP thinks that he might have appendicitis. The doctor at the hospital thinks that this is likely, but as Jamie's condition has improved since his arrival, she is going to observe him for a while and do some more tests. Jamie's mum was able to come to the hospital with him and they are waiting for his dad to come. Jamie is feeling a bit better and tells his mum about how he had played at hospitals at his nursery and how one of his friends had told all the children about how he had been into the hospital when he broke his arm. He remembered how they had all done drawings on his plaster. After a while Jamie became anxious and told his mum that he didn't want to stay in hospital and wanted to go home. He said the hospital pyjamas were uncomfortable and that his pet rabbit would be missing him. Jamie's mum comforted him and said that the nurses had told her that she could stay all the while and that she would be sleeping at the hospital with Jamie. She said that when his dad came he would be bringing Jamie's own pyjamas and his favourite teddy and that Roy from next door was going to take special care of his rabbit. After this, Jamie settled down and even had a little sleep until his dad came.

1 What had happened at nursery that helped Jamie to feel more familiar with hospital?
2 What did his mum do to help him settle down more easily?
3 If Jamie has to have an operation for his appendicitis, how will the staff help him to understand what is going to happen?

In hospital

Positive reminders

Continuing links with home are important even when a child has parents or carers who are resident or visit frequently. There are ways to provide children with reminders of home:

- familiar possessions – clothes, toys, cuddlies
- a photograph for the child's locker
- something familiar belonging to the mother, father, and other carers
- letters and cards, to be put up where the child can see them.

Emotional reactions

Children's reactions to being in hospital will be affected by the severity of their illness. The acutely ill child may have little awareness of their surroundings; the less ill child will react sensitively to the environment. The two factors that most affect the child's feelings are age and degree of dependence on parents or carers. Babies and pre-school children are most secure if the parent or carer is with them for all or most of the time; 4–8-year-olds are beginning to be independent, but need a lot of reassurance. They need to have a parent or carer with them, particularly during the more stressful parts of their hospital stay.

Children who are separated from their parent or carer during a stay in hospital may show all the signs of acute distress. These are:

- a period of distress or protest shown by crying, and expressions of anger about being left
- followed by a period of despair where the child fears that their carer might not return and becomes listless, disinterested and refuses to play
- which may give way to detachment where the child becomes convinced that their carer will never return and their behaviour becomes erratic.

Play

Any severe anxiety may have short-term or longer lasting effects on a child's emotional development. Anxiety associated with being in hospital must be anticipated, recognised and reduced to a minimum. Play can be a valuable way of doing this and there are a variety of opportunities, some of which are outlined below.

- *In the community* Parent and toddler groups, playgroups, nurseries and primary schools can provide play, a hospital box, toys and books. Children can be encouraged to act out their experiences, in imaginative play, role-play. Topics such as 'People who help us'; visits from the school nurse, health visitor or other health personnel will be helpful familiarisation for children. The National Association for the Welfare of Children in Hospital (NAWCH) provides information for parents and children about local facilities
- *In out-patients* Play should be available in out-patients, and children attending can be encouraged to participate by attractive and interesting provision; this helps to reduce their own anxiety level and that of their parents

■ *In the ward* When settling in, familiar favourite toys and treasured objects should always be brought in to the ward and kept with the child. Most children's wards in hospital have a playroom where a qualified play leader will provide suitable activities, stories, videos, etc., either in the playroom and at the bedside.

Planning play

Sick children need to play. but they may not make the effort or have the ability to create suitable play activities for themselves. As mentioned in the section on caring for sick children at home, concentration may be lacking, they may tire easily and **regression** to a former level of behaviour may occur.

regression
Responding in a way that is appropriate to an earlier stage of development

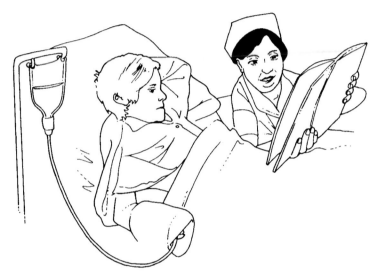

Sick children may lack concentration and tire easily

A variety of play needs to be offered. Some children, because of their previous experience, may need support to play and to be messy. Those who are immobile will need individual play. The child should be able to take part fully in the activity. The best play builds on the familiar, fits the child's abilities and stimulates with something new.

The child confined to bed

Children who have to stay in bed, because they are very ill or because their treatment means that they cannot get up, will need appropriate activities that will interest them. These could include, talking, reading, being read to, board games, tapes of stories, videos, hand-held computer games. Variety is the essential ingredient as children who are ill frequently have short attention spans.

Supine

supine
Lying on the back

Lying **supine** means that vision is restricted. Mirrors can help here, and pictures, posters and mobiles will make the area above the child's head more interesting. Books, listening to stories, tapes, and talking and some board games will be possible, but using the arms for all activities in this position is very tiring.

On the side

If the child has to lie on their side, then activities with play people, animals, board games or trains are possible.

Prone

> **prone**
> Lying face down

In **prone** more activities are possible, especially if the child is supported on a special frame. The child can then paint, read or play board games.

Sitting up

Children may be confined to bed but able to sit up, for example if they are on traction. They may have lots of energy which can be released through clay and dough play or a hammering activity.

The child with an intravenous infusion (IV)

An IV may limit mobility but not confine the child to bed. When the IV is set up, care is taken not to use the dominant arm. This leaves the more skilful hand free for play. Wherever possible, move the child to where the activities are going on. Suitable activities will include painting, board games, small toys, anything that does not require two hands. If in doubt, try it out one-handed yourself first.

The child needing intensive care

Very ill children may show little interest in play, but it is still important to continue visual and aural stimulation. Singing, reading, mobiles, pictures and talking to the child about everyday things are very important. A favourite comfort object needs to be in sight, even if it cannot be held.

The child requiring isolation

A child being nursed in a cubicle may see little of other children. Any visitors, usually adults, may have to wear gowns and masks. As a result, the child will need the carers to spend much more time in the cubicle initiating and joining in with the play. Toys and games will have to stay in the cubicle. Washable toys and water play are especially useful.

The ward playroom

Many children's wards and departments have their own playrooms with a qualified child-care worker, who will provide play to meet the needs of the children who use it. A full range of play and learning opportunities will be available with skilled staff to support the children and their parents and carers. In many hospitals there will be a qualified teacher to support the continued learning of school aged children.

Children with life-threatening or terminal illness

The death of a child seems to be more difficult to accept than the death of an adult. Many people feel that children, with all their future before them, are a far greater loss than an adult who has already lived a full and useful life. The death of a child today, when there are so many ways of preventing death, is far more of a tragedy than in the days when many children died in infancy.

A child's perception of death

Children have many experiences of death in a broad sense. Loss and separation are also a part of many of their experiences. How they think about these things depends on how the adults close to them react and on the explanations they give. Death is often a subject which is not spoken about and the thought is pushed away, when the need is to think through ideas in order to be able to answer children's questions. The idea of death is complex and is built up over many years. The child's understanding will be limited by:

- previous experience
- language development
- grasp of the concept of time
- intellectual development.

Children who are dying often have very clear images, fears and concerns about death. Adults may say that a child does not know, but many children do realise they are dying and the crucial difference is whether they have the chance to express their feelings or not. To say that a child does not talk about death could mean that the child has had no *chance* to talk, usually because the adults are finding this too difficult.

The young child, under 7, thinks that death is reversible, a state of sleep or separation, from which the person could return. Perhaps the main fear for the young child who is dying is thinking about separation and going into a darkness where there is no one familiar to give love and comfort. Children will express their fears in different ways; they may want close physical comfort and someone to listen and talk to them. At other times, they may express their fears in anger. Their anger can often be directed at the person they love and trust the most. This can often be very hard for loving parents and carers to understand, but it is an indication of the child's feelings of trust in them.

Adult reactions to the death of a child

Parents' emotions affect the care they give to their dying child and to the rest of the family. Frequently parents experience a range of emotions.

- *Initial shock* Parents and carers may suspect that their child has a life-threatening illness, but the confirmation of this will produce the reactions of shock, disbelief, numbness and panic; they may not take in any of the explanations and afterwards may say that no one explained.

- *Confusion* This is a common reaction, often caused by parents or carers suddenly losing the role they thought they had, that of bringing up a child.
- *Fear* Part of the confusion is because of a gripping physical, emotional fear; there is a feeling of being trapped and being unable to cope with the unknown.
- *Anger* This arises from the feelings of unfairness that the child is dying; the feelings of anger are often very powerful and it can take very little to trigger them off.
- *Guilt* Parents and carers often take the death of a child as a punishment for something they have done, but this is often unrelated to the child's illness.

Staying in the family

Children with terminal illness very rarely die in hospital. Families are supported so that they can care for their child at home. Each family can decide upon their own plan of care in consultation with the care team. The family can be in frequent contact with the home-care nurse who acts as the consultant to the family in providing care for their child. During the home visits, home-care nurses also provide emotional support to the child's family. Although families are apprehensive about their child dying at home, good support and a feeling of being in control in familiar surroundings will often create the best and most comfortable circumstances for all the family.

Think about it

Think of all the fears that a 5-year-old might have if left alone in hospital.

✓ Progress check

1 In what ways can you raise children's awareness of hospitals?
2 What are the advantages of a planned admission to hospital?
3 List some of the ways in which children might express their fear of hospital.
4 What is the role of the home-care nurse?
5 Describe suitable play for a child who has to stay in bed.
6 Why is it important for a child's parent or carer to remain with them while they are in hospital?

Do this! 23.2

1 Plan two activities for a 6-year-old who has one arm out of action because of an IV in place.

2 It is Monday morning and children aged from 3 to 10 will be admitted for their operations tomorrow. You are in charge of the play room. Decide what activities you will set out to encourage the children to come in and participate. Give reasons for your choices.

Key terms

You need to know what these words mean. Go back through the chapter to find out.
dose
prone
regress
supine

Now try these questions

1 Describe how you would care for a child at home who is recovering from measles.

2 What important points need to be considered if medicines are being given to a child who is ill at home?

3 How can children be prepared for a planned admission to hospital?

4 What action would you take if a child was taken ill in the child-care setting?

5 How would you take a child's temperature using a mercury thermometer?

24 Responding to emergencies

This chapter includes:

- First aid in emergencies
- Examining a casualty
- ABC of resuscitation
- Recovery position
- First aid for minor injuries
- First aid box
- Asthma
- Diabetes
- Febrile convulsions
- Workplace policies and procedures

With good supervision in a safe environment, accidents and injuries will be kept to a minimum. All child-care establishments should have at least one qualified first aider. Ideally, everyone who works with children should have completed a recognised first aid course. It is vital for all child-care workers to know how to deal with emergency situations and when to call for medical assistance.

This chapter provides a basic overview of emergency aid for children, but does not offer a replacement for a recognised first aid course.

You may find it helpful to read this chapter in conjunction with:

▶ **Book 2, Chapter 20**   Safety

First aid in emergencies

First aid is the assistance given to casualties before an ambulance arrives or the casualty arrives at a hospital. The principles are to:

- **p**reserve life
- **p**revent the worsening of the condition
- **p**romote recovery.

It is important to act logically and calmly in any emergency situation and remember the following four actions.

- *Assess the situation* If you are the first person to arrive at the scene of any accident, it is vital to assess quickly what happened and how it occurred. Find out how many children are injured and whether there is

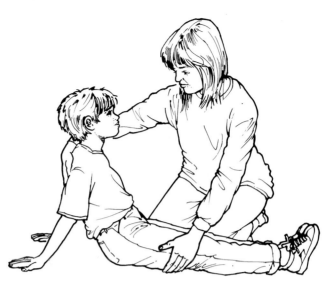

Assess the situation

any continuing danger. Are there any other adults who can help? Is an ambulance required?

■ *Safety first* Thinking of safety includes the safety of all children and adults, including yourself. You cannot help if you are injured too. Remove any dangerous hazards from the child and move the child only if it absolutely essential. Try to make the area safe.

■ *Priorities* Treat the serious injuries first. Generally this means the quietest casualty is in most need of help – they may be unconscious. Conditions which are immediately life-threatening in children are:
 – severe bleeding
 – inability to breathe.

■ *Seek help* Shout for help or ask others to get help, for example if a playground accident occurs another child may be sent to fetch the first aider or another adult from the establishment. Call an ambulance and administer first aid. Move the child to safety if this is required.

Examining a casualty

unconscious
Showing no response to external stimulation

It is vital to find out if the child is conscious or **unconscious**. This can usually be done by gently talking to the child to assess their condition.

■ Check for response – call the child's name, pinch the skin.
■ Shout for help.
■ Open the airway and check for breathing.
■ Check the pulse.
■ Act on your findings according to the chart on page 444.

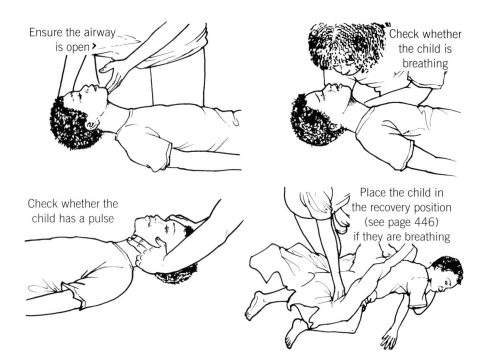

Ensure the airway is open ➤

Check whether the child is breathing

Check whether the child has a pulse

Place the child in the recovery position (see page 446) if they are breathing

The unconscious child

How to deal with an unconscious casualty

Unconscious Breathing Pulse present	Unconscious Not breathing Pulse present	Unconscious Not breathing No pulse
1 Treat life-threatening injuries, e.g. bleeding, burns	1 Artificial ventilation (see opposite) – about 20 breaths of mouth-to-mouth ventilations for 1 minute	1 Cardiopulmonary resuscitation (CPR) (see opposite) – 5 chest compressions – 1 breath of mouth-to-mouth ventilations Repeat for 1 minute
2 Place in recovery position (page 446)	2 Call an ambulance	2 Call an ambulance
3 Call an ambulance	3 Continue ventilations	3 Continue CPR until help arrives
	4 Check for pulse each minute	

✓ *Progress check*

1 What are the principles of first aid?
2 Which four steps should the child-care worker remember if an accident occurs?
3 Explain why it is important to remain calm in the event of an accident.
4 How can you find out whether the child is conscious?
5 What steps should be taken for a child who is unconscious, breathing and with a pulse?
6 What is CPR?

ABC of resuscitation

If a child stops breathing, they will quickly become unconscious because no oxygen can reach the brain. The heartbeat will slow down and eventually stop because of lack of oxygen.

The ABC of resuscitation

A is for **airway**

Is it clear?

Open the airway (mouth) and remove any obstructions. Lift the head and tilt the chin to bring the tongue away from the back of the throat.

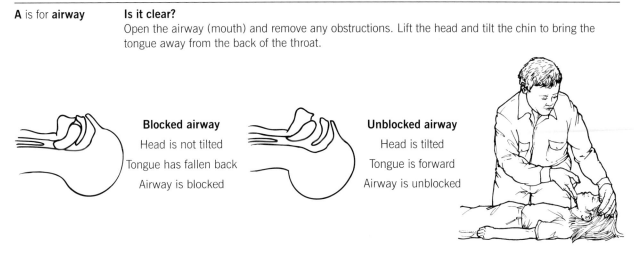

Blocked airway

Head is not tilted

Tongue has fallen back

Airway is blocked

Unblocked airway

Head is tilted

Tongue is forward

Airway is unblocked

B is for **breathing**

> **artificial ventilation**
> Mouth-to-mouth breathing to get oxygen into the lungs of the casualty

Is she breathing?

Putting your cheek close to the child's mouth and nose should enable you to feel their breaths. Look for the rise and fall of the chest. If breathing has stopped **artificial ventilation** should be started, by blowing your breaths into the child's lungs so that oxygen can continue to circulate around the body.

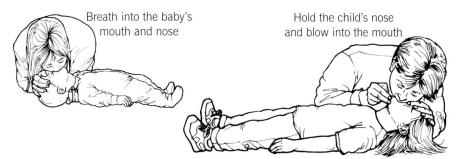

Breath into the baby's mouth and nose

Hold the child's nose and blow into the mouth

C is for **circulation**

> **cardiopulmonary resuscitation (CPR)**
> Chest compressions and artificial ventilation to get oxygen circulating around the body

Is her heart beating?

Feeling for the pulse for 5–10 seconds will detect whether or not the heart has stopped. Use the first two fingers (not the thumb) to feel the carotid pulse in the hollow of the neck between the Adam's apple and the large neck muscle at the side of the neck. If there is no pulse, start **cardiopulmonary resuscitation (CPR)**.

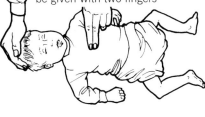

For a baby, chest compressions should be given with two fingers

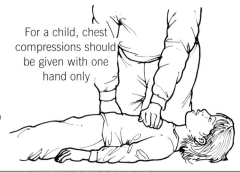

For a child, chest compressions should be given with one hand only

Recovery position

An unconscious child who is breathing and has a pulse should be put into **recovery position** to keep the airway clear by preventing choking on the tongue or vomit. Check for breathing and the pulse until medical help arrives.

> **recovery position**
> Safe position to place an unconscious casualty in if they are breathing and have a pulse

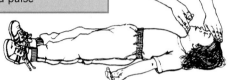

1 Lay the child on their back
Tilt the head back
Lift the chin forward
Ensure the airway is clear

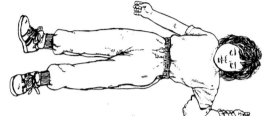

2 Straighten the child's legs
Bend the arm nearest to you at a right angle

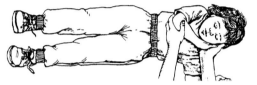

3 Take the arm furthest away from you and move it across the child's chest, bend it and place it on the cheek

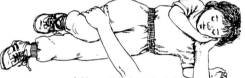

4 Keep this leg straight
Place foot flat on ground
Clasp under the thigh of the outside leg and bend it at the knee

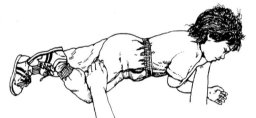

5 Pull the bent leg towards you to roll child onto their side
Use the knees to stop the child rolling onto their front
Keep hand against cheek

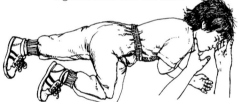

6 Bend top leg into a right angle to prevent child rolling forward
Tilt head back to keep airway open
Adjust hand under child's cheek

The recovery position

✓ Progress check

1 Why does a child quickly become unconscious when they stop breathing?
2 What does ABC stand for?
3 How can you check the airway?
4 How can you tell if a child is breathing?
5 Where can the pulse be most easily felt in a child?

Do this! 24.1

1 Practise putting a child in the recovery position.

2 Practise checking the carotid pulse of colleagues and family – with their co-operation!

First aid for minor injuries

It is essential to remain calm when dealing with an injured child. They need to be reassured that they are in safe hands and everything will be alright.

Burns/scalds

- Do not remove any fabric that may be sticking to the area.
- Use cold water to cool the burn or scald for at least 10 minutes. (Use another cool liquid, such as milk, if cold water is unavailable.)
- Avoid touching burn or blisters.
- Avoid immersing the child in cold water.

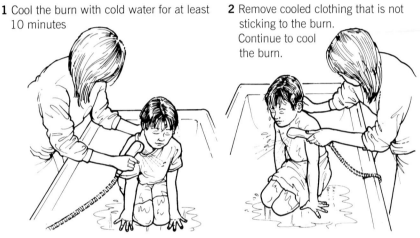

1 Cool the burn with cold water for at least 10 minutes

2 Remove cooled clothing that is not sticking to the burn. Continue to cool the burn.

Dealing with burns and scalds

Bleeding

- Minor bleeds must be cleaned and covered.
- Major bleeds must be stopped by direct pressure as quickly as possible.
  - If possible, keep the injured part raised.
  - Lay the child down to keep the head low.
  - Cover the wound with a firm, sterile dressing and a bandage.

Remember that you should always wear gloves when dealing with blood or any other body fluids.

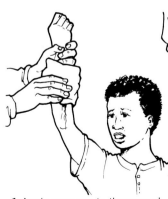
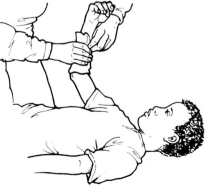

1 Apply pressure to the wound and raise the injured part

2 Lay the child down, while continuing to apply pressure and keep the injured part raised

3 Keeping the injured part raised, cover the wound with a firm, sterile dressing and a bandage.

Dealing with bleeding

Nose bleeds

■ Sit the child leaning forwards and pinch the soft part of the nose above the nostrils for 10 minutes.

■ Allow the child to spit or dribble into a bowl.

■ Continue to pinch the nose until the bleeding has stopped, checking after 10 minutes.

■ Clean the child gently and tell them not to blow their nose, and breathe through their mouth.

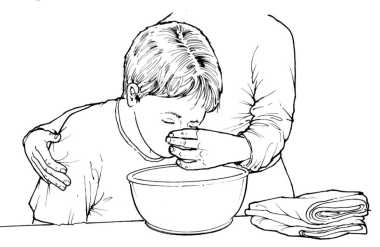

Dealing with a nose bleed

Sprains

■ Raise and support the injured limb to minimise swelling. Remove shoe and sock if it is a sprained ankle.

■ Apply a cold compress – a polythene bag of ice or a pack of frozen peas would do, if available.

■ Wrap the limb in cotton wool padding and then bandage firmly.

■ Keep the limb raised.

RICE will help you remember what to do:

■ **R**est

■ **I**ce

■ **C**ompression

■ **E**levation

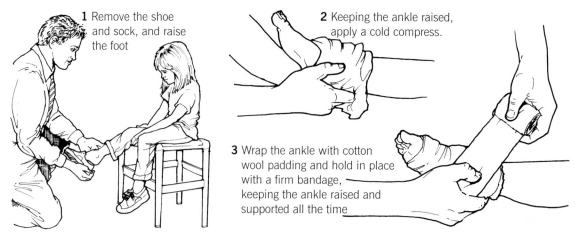

1 Remove the shoe and sock, and raise the foot

2 Keeping the ankle raised, apply a cold compress.

3 Wrap the ankle with cotton wool padding and hold in place with a firm bandage, keeping the ankle raised and supported all the time

Dealing with a sprained ankle

Foreign body

Children who have poked an object into their nose or ears should be taken to the nearest Accident and Emergency Department where the object can be safely removed.

Choking

If you are dealing with a young child:

- Put the child over your knee, head down.
- Slap sharply between the shoulder blades up to five times.
- Turn the child over, and give five downward thrusts – place the heel of your hand on the child's lower breastbone (at the base of the sternum). Push sharply downwards five times.

a For a small child

1 Bend the child over your knees, face down, and give five sharp slaps between the shoulder blades

b For an older child

1 Bend the child forwards and give five sharp slaps between the shoulder blades

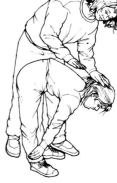

2 Turn the child over, support their back on your thigh, and give five downward thrusts (see text above)

2 Lay the child on their back and give five downward thrusts (see text above)

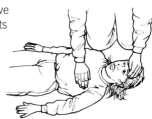

3 Check the mouth and remove object if possible. If not, continue by giving five upward thrusts (see page 450)

3 Check the mouth and remove object if possible. If not, continue by giving five upward thrusts (see page 450)

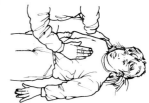

4 Check the mouth and remove object if possible

4 Check the mouth and remove object if possible

5 If object cannot be removed, call for medical aid. Continue the process, starting with 1 again, until the object can be removed or help arrives. (With an older child, the back slaps can given by turning them onto their side.)

Dealing with (a) a small child and (b) an older child who is choking

- Check to see if the object has become dislodged and is in the mouth.
- If the object cannot be removed, give five upward thrusts – place the heel of your hand on the abdomen just below the ribcage. Push firmly upwards five times. Then check the mouth again.
- Call for medical aid – take the child to the phone with you if you are alone.
- Check ABC.

Repeat the process again until help arrives or the object can be removed.

If you are dealing with an older child, start by giving back slaps with the child standing and bent forwards. Then lie the child on the floor and continue as for the young child.

First aid box

All establishments and homes should have a first aid box that is easily accessible and contains all the items shown in the illustration below.

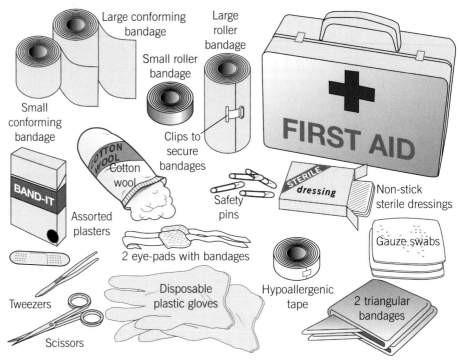

The contents of a first aid box

Progress check

1 What should the first aid box in a child-care establishment contain?
2 What is the emergency procedure for dealing with a child who is choking?
3 What is the first aid treatment for a nose bleed?
4 How long should burns be cooled with cold water?
5 What does RICE stand for in connection with the treatment of sprains?

> ### *Do this!* 24.2
>
> Look at the prices of all the vital items that should be in a first aid box. Make a chart of all the items and their cost.
>
> How much would it cost an establishment to provide all the required items?

Asthma

Asthma attacks are very frightening for children – the airways go into spasm making breathing difficult, especially breathing out. The typical picture is of a child leaning forwards with a hunched posture, gasping for breath – taking air in but unable to blow it out. Speech is impossible during an attack.

Immediate action

If a child is suspected of having asthma, a doctor should be seen within 24 hours.

If an undiagnosed child has an asthma attack, call an ambulance, In the meantime, follow the steps below.

Management of an asthma attack

- Reassure the child.
- Encourage relaxed breathing – slowly and deeply.
- Loosen tight clothing around the neck.
- Sit the child upright and leaning forward against a support, such as a table, supporting themselves with their hands in any comfortable position.
- Stay with the child.
- Give the child their bronchodilator to inhale – two doses – if they are known asthmatics.
- Offer a warm drink to relieve dryness of the mouth.
- Continue to comfort and reassure and *do not panic*. Your panic will increase the child's anxiety which will impair their breathing even more.
- When the child has recovered from a minor attack they can resume quiet activities.
- If the condition persists, call for an ambulance and contact parents.
- Report the attack to the parents when the child is collected. If the child is upset by the episode, they should be contacted immediately.

When to call an ambulance

Call an ambulance immediately, or get someone else to do so if:
- this is the first asthma attack
- the above steps have been taken and there is no improvement in 5–10 minutes.

- the child is exhausted
- the lips, mouth and face are turning blue.

> ✓ **Progress check**
>
> 1 What happens during an asthma attack?
> 2 How would you recognise an asthma attack in a young child?
> 3 How would you deal with a child who is having an asthma attack?
> 4 When would you consider it necessary to call an ambulance?

Diabetes

hypoglycaemia
Low levels of glucose in
the blood

Because this condition arises when there is a disturbance in the way the body regulates the sugar concentrations in the blood, **hypoglycaemia** (too little sugar in the blood) or hyperglycaemia (too much sugar in the blood) may occur. Both conditions will eventually lead to unconsciousness, but hyperglycaemia usually develops slowly, so it most likely that a diabetic child will experience episodes of hypoglycaemia.

Hypoglycaemia

This may result from too much insulin, not enough food, illness or unusually vigorous exercise. Signs include:
- irritability and confusion
- loss of co-ordination and concentration
- rapid breathing
- sweating
- dizziness.

Management of a hypoglycaemic attack

If the child is conscious:
- Sit the child down and stay with them.
- Give sugar, for example glucose tablets, chocolate or a sugary drink, such as lucozade.
- The condition should improve within a few minutes.
- If so, offer more sweetened food or drink.
- Inform parents who should seek necessary advice to stabilise the condition. Parents must be informed of any hypoglycaemic attack because it could indicate the need for adjustment to the diet and/or insulin.

If the child is unconscious:
- put them in recovery position (see page 446).
- call an ambulance, ensuring that somebody stays with the child at all times.

It is good practice to carry glucose tablets or a sweetened drink when accompanying a child with diabetes on a school trip or a swimming lesson.

Case study: A hypoglycaemic attack

Sally is 6 years old and she is diabetic. Her condition is controlled by insulin injections in the morning before school and in the afternoon after school. She is aware of controlling her diet and knows which foods she can eat and when.

Sally's class have just started to go swimming on Tuesday afternoons and she is very excited. She is so busy chatting about swimming at lunch time that she only eats a small amount of her school dinner. Sally trips up the top step when getting out of the pool, and is very slow to get her clothes on, buttoning her blouse the wrong way. The teacher, Miss Brown, notices that her face looks damp when she gets on the bus and that she is breathing quickly. She looks pale and starts to cry quietly. Miss Brown always carries a packet of dextrose tablets in her bag and she offers them to Sally. After sucking two tablets, Sally seems more in control. She stops sweating and by the time the bus arrives back at school, she feels much better. Sally climbs down the bus steps and into the classroom to eat some digestive biscuits and drink a carton of milk.

1 What signs of hypoglycaemia was Sally displaying?
2 What did the child-care worker do to remedy the situation?
3 What caused this attack?

✓ Progress check

1 What is the role of the child-care worker during a hypoglycaemic attack?
2 What action should be taken if you are not sure whether the child is hyperglycaemic or hypoglycaemic?
3 Why is it so important to report any hypoglycaemic episodes to parents?

Febrile convulsions

A febrile convulsion is a type of fit or seizure which occurs as a direct result of a raised body temperature. They usually occur in children between the ages of 6 months to 5 years at the beginning of an illness – children are vulnerable because the developing brain cannot cope with the sudden increase in temperature. A child who has had one febrile convulsion is more likely to have another one.

Signs

- Loss of consciousness
- Rigidity (stiffness) of the body
- Twitching movements of the body and/or face – eyes may roll back
- Possible incontinence of urine or faeces

The child may regain consciousness briefly and then sleep or lapse straight into a deep sleep. They will probably be confused and irritable when they wake up.

Management of a febrile convulsion

■ Stay with the child throughout the convulsion and prevent them damaging themselves, by falling out of bed for example. *Do not interfere* with the process of the convulsion – allow it to take its course.

■ Ask a colleague to send for the doctor if possible.

■ Put the child into recovery position when movements have stopped – loosen tight garments.

■ Gently reassure the child if they regain consciousness before sleeping.

■ Call the doctor when the convulsion is over, if this has not been done already.

■ Continue efforts to reduce the temperature, i.e. tepid sponging and removing clothing.

The doctor may prescribe antibiotics to fight bacterial infections and may prescribe sedatives to be given if the temperature increases again to prevent future attacks.

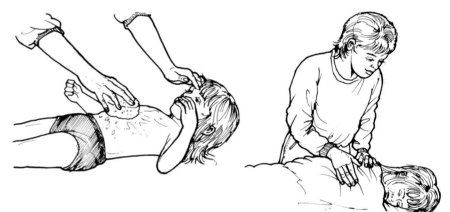

Dealing with a febrile convulsion

Cool the child by removing clothing and bedclothes. Sponge with tepid water until temperature falls

Roll the child onto their side and cover with a sheet

Case study: Febrile convulsion

Geraldine had completed a first aid course for children at her local college before taking up her new post as playworker at the local out-of-school club. She thought she should be prepared for any accidents the children may have in the playground or elsewhere. She thoroughly enjoyed the new job. At the end of the first month she joked with her colleagues that she was pleased not to have found any need for her first aid skills.

One evening, a few of the children were watching a video, sitting on beanbags on the school hall floor. Frazer, who had seemed a little under the weather, suddenly rolled off his cushion onto the floor and began to convulse. Geraldine immediately went to his side and stayed with him. She checked his airway was clear, but did not interfere with the progress of the convulsion. One of her colleagues reassured the other children and took them into another play area. Another child-care worker telephoned Frazer's parents to tell them what was happening and request that they come to collect him as soon as possible. The parents agreed that the doctor should be contacted. Frazer had never had a convulsion before and although Geraldine had not taken his temperature, she could feel that Frazer was hot. He settled off to sleep on the beanbags when the convulsion was over.

1 What had happened to Frazer?
2 What did Geraldine do immediately to help Frazer?
3 How did her colleagues support her?
4 What else could be done to reduce Frazer's temperature?

✔ *Progress check*

1 What is a febrile convulsion?
2 What are the possible signs of a febrile convulsion?
3 What action should the child-care worker take?
4 How can a child's temperature be reduced?

Workplace policies and procedures

Informing parents

Parents must be informed of all injuries, however minor, which occur to their child, with as much detail as possible about how the injury happened. This ensures continuity of care between the establishment and home – the child may need to talk about their experiences with their parents who are then prepared to deal with any consequences.

Accident book

accident book
Legal documentation of all accidents and injuries occurring in any establishment

Every accident should be recorded in an **accident book** to comply with health and safety regulations.

The information recorded in the accident book should include:

- time and date of the accident
- name and address of the injured child or adult
- the location of the accident
- who was involved and what happened (details of witnesses)
- details of the injury
- any treatment that was given
- who was informed of the accident.

Accident books should be kept safely for at least three years.

✔️ *Progress check*

1 Why is it important to inform parents about any accidents which their child is involved in?
2 What information should be recorded in an accident book?
3 How long should accident books be kept for?

Do this!   *24.3*

1 Find out the policy in your setting for reporting and recording accidents.

2 Ask to see the accident book in your placement.
   a) What are the most common accidents?
   b) Could they be prevented?

3 Find out who the first aiders are in each establishment you are placed in.

4 In each establishment, check the location of :
   ■ fire alarms
   ■ fire extinguishers
   ■ fire exits
   ■ first aid box.
   Make a plan of the location of all the vital safety equipment.

Key terms

You need to know what these words and phrases mean. Go back through the chapter to find out.
accident book
artificial ventilation
cardiopulmonary resuscitation (CPR)
hypoglycaemia
recovery position
unconscious

Now try these questions

1 What action should a child-care worker take if they found an unconscious child in the playground?

2 Explain why a comprehensive knowledge of first aid is important for child-care workers.

3 Describe the workplace health and safety policies and procedures in your establishment.

Glossary

ABC of behaviour The pattern of all behaviour: *Antecedent* – what happens before the behaviour occurs; *Behaviour* – the resulting behaviour, acceptable or unacceptable; *Consequence* – the result of the behaviour, positive or negative

absolute poverty Not having enough provision to maintain health and working efficiency

accessible Easy to reach or approach

accident An unexpected and unforeseen event

accident book Legal documentation of all accidents and injuries occurring in any establishment

accommodation away from home A placement with a foster carer or in a residential setting arranged by the local authority social services department

achievement The emotional need for the satisfaction gained from success

active immunity The body's ability to resist a disease that has been acquired by having the disease or by having a specific immunisation

advocacy Speaking on behalf of, or in favour of disabled people

affection The emotional need to feel loved by parents, carers, family, friends and the wider social community

AIDS Acquired Immune Deficiency Syndrome, results from infection with Human Immunodeficiency Virus (HIV) and damages the immune system

amino acid A part of protein

amniocentesis A sample of amniotic fluid is taken via a needle inserted into the uterus through the abdominal wall; used to detect chromosomal abnormalities

amnion The membranes that make up the sac containing the developing baby

anaemia A condition in which the blood lacks adequate amounts of haemoglobin

anatomically correct dolls Dolls with accurately reproduced body parts including sexual organs

animism The belief that everything that exists has a consciousness

anoxia A deficiency of oxygen

antecedent *See* **ABC of behaviour**

antenatal The period of time from conception until the baby is born

antenatal care Care of the pregnant mother and developing fetus during pregnancy

anterior fontanelle A diamond-shaped area of membrane at the front of the baby's head. It closes between 12 and 18 months of age

antibody A substance made by white cells to attack pathogens

anti-convulsant A drug that is given to prevent fits

anti-discriminatory practice Practice that encourages a positive view of difference and opposes negative attitudes and practices that lead to unfavourable treatment of people

Apgar score A method of assessing the newborn baby's condition by observing the vital signs

Area Child Protection Committee (ACPC) Writes, monitors and reviews the child protection procedures for its area, and promotes co-ordination and communication between all workers

artificial ventilation Mouth-to-mouth breathing to get oxygen into the lungs of the casualty

associative play Play with other children; intermittent interactions and/or involvement in the same activity although their play may remain personal

asthma Difficulty in breathing when the airways in the lungs become narrowed; triggered by allergies, infections, exercise, emotional upset

attainment targets Different elements of a curriculum area. For example, the attainment targets for English are speaking, reading and writing

audiometry A method of testing hearing using sound produced by a machine called an audiometer

autism Difficulty in relating to other people and making sense of the social world

average A medium, a standard or a 'norm'

baseline assessment An assessment of a child's capabilities on entry to school at 5 years

bedtime routine A consistent approach to putting children to bed which encourages sleep by increasing security

behaviour Acting or reacting in a specific way, both unacceptably and acceptably

behaviourists Psychologists whose work demonstrates that learning takes place because actions are reinforced positively, through reward, or negatively, by punishment

behaviour modification Techniques used to bring about changes in unacceptable behaviour so that it becomes acceptable

belonging The emotional need to feel wanted by a group

bilingual Speaking two languages

biological theories Our temperament, sociability, emotional responses and intelligence are determined by what we inherit genetically from our biological parents

birth asphyxia Failure of the baby to establish spontaneous respiration a birth

bond of attachment An affectionate two-way relationship that develops between an infant and an adult

booking clinic The first visit to the hospital antenatal clinic

booster An additional dose of a vaccine given after the initial dose

braille A system of printing in relief (raised dots in combination) for use by people with impaired sight.

British Sign Language (BSL) The visual, gestural language of the British deaf community

bronchitis A chest infection caused by infection of the main airways

bronchodilator A drug that helps the airways to expand, used to treat asthma

Caesarian Delivery of the fetus via an abdominal incision

calorie A unit of energy

capillaries Very small blood vessels

cardiopulmonary resuscitation (CPR) Chest compressions and artificial ventilation to get oxygen circulating around the body

central nervous system The brain, spinal cord and nerves

cerebral palsy A disorder of movement and posture; part of the brain that controls movement and posture is damaged or fails to develop

cerebro-spinal fluid The fluid surrounding the brain and spinal cord

cervix The narrow entrance to the uterus from the vagina

child-centred With the child at the centre, taking into account the perspective of the child

child protection register Lists all the children in an area who are considered to be at risk of abuse or neglect

children in need A child is 'in need' if they are unlikely to achieve or maintain a reasonable standard of health or development without the provision of services, or if they are disabled

chorionic villus sampling (CVS) A small sample of placental tissue is removed via the vagina; used to detect chromosomal and other abnormalities

chromosome Long threads of DNA carrying hundreds of genes present in every human cell

chronological age The age of a child in years and months

cleft lip or palate A structural impairment of the top lip, palate or both

coeliac condition A metabolic disorder involving sensitivity to gluten; there is difficulty in digesting food

cognitive development The development of thinking and understanding, which includes problem-solving, reasoning, concentration, memory, imagination and creativity; *also called* intellectual development

coherent self-image and self-concept A view of themselves that fits together and makes a complete whole

colostrum The first breast milk containing a high proportion of protein and antibodies

compensatory education A programme or initiative that is offered to those who might be likely to experience disadvantage in the education system

complementary feeds Additional feeds as well as breast feeds

complete protein A protein containing all the essential amino acids; *also called* first-class proteins

concentration The skill of focusing all your attention on one task

concept The way in which a range of knowledge and experiences can be organised, understood and referred to. Concepts can be simple, for example *wet*, *long*, *red*, or complex and abstract, such as *love*, *freedom*, *justice*

conception Occurs when sperm fertilises a ripe ovum

condition Medically-defined illness

conductive deafness Deafness caused by an interruption to the process of sounds passing through the eardrum and the middle ear

conductive education A teaching method aimed at enabling motor-impaired children to function in society; *see* **orthofunction**

congenital A disease or disorder which occurs during pregnancy and is present from birth

congenital deformity A term used in the Children Act 1989; a disability evident at the time of birth

congenital dislocation of the hip The hip joint is unstable or dislocated because it fails to develop properly before birth

conscience The faculty by which we know right from wrong

conscientious objections Not to do something on the grounds of belief

consequence *See* **ABC of behaviour**

conservation In Piaget's concrete operations stage, an understanding that the quantity of a substance remains the same if nothing is added or taken away, even though it may appear different

consistency The emotional need to

feel that things are predictable

contract In the context of unacceptable behaviour, an agreement between an adult and child with the aim of modifying behaviour

contraction Involuntary, intermittent muscular tightenings of the uterus

co-operation card A record of pregnancy carried by the mother and used at each antenatal appointment

co-operative play Children play together co-operatively; able to adopt a role within the group and to take account of others' needs and actions

cradle cap A scaly, dry crust on the scalp and/or forehead

creativity The expression of ideas in a personal and unique way, using the imagination

critical or sensitive period A period of time vital for the achievement of a particular skill

cultural background The way of life of the family in which a person is brought up

culture The way of life, the language and the behaviour that is acceptable and appropriate to the society in which a person lives

curiosity An inquisitive interest

curriculum The content and methods that comprise a course of study

customs Special guidelines for behaviour which are followed by particular groups of people

cystic fibrosis An hereditary, life-treatening condition affecting the lungs and digestive tract

day care The provision of care during the day in a variety of settings outside people's own homes with people other than close relatives, either full- or part-time

decentre Being able to see things from another's point of view

demand feeding Feeding babies when they are hungry in preference to feeding by the clock

dental caries Tooth decay

deep relaxing sleep (DRS) Periods of unconsciousness during the sleep cycle

designated member of staff The person identified in an establishment to whom allegations or suspicions of child abuse should be reported

Desirable Outcomes Curriculum The curriculum that must be provided by all centres receiving government funding for the education of 4-year-olds

development centile charts A way of recording development so that the child's performance can be seen visually

developmentalists Psychologists whose work demonstrates that learning is linked to clearly defined stages of development and that children proceed through these at varying speeds

diabetes A condition in which the body cannot metabolise carbohydrates, resulting in high levels of sugar in the blood and urine

differentiate To distinguish and classify as different

differentiation (in biology) The term used to describe how cells in the body develop and take on different functions

differentiation (in education) The matching of provision to the individual needs and develop-mental level of the child

diffuse bruising Bruising that is spread out

digestion The process of breaking down food so that it can be absorbed and used by the body

disability The disadvantage or restriction of activity caused by society which takes litle or no account of people who have physical or mental impairments and thus excludes them from the mainstream of social activities. According to the social model, disability is defined as 'socially imposed restriction' Oliver (1981)

disclosure (of abuse) When a child tells someone (they have been abused)

discrimination Behaviour based on prejudice which results in someone being treated unfairly

distraction test A hearing test carried out at about 7 months

distress syndrome The pattern of behaviour shown by the children who experience loss of a familiar carer with no one to take their place

DNA (deoxyribonucleic acid) A chemical messenger containing genetic information found in the nucleus of every cell

domiciliary services Services provided in the home

dominant gene A powerful gene which dominates other genes at fertilisation

dose The prescribed amount of medicine to be taken

Down's syndrome A condition caused by an abnormal chromosome, which affects a person's appearance and development

eczema An irritating dry skin rash often caused by an allergy

egocentric Self-centred, from the words *ego* meaning self and *centric* meaning centred on; seeing things only from one's own viewpoint

embryo The term used to describe the developing baby from conception until eight weeks after conception

Emergency Protection Order A court order which enables a child to be removed to safe accommodation or kept in a safe place

emergent writing An approach to writing that encourages children to write independently; *also known as* developmental writing

emotional development The growth of the ability to feel and express an increasing range of emotions appropriately, including those about oneself

empathy An understanding of how other people feel

empower To enable children to take part in the world

encopresis Deliberate soiling into the pants, onto the floor or other area after bowel control has been established

endocrine gland A ductless gland which produces and stores hormones, releasing them directly into the bloodstream

endometrium The lining of the uterus

enquiry (into suspected abuse) A local authority has a duty to carry out an enquiry if there are reasonable grounds to suspect that a child is suffering or is likely to suffer significant harm

E number A number given to an additive approved by the European Union

enuresis Involuntary bedwetting during sleep

environmental aids and adaptations For example, a flashing light doorbell for deaf people, modified utensils and eating tools, bathing aids, etc.

enzyme A substance that helps to digest food

epidural Anaesthetic injected into the epidural space in the spine to numb the area from the waist down

epilepsy Recurrent attacks of temporary disturbance of the brain function

episiotomy A cut to the perineun to assist the delivery of the fetus

equal opportunities All people participating in society to the best of their abilities, regardless of race, religion, disability, gender or social background

equal opportunities policies Policies designed to provide opportunities for all people to achieve according to their efforts and abilities

ethnic group A group of people who share a common culture

ethnic minority group A group (of people with a common culture) which is smaller than the majority group in their society

ethologist A person who studies human nature, intellect and character systematically

experiential Achieving through experience

extended family A family grouping which includes other family members who live either together or very close to each other and are in frequent contact with each other

failure to thrive Failing to grow normally for no organic reason

family of origin The family a child is born into

fat-soluble vitamin A vitamin that can be stored by the body, so it need not be included in the diet every day

febrile convulsion A fit or seizure that occurs as a result of a raised body temperature

femur The long bone in the thigh

fetal alcohol syndrome A condition affecting babies whose mothers are alcoholic or 'binge' drinkers in pregnancy

fetal distress A condition of the fetus resulting from lack of oxygen, usually occurring during labour

fetus The term used to describe the baby from the eighth week after conception until birth

fine motor skills Small finger movements, manipulative skills and hand–eye co-ordination

flammable Material which burns easily

fluoride A mineral which helps to prevent dental decay

fontanelles The areas on the baby's head where the skull bones have not joined together

food allergies Reactions to certain foods in the diet

forceps Spoon-shaped implements to protect the head and assist in the delivery of the fetus

frenulum The web of skin joining the gum and the lip

frozen awareness/frozen watchfulness Constantly looking around, alert and aware (vigilant), while remaining physically inactive (passive), demonstrating a lack of trust in adults

functions of the family The things the family does for its members

gender Being either male or female

gene Detailed unit of inheritance carrying genetic information which is responsible for passing characteristics from generation to generation

genetic counselling Specialist service to provide advice and support for parents who may carry genetically inherited conditions

genital Sexual organs

glue ear Where infected material builds up in the middle ear following repeated infections

gluten A protein found in wheat, rye, barley and oats

grant-maintained status Schools which receive their money (grant) directly from the government, not from their local authority

grief Feelings of deep sorrow at the loss, through death, of a loved person

gross motor skills Whole body and limb movements, co-ordination and balance

guardian *ad litem* Person appointed by the courts to safeguard and promote the interests and welfare of children during court proceedings

Guthrie test On the sixth day after birth, sample of the baby's blood is taken, usually by pricking the heel, to test for phenylketonuria, cystic fibrosis and cretinism

haemoglobin A red oxygen-carrying protein containing iron present in the red blood cells

haemophilia An inherited blood disorder where there is a defect in one of the clotting factors

head lag The baby's head falls back when pulled to sit

health visitor A trained nurse who specialises in child health promotion

hearing impairment Either conductive deafness or nerve deafness; ranges from slight hearing difficulty to profound deafness

hearsay What you are told by others

heat rash Pin-point red skin rash

heredity The transmission of characteristics from one generation to the next

hidden curriculum Messages, often unintended, that are communicated to children as a consequence of the attitudes and values of the adults who deliver the curriculum

HIV Human immunodeficiency virus; *see* **AIDS**

hormones Chemical messengers produced in endocrine glands and carried in the bloodstream to their target organ to stimulate a specific action

housing associations Non-profit-making organisations that exist to provide homes for people in need of housing from a variety of social and cultural backgrounds

Human chorionic gonadaotrophin (HCG) A hormone produced by the implanted embryo, which is excreted in the mother's urine; its presence confirms pregnancy

hydrocephalus A condition involving an increase in the fluid surrounding the brain, often associated with spina bifida

hygiene The study of the principles of health

hypertension High blood pressure

hypoglycaemia Low levels of glucose in the blood

hypothermia A body temperature of less than 35° C

hypothesis The provisional explanation or solution to a problem reached by assessment of the observed facts.

identification Making oneself the same as those who are significant to us

imagination The ability to form mental images, or concepts of objects not present or that do not exist

imitate To copy closely, take as a model

immunity The presence of antibodies which protect the body against infectious disease; *see* **active immunity**; **passive immunity**

impairment Lacking part or all of a limb, or having altered or reduced function in a limb, organ or mechanism of the body. According to the social model, impairment is defined as 'individual limitation' (Oliver 1981)

implantation Occurs when the fertilised ovum settles into the lining of the uterus; *see* **ovum**

imprinting An attachment that forms rapidly

inclusive Organised in a way that enables all to take a full and active part; meeting the needs of all children

incomplete protein A protein containing some essential amino acids; *also called* second-class proteins

incubation period The time from when pathogens enter the body until the first signs of infection appear

incubator An enclosed cot which regulates temperature and humidity

independence The development of skills that lead to less reliance on other people for help or support; the emotional need to feel you are managing and directing your own life

independent life skills Skills needed to live and care for oneself

indicators Signs and symptoms

Individual Education Plan (IEP) An outline of short- and long-term aims and objectives with targets for achievement of goals by children with special educational needs

induction Starting labour by artificial means, for example by breaking the waters or giving hormones to stimulate contractions

infant mortality rate The number of deaths in the first year of life calculated per 1,000 live births

inherit The passing of a characteristic or set of characteristics from one generation to the next

initial child protection conference Brings together the family, professionals concerned with the child and other specialists to exchange information and make decisions

innate Existing from birth

innate ability Natural ability

instincts Patterns of behaviour that are not learned

institutionalised care Care where the needs of the institution and carers are more important than the needs of the individuals being cared for within it

institutionalised discrimination Unfavourable treatment occurring as a consequence of the procedures and systems of an organisation

institutional oppression The power of organisations brought to bear on an individual to keep them in their place

insulin A hormone produced in the pancreas to metabolise carbohydrate in the bloodstream and regulate glucose

intellectual development *See* **cognitive development**

internalise To understand the things that adults think are important and begin to believe and behave similarly

jargon Terminology that is specific to a particular professional background

jaundice Yellowing of the skin and whites of the eyes as a result of too much bilirubin in the blood

Job Seekers' Allowance Benefits paid to people who are registered as unemployed

ketones Excreted in the urine as a result of the breakdown of body cells to provide energy

key worker Works with, and is concerned with the care and assessment of, particular children

labelling Giving a reputation (or label) to someone based upon a small part of their behaviour. For example, a child who is very noisy may be labelled as disruptive. This creates a prejudiced view of the child

labour The process by which the fetus, placenta and membranes are expelled from the birth canal

lacerations Tears in the skin

Language Acquisition Device (LAD) The name Chomsky gives to our innate physical and intellectual abilities that enable us to acquire and use language

language development The development of communication skills, which includes non-verbal communication, reading nd writing skills, as well as spoken language; *also called* linguistic development

lanugo The fine hair found on the body of the fetus before birth andon the newborn infant; mainly associated with pre-term babies

layette First clothes for a baby

learning theories Children develop as they do because they have contact with other people and learn from them

legislation Laws that have been made

lethargy Lacking energy, tired and unresponsive

light-for-dates A baby who is smaller than expected for the length of pregnancy (gestation)

line manager The person to whom you are responsible in the organisation

linguistic development *See* **language development**

listeriosis A disease resulting from infection with the listeria virus which may damage the fetus

literacy The aspects of language concerned with reading and writing

localising Searching for and locating the source of a sound

local management of schools (LMS) Enables a head teacher and the governors of a school to decide how to spend their money and staff a school

locomotion The developing ability to move from one place to another, usually by crawling, walking, running

look and say An approach to reading that relies on recognition of the shape or pattern of a word

low birth-weight Babies born prematurely (pre-term) or below the 10th centile for their gestation, usually weighing less than 2.5 kg at birth

mainstream setting *Not* special provision for disabled children but what is available for *all* children

Makaton A system of simple signs used with people who have limited language skills

marginalise To categorise and put to one side

maternal deprivation 'The prolonged deprivation of young children of maternal care' (Bowlby)

maternal mortality rate The number of women who die as a result of pregnancy within a year of the birth

matriarchal family A family in which women are important and dominant

maturity Complete in natural and expected development for age; being fully developed and capable of self-control

means test An assessment of a person's income and savings, made by completing a form (test) about their income (means) to determine whether they are eligible to receive certain benefits

meconium The first stool passed by the newborn infant – a soft black/green motion which is present in the fetal bowel from about the sixteenth week of pregnancy

medical model A view of disability as requiring medical intervention

melanocytes Pigmented cells

memory The part of the brain where information is stored and retrieved from

menstrual cycle The process of ovulation and menstruation in sexually mature, non-pregnant women

metabolic Related to the process of digesting, absorbing and using food

migration The movement either to or from a country

milestones Important skills which the average child should have accomplished within a specified time

milia 'Milk spots' – small white spots on the nose of newborn babies caused by blocked sebacious glands

milk teeth The first 20 (deciduous) teeth

mongolian blue spot Smooth, bluish grey to purple skin patches consisting of an excess of pigmented skin cells

moral conscience An understanding of right and wrong

motor development The process of muscular movements becoming more complex

motor-impaired An impairment of a function of movement

moulding The process during birth where the shape of the baby's head is changed to make the birth easier

multiability society A society where people have a variety of differing abilities and disabilities

multicultural society A society whose members have a variety of cultural and ethnic backgrounds

multi-disciplinary Made up of different professionals

multilingual Speaking many languages

multiple deprivation The concentration of social problems in one area

multi-professional assessment A measuring of the childs

performance by professional from different backgrounds, e.g. health care, social work, psychology, etc.

muscular dystrophy; Duchenne A condition involving progressive destruction of muscle tissue, which only affects boys

nappy rash Soreness of the skin in the nappy area

narrative A piece of factual writing

National Childcare Strategy A strategy introduced by the UK government in May 1998 to ensure good quality, accessible, affordable child care for children aged up to 14

National Curriculum A course of study, laid down by government, that all children between 5 and 16 in state schools in the UK must follow

nature–nurture debate Discussion as to whether genetic factors (nature) or environmental factors (nurture) are more important in influencing behaviour and achievement

negative self-image A view of oneself as not worthwhile or valuable

neonate A newborn baby

nerve deafness Deafness caused by damage to the inner ear, or to the nerves, or hearing centres in the brain

neural tube Cells in the embryo that will develop into the baby's spinal cord

non-judgemental Not taking a fixed position on an issue

non-verbal communication Non-spoken communication, for example, bodily movements, eye contact, gestures and facial expression; sometimes used to enhance or replace speech

norm Developmental skill achieved within an average time-scale

normative measurements An average or norm against which any individual child's

development can be measured

norms The rules and guidelines that turn values into action

nuclear family A family grouping where parents live with their children and form a small group with no other family members living near to them

nutrient A substance that provides essential nourishment

object permanence An understanding that objects continue to exist when not in view

oedema Swelling of the tissues with fluid

oestrogen A hormone produced by the ovaries

orientate To determine the position of things

orthofunction A teaching method used in conductive education that involves the whole person physically and mentally and 'instils in children the ability to function as members of society, and to participate in normal social settings appropriate to their age'

ossification The process by which the bones become hardened

otitis media An infection of the middle ear

over-compliant Too easily changed in response to the wishes of others

ovum Egg produced by the ovary

palmar grasp Whole-hand grasp

pancreas A gland that secretes insulin and enzymes that aid digestion; *see* **enzyme**; **insulin**

parasite Lives on and obtains its food from humans

parallel play A child plays side-by-side with another child, but without interacting; their play activities remain separate

paramount Of first importance

parental responsibility The duties, rights and authority that parents have towards their children

partnership with parents A way of working with parents that recognises their needs and their entitlement to be involved in decisions affecting their children

passive immunity The body's ability to resist a disease, acquired from antibodies given directly into the body, for example the antibodies passed on in breast milk.

pathogen Germs such as bacteria and viruses

patriarchal family A family in which men are dominant and make the important decisions

peer group (or **peers**) A child's equals, i.e. other children

pelvis The bones that make up the hip girdle

percentile charts/centile charts Specially prepared charts that are used to record measurements of a child's growth. There are centile charts for weight, height and head circumference.

perinatal The period of time during birth

peripatetic Travelling to see those they work with

personal identity (or **self-identity**) One's own individuality, the characteristics that make us separate and different from others, our personality

personality *See* **personal identity**

personal continuity A sense of having a past, a present and a future

phagocytosis The process by which white cells absorb pathogens and destroy them

phenylketonuria (PKU) A metabolic impairment that prevents the normal digestion of protein; recessively inherited

phonics An approach to reading that is based on recognition of sounds

physical development The development of bodily movement and control

pincer grasp Thumb and first finger grasp

pinpoint haemorrhages Small areas of bleeding under the surface

placenta The structure that supports the baby as it develops in the uterus

placental barrier The placenta's function in allowing the exchange of materials between mother and fetus

Portage Home Teaching scheme A scheme to help parents/carers to teach their children with learning difficulties in their own homes, by setting short-term, achievable goals

positive action Taking steps to ensure that a particular individual or groups has an equal chance to succeed

positive image The representation of a cross-section of a whole variety of roles and everyday situations, to challenge stereotypes and to extend and increase expectations

positive self-image A view of oneself as worthwhile and valuable

postnatal Describes the period of time after the birth

posture Position of parts of the body

poverty trap Experienced by people if they are receiving state benefits and they find that by earning a small amount more they lose most of their benefits and become worse off

preconceptual The time between a couple deciding they would like to have a baby and when the baby is conceived

preconceptual care Attention to health before pregnancy begins

predisposing factors Factors that make abuse or neglect more likely to occur – usually the result of a number of these factors occurring together

pre-eclampsia *See* **toxaemia of pregnancy**

prejudice An opinion, usually unfavourable, about someone or something, based on incomplete facts

premature A baby born before 36 completed weeks of pregnancy; also referred to as pre-term

prescribed roles Duties laid down by others

pre-term A baby born before 36 completed weeks of pregnancy; also referred to as premature

primary health care team A group of professionals who are concerned with the delivery of first-line health care and health promotion

primitive reflex An automatic response to a particular stimulus in a neonate

primitive tripod grasp Thumb and two finger grasp

principle A basic truth which underpins an activity

private sector *See* **private services**

private services Services provided by individuals, groups of people, or companies to meet a demand, provide a service, and make a financial profit; *also known as* the private sector

problem-solving The ability to draw together, and assess information about a situation in order to find a solution

procedure A pre-set agreed way of doing something

process A continuous series of events which leads to an outcome

professional approach How workers deal with and relate to people – they must not allow personal responses to affect their work

progesterone A hormone produced by the ovaries

prone Lying face down

psychoanalytical theory A mixture of biological and learning theories, involving the idea that a child's development can be badly affected if at any stage their needs are not met appropriately

psychological From the study of the mind

psychopathic events Actions by people who are unable to put themselves in another person's place and empathise with how that person might feel

pyloric stenosis A thickening of the muscle at the outlet of the stomach to the small intestine – milk cannot pass through the narrowed outlet into the small intestine

rapid eye movements (REM) Periods of dream sleep

ratio The numerical relationship or proportion of one quantity to another

recessive gene The weaker gene of a pair at fertilisation

reconstituted family A family grouping in which the adults and children who have previously been part of a different family

recovery position Safe position to place an unconscious casualty in if they are breathing and have a pulse

referral The process by which suspected abuse is reported by one person to someone who can take action if necessary

reflective practitioners Workers who think about what they have done/said with a view to improving practice

reflex An involuntary response to a stimulus

regression Responding in a way that is appropriate to an earlier stage of development

regulations Formal rules that must be followed

reinforcement Responding to an action or behaviour so that a particular consequence – a reward or punishment – is associated with the action and it is repeated (positive reinforcement) or not (negative reinforcement)

relative poverty Occurs when people's resources fall seriously short of the resources commanded by the average individual or family in the community

residential care The provision of care both during the day and the night outside people's homes with people other than close relatives

respite care Short-term care for a child to receive training and assessment and/or to allow their family to have a break

Rhesus factor A specific factor in the blood of about 85 per cent of humans

rights of children The expectations that all children should have regarding how they are treated within their families and in society; *see* **universal needs of children**

rights of parents To bring up their children and make decisions on their behalf, but they also have duties and responsibilities towards their children; *see* **parental responsibility**

rituals Sets of activities

role model A person whose behaviour is used as an example by someone else as the right way to behave

role-play Acting out a role as someone else

rubella German measles, a mild viral infection which damages the fetus in the first 12 weeks of pregnancy

sacrum Base of the spine

safety legislation Laws which are created to prevent accidents and promote safety

sanction A negative outcome attached to a specific behaviour

saturated fats Solid at room temperature and come mainly from animal fats

schema Piaget's term for all the ideas, memories and information that a child might have about a concept or experience

screening Checking the whole population of children at specific ages for particular abnormalities

sebum An oily substance which lubricates the skin, it is produced by the sebaceous glands and secreted through the hair shaft

Section 8 Orders Passed by a court when there is a dispute about whom a child should live with, who they can have contact with, and some of the steps and decisions adults can take about them

self-acceptance Approving of oneself, not constantly striving to change oneself

self-advocacy Putting forward one's own viewpoint

self-approval Being pleased with oneself

self-awareness A knowledge and understanding of oneself

self-concept See **self-image and self-concept**

self-esteem Liking and valuing oneself; *also referred to as* self-respect

self-identity See **personal identity**

self-image and self-concept The picture we have of ourselves and the way we think other people see us

self-reliance The ability to depend on oneself to manage

self-worth Thinking of oneself as having value and worth

sensory impairment Hearing or sight loss

separation distress Infants becoming upset when separated from the person to whom they are attached

sequence The order in which a series of milestones occur

serum alpha-fetoprotein (SAFP) A protein found in the maternal blood during pregnancy; a high level requires further investigation

sex-linked disorders Characteristics and diseases inherited via the X (female) chromosome

sickle cell anaemia An inherited condition of haemoglobin formation

skill An ability that has been practised

social approval When a person's conduct and efforts are approved of by others

social creation Brought about by society

social development The growth of the ability to relate to others appropriately and become independent, within a social framework

social emotions Empathy with the feelings of others; the ability to understand how others feel

socialisation The process by which children learn the culture (or way of life) of the society into which they are born

socially deviant behaviour Behaviour that is socially different and does not follow the rules of the dominant group in a society

social mobility The movement of a person from one social group (class) to another

social model A view of disability as a problem within society

social role A position in society that is associated with particular group of expected behaviours

social status The value that a society puts on people in particular roles in society

socio-economic group Grouping of people according to their status in society, based on their occupation, which is closely related to their wealth/income; another way of referring to someone's social class

solitary play A child plays alone

spatial awareness A developing knowledge of how things move and the effects of movement

special educational needs Learning difficulties requiring special educational provision to be made

specific learning difficulties Difficulties learning to read, write or spell or in doing mathematics, not related to generalised learning difficulties

specific therapeutic goals Identified objectives to counteract the effects of the condition or impairment

sperm (spermatozoa) The mature male sex cell

spina bifida A condition in which the spine fails to develop properly before birth

spinal cord Nerve tissue which carries messages from the brain to the rest of the body, and vice versa

spiritual beliefs What a person believes about the non-material world

Statement of Special Educational Needs A written report setting out a disabled child's needs and the resources needed to meet these needs

statutory child protection Those aspects of protecting children that are covered by legislation

statutory duty Duty required by law

statutory school age The age at which a child legally has to receive education: from the beginning of the term after their fifth birthday, until the end of the school year in which they have their sixteenth birthday

statutory sector Care establishments provided by the state; *also known as* the state sector

statutory service A service provided by the government after a law (or statute) has been passed in parliament; *also referred to as* the state sector

stereotyped roles Pre-determined, fixed ideas that individuals are expected to conform to

stereotyping When people think that all the members of a group have the same characteristics as each other; often applied on the basis of race, gender or disability

sticky eyes A discharge from the eyes in the first three weeks of life

stimulus Something that arouses a reaction

stools Faeces, the product of digested food

stranger anxiety Fear of strangers

subconscious Thoughts and feelings that a person is not fully aware of

subdural haematoma Bleeding into the brain

substitute care The care given to children during periods of separation from their main carers

sudden infant death syndrome (SIDS) The unexpected and usually unexplained death of a young baby

suffocation Stopping respiration

supine Lying on the back

sweat Liquid produced in the sweat glands and secreted through the pores onto the surface of the skin

talipes An abnormal position of the foot caused by the contraction of certain muscles or tendons

term Between the 38th and 42nd week of pregnancy

theories of development Ideas about how and why development occurs

threshold of acceptability The behaviour towards children that is believed to be acceptable by a society at a certain time

thrush A fungal infection of the mouth and/or nappy area

tokenistic A superficial representation of minority or disadvantaged groups, for example including a single black child in a school brochure, a single woman on a board of directors

toilet training Teaching young children the socially acceptable means of emptying the bladder and bowels into a potty and/or toilet

toxaemia of pregnancy A serious condition which only occurs in pregnancy and may damage the health of the fetus and the mother, also known as pre-eclampsia or, in its severe form, as eclampsia

toxin A poisonous substance produced by pathogens

transcutaneous nerve stimulation (TENS) An electronic device to control pain in labour

transition In the context of child care, the movement of a child from one care situation to another

trial-and-error learning The earliest stage in problem-solving. Young children randomly try out solutions to a problem, often making errors, until finding a solution or giving up

triple test An antenatal blood test to measure levels of serum alpha-fetoprotein (SAFP), human chorionic gonadotrophin (HCG) and oestriol

ultrasound scan A check made during pregnancy using an echo-sounding device to monitor the growth and development of the fetus

umbilical cord Contains the blood vessels that connect the developing baby to the placenta

unconscious Showing no response to external stimulation

undescended testicles When the testes remain located in the body instead of coming down into the scrotum

universal needs of children All children have certain needs, whatever their culture, ethnic origin, social class or family background, and are entitled to have them met

unsaturated fats Liquid at room temperature and come mainly from vegetable and fish oils

uterus Part of the female reproductive tract; the womb

vaccine A preparation used to stimulate the production of antibodies and provide immunity against one or several diseases

values Beliefs that certain things are important and to be valued, for example a person's right to their own belongings

vascular Well supplied with blood vessels

ventouse A suction cup applied to the fetal head to assist delivery

ventral suspension When the baby is held in the air, face down

vernix caseosa White creamy substance found on the skin of the fetus, in the skin creases of mature babies and on the trunk of pre-term infants

viable Capable of surviving outside the uterus

villi Finger-like projections of the placenta that fit into the wall of the uterus

visual impairment Impairment of sight, ranging from blindness to partial sight

voluntary action An intentional act that a child chooses to do

voluntary sector Care establishments provided by voluntary organisations

voluntary services Services provided by voluntary organisations which are founded by people who want to help certain groups of people they believe are in need of support; *also referred to as* the voluntary sector

weals Streaks left on the flesh

weaning The transition from milk feeds to solid foods

womb *See* **uterus**

zone of proximal development Vygotsky's term for the range of learning that the child is incapable of achieving alone but that is possible with assistance

Index

Page references in blue are to this book; those in black refer to Book 1. Page references in italic indicate illustrations or tables.